Soft Tissue Balancing in Total Knee Arthroplasty

Shuichi Matsuda • Sébastien Lustig
Willem van der Merwe
Editors

Soft Tissue Balancing in Total Knee Arthroplasty

Springer

Editors
Shuichi Matsuda
Department of Orthopaedic Surgery
Kyoto University Department of
Orthopaedic Surgery
Kyoto, Japan

Sébastien Lustig
Department of Orthopedic Surgery
Lyon University - Croix Rousse Hospital
Department of Orthopedic Surgery
Lyon, France

Willem van der Merwe
Sports Science Institute of South Africa
Orthopaedic Clinic
Cape Town, South Africa

ISBN 978-3-662-54081-7 ISBN 978-3-662-54082-4 (eBook)
DOI 10.1007/978-3-662-54082-4

Library of Congress Control Number: 2017937383

Printed on acid-free paper

This Springer imprint is published by Springer Nature
The registered company is Springer-Verlag GmbH Germany
The registered company address is: Heidelberger Platz 3, 14197 Berlin, Germany

Preface

Total knee arthroplasty is one of the most successful procedures in orthopedic surgery. However, about 20% of patients are not satisfied with the results of knee arthroplasty. Factors affecting clinical results include soft tissue balancing, knee alignment, implant design, and fixation. Although every surgeon understands that soft tissue balancing is very important during knee arthroplasty, it has been difficult to accurately evaluate, intraoperatively. Moreover, questions remain regarding appropriate soft tissue conditions needed to improve clinical results.

Extensive anatomical, clinical, and biomechanical studies have enabled more accurate evaluation of soft tissue conditions, and we are getting closer to achieving "appropriate soft tissue balancing" based on clinical evidence. This book provides an excellent summary of the current knowledge regarding soft tissue balancing in total knee arthroplasty, focusing on primary knee arthroplasty.

In this book, experts from around the world, including members of the ISAKOS Knee Arthroplasty Committee, offer clear, up-to-date guidance on all aspects of soft tissue or ligament balancing during primary knee arthroplasty, with the aim of enabling the reader to achieve optimal patient outcomes. The book has seven sections, with an introduction explaining the normal soft tissue conditions and knee kinematics in the native knee, followed by descriptions of surgical procedures, including cruciate-retaining, cruciate-substituting, and bicruciate-retaining total knee arthroplasty. In the next section, techniques for the management of severe deformity are introduced, including tips for increasing range of motion. The most striking feature of the book is the many pages devoted to the accurate evaluation and clinical relevance of ligament balancing. Different techniques and devices for intraoperative soft tissue assessment are discussed, highlighting, for example, the use of gap-measuring devices or trial liners with load-bearing sensors to achieve more objective evaluation. Above all, special attention is devoted to the crucial issue of the impact of intraoperative soft tissue balance on postoperative results. In the closing section, highly experienced surgeons introduce intraoperative troubleshooting to assist successful completion of arthroplasty.

Many thanks to all our contributors for their efforts, with the hope that knee surgeons truly gain from the text and updates in this book.

Kyoto, Japan — Shuichi Matsuda
Cape Town, South Africa — Willem van der Merwe
Lyon, France — Sébastien Lustig

Contents

Contributors

Mohamed Adi Strasbourg University, Strasbourg, France

Shaw Akizuki, MD Center for Joint Reconstruction, Nagano-Matsushiro General Hospital, Nagano, Japan

Michel Bonnin Centre Orthopedique Santy, Lyon, France

Nicolaas C. Budhiparama Nicolaas Institute of Constructive Orthopaedic Research & Education Foundation, Jakarta, Indonesia

Jorge Chahla Steadman Philippon Research Institute, Vail, CO, USA

Myles R.J. Coolican, FRACS, FAOrthA Sydney Orthopaedic Research Institute, Chatswood, NSW, Australia

Jaroslaw Czekaj Albert TRILLAT Center, Lyon North University Hospital, Lyon, France

Carlos Eduardo da Silveira Franciozi, PhD, MD Federal University of São Paulo, São Paulo, Brazil

Rogério Teixeira de Carvalho, MD Federal University of São Paulo, São Paulo, Brazil

Ricardo Telles de Freitas, MD Knee, Ankle and Sports Trauma Unit, Orthopedic Department, Hospital Cuf Descobertas, Lisbon, Portugal

Ahmed El-Naggar Dubai Hospital, Dubai, United Arab Emirates

David Figueroa, MD Facultad de Medicina Clínica Alemana, Universidad del Desarrollo, Concepción, Chile

Francisco Figueroa, MD Facultad de Medicina Clínica Alemana, Universidad del Desarrollo, Concepción, Chile

Hiroshi Horiuchi, MD, PhD Center for Joint Reconstruction, Nagano-Matsushiro General Hospital, Nagano, Japan

Stephen M. Howell Biomedical Engineering Graduate Group, University of California, Davis, CA, USA

Nadia N. Ifran Nicolaas Institute of Constructive Orthopaedic Research & Education Foundation, Jakarta, Indonesia

Yasuo Itami, PhD, MD Osaka Medical College, Takatsuki, Japan

Ryosuke Kuroda, MD, PhD Department of Orthopaedic Surgery, Kobe University Graduate School of Medicine, Kobe, Japan

Robert F. LaPrade Steadman Philippon Research Institute, Vail, CO, USA

The Steadman Clinic, Vail, CO, USA

Myung Chul Lee Department of Orthopaedic Surgery, Seoul National University Hospital, Seoul, South Korea

Hong-Ahn Lim, MD Department of Orthopaedic Surgery, Kyoto University Department of Orthopaedic Surgery, Kyoto, Japan

Timothy Lording Melbourne Orthopaedic Group, Melbourne, VIC, Australia

Sébastien Lustig Albert TRILLAT Center, Lyon North University Hospital, Lyon, France

Marcus Vinicius Malheiros Luzo, PhD, MD Federal University of São Paulo, São Paulo, Brazil

Shuichi Matsuda Department of Orthopaedic Surgery, Kyoto University, Kyoto, Japan

Tomoyuki Matsumoto, MD, PhD Department of Orthopaedic Surgery, Kobe University Graduate School of Medicine, Kobe, Japan

Rob Middleton Nuffield Orthopaedic Centre, Nuffield Department of Orthopaedics Rheumatology and Musculoskeletal Science, University of Oxford, Oxford, UK

Kyle Muckenhirn Steadman Philippon Research Institute, Vail, CO, USA

Jacobus H. Müller, MD, PhD Biomedical Engineering Research Group, Department of Mechanical and Mechatronic Engineering, Stellenbosch University, Stellenbosch, South Africa

Hirotsugu Muratsu, MD, PhD Department of Orthopaedic Surgery, Steel Memorial Hirohata Hospital, Himeji, Japan

Alexander J. Nedopil Department of Orthopaedics, University of California, Sacramento, CA, USA

Sebastien Parratte Institute for Locomotion, Sainte Marguerite Hospital, Aix-Marseille University, Marseille, France

Andrew Price Nuffield Orthopaedic Centre, Nuffield Department of Orthopaedics Rheumatology and Musculoskeletal Science, University of Oxford, Oxford, UK

Gianmarco V.M. Regazzola, MD Sydney Orthopaedic Research Institute, Chatswood, NSW, Australia

Joshua D. Roth Biomedical Engineering Graduate Group, University of California, Davis, CA, USA

Mechanical Engineering Department, University of Wisconsin-Madison, Madison, WI, USA

Hitoshi Sekiya Department of Orthopaedic Surgery, Shin-Kaminokawa Hospital, Kaminokawa-town, Tochigi, Japan

Jong-Keun Seon, MD Department of Orthopaedic Surgery, Kyoto University Department of Orthopaedic Surgery, Kyoto, Japan

Young-Joo Shin, MD Department of Orthopaedic Surgery, Kyoto University Department of Orthopaedic Surgery, Kyoto, Japan

Eun-Kyoo Song, MD Department of Orthopaedic Surgery, Kyoto University Department of Orthopaedic Surgery, Kyoto, Japan

Samih Tarabichi Burjeel Hospital for Advanced Surgery, Dubai, United Arab Emirates

Mário Vale, MD Knee, Ankle and Sports Trauma Unit, Orthopedic Department, Hospital Cuf Descobertas, Lisbon, Portugal

Willem van der Merwe Sports Science Institute of South Africa Orthopaedic Clinic, Cape Town, South Africa

Ricardo Varatojo, MD Knee, Ankle and Sports Trauma Unit, Orthopedic Department, Hospital Cuf Descobertas, Lisbon, Portugal

Jan Victor, MD, PhD Ghent University, Ghent, Belgium

Kelly Vince, MD FRCS(C) Department of Orthopedic Surgery, Whangarei Hospital, Northland District Health Board, Whangarei, New Zealand

Part I

Native Knee

Anatomy and Biomechanics of the Native Knee and Its Relevance for Total Knee Replacement

1

Kyle Muckenhirn, Jorge Chahla, and Robert F. LaPrade

Contents

1.1 Introduction

The knee is a complex joint that primarily allows the leg to flex and extend while also accommodating rotational, angular, and translational forces. Structurally, the femoral and tibial bony articulation surfaces offer little inherent stability. The intimate relationship between the ligaments, capsule, and muscles surrounding the joint is required to reinforce it. If any of these structures are compromised, the subsequent biomechanical imbalance can increase the likelihood of additional injury or increased joint loading, making it essential to recognize and treat these pathologies. Nonetheless, a history of knee trauma or reconstructive surgery significantly increases the likelihood of developing osteoarthritis [1], which is one of the leading causes of chronic disability [2]. In cases of severe pain and debilitation along with

K. Muckenhirn • J. Chahla
Steadman Philippon Research Institute, Vail, CO, USA

R.F. LaPrade (✉)
Steadman Philippon Research Institute, Vail, CO, USA

The Steadman Clinic, Vail, CO 81657, USA
e-mail: drlaprade@sprivail.org

S. Matsuda et al. (eds.), *Soft Tissue Balancing in Total Knee Arthroplasty*,
DOI 10.1007/978-3-662-54082-4_1

joint osteoarthritis, total knee arthroplasty (TKA) can be indicated. However, up to one-quarter of patients have reported dissatisfaction following TKA [3, 4], often as a result of anterior knee pain, stiffness, unexplained swelling, loss of range of motion, changes in proprioception, or loss of preoperative function mainly in the younger and more active population [1]. Poor outcomes can also stem from improper TKA alignment, leading to increased wear, poor functionality, and early failure [5–10], which advocates more closely reproducing the native kinematics which requires a detailed knowledge of the anatomy and biomechanics. Thus, the purpose of this chapter was to perform a detailed description of the ligamentous anatomy of the knee and the most important bony and soft tissue landmarks to consider for a total knee replacement.

1.2 Anterior Cruciate Ligament

The anterior cruciate ligament (ACL) is an intra-articular ligament mainly composed of type 1 collagen that receives its blood supply from the middle genicular artery [11]. There are two functional bundles of the ACL, an anteromedial bundle (AMB) and posterolateral bundle (PLB), named for the relationship of their insertion on the tibial plateau [11, 12]. Both bundles also attach to the posteromedial aspect of the lateral femoral condyle, with reliable bony landmarks providing useful references for identification at both attachments. The bifurcate ridge (BR) separates the proximal AMB and the distal PLB, while the lateral intercondylar ridge (LIR) or "resident's ridge" serves as the anterior femoral margin of both bundles. Coursing anteromedially from the femoral attachment, the anterior-most border of the ACL tibial attachment is demarcated by the ACL ridge [13]. In close proximity is also the anterior root attachment of the lateral meniscus, with consequent overlap reported between the deep anterolateral meniscal root fibers and the broad tibial ACL attachment [14, 15].

The role of the cruciates in TKA is debated with most prosthetic designs requiring complete excision of the ACL. One exception is unicompartmental knee arthroplasty (UKA), which requires an intact ACL and has been reported to produce worse outcomes in ACL-deficient knees (survival rate of 95% versus 81% at 9 years follow-up) [17, 18]. UKA offers several potential advantages to TKA [19] when indicated, but as a prerequisite, the ACL may need to be reconstructed concurrently or in a staged fashion in some cases requiring a thorough understanding of its anatomy to best restore its overall function (Fig. 1.1).

Biomechanically, the ACL is the primary static stabilizer to anterior tibial translational forces [20–26], and it resists internal and external tibial rotation in flexion and extension [16, 27]. Cadaveric studies have demonstrated that in extension the PLB is taut and experiences the greatest force, whereas the AMB is taut in flexion with the highest transmission of forces at 60° [23]. In addition to resisting external forces, sensory and mechanoreceptors within the ligament contribute to proprioception and also assist in initiating important secondary stabilizing muscular reflexes [28, 29].

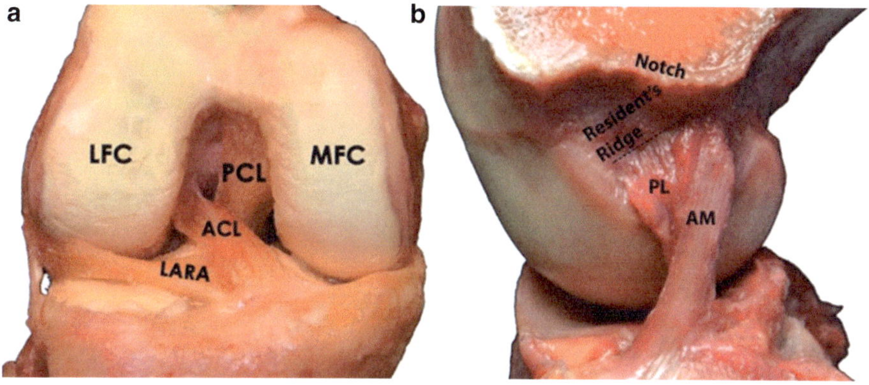

Fig. 1.1 (**a**) Anterior view of a right cadaveric knee demonstrating the anterior cruciate ligament (*ACL*), posterior cruciate ligament (*PCL*), and lateral meniscal anterior root attachment (*LARA*). (**b**) Sagittal cross section of a right femur demonstrating the anteromedial (*AM*) and posterolateral (*PL*) bundle of the ACL in relation to resident's ridge

Loss of proprioception following TKA is one factor contributing to patient dissatisfaction [1], which may be avoided in cruciate-retaining knee implants. Furthermore, sagittal plane kinematics have been preserved in 10-year follow-up studies after UKA [30], which contrasts with many current TKA designs that can result in anterior tibial subluxation in full extension [31–33] and paradoxical anterior femoral translation during flexion [34].

1.3 Posterior Cruciate Ligament

The posterior cruciate ligament (PCL) is an intra-articular, extra-synovial [35] ligament comprised of two bundles. There is a larger anterolateral bundle (ALB) and a smaller posteromedial bundle (PMB) [16, 36–38], which are named for their respective attachments onto a depression on the posterior aspect of the tibia. An important landmark of the tibial PCL attachment is an anterior relation with the shiny white fibers of the posterior horn of the medial meniscus [39]. The center is located 1.3 ± 0.5 mm proximal to the bundle ridge, which is a bony prominence separating the ALB and PMB with an average distance of 8.9 ± 1.2 mm between their individual centers [39]. At the posterior aspect of the tibial plateau, a bony ridge marks the distal border of the PCL [40]. The two PCL bundles can often be distinguished more easily at their attachment to the lateral aspect of the medial femoral condyle, adjacent to the articular cartilage margin. The ALB is 12.1 ± 1.3 mm proximomedial to [39] and twice the size of the PMB [41]. Additionally, there are two meniscofemoral ligaments, an anterior (Humphry) and posterior (Wrisberg) that can often be found adjacent to the PMB at its femoral attachment [42]. Both of these structures may be present in up to 60% of knees, while 95% contain at least one [43].

The anatomy of the posterior cruciate ligament is relevant for cruciate-retaining prosthetic designs for which potential advantages are preservation of bone

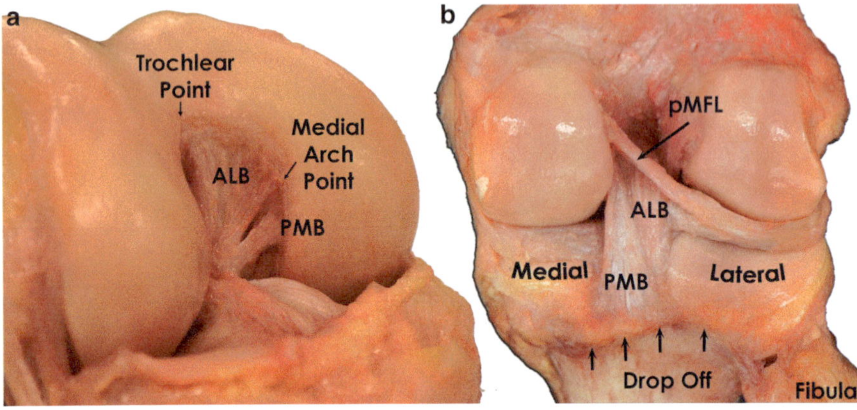

Fig. 1.2 (**a**) Anteromedial view of a cadaveric knee demonstrating bony landmarks of the femoral attachments of the anterolateral bundle (*ALB*) and posteromedial bundle (*PMB*). (**b**) Posterior view of a cadaveric right knee demonstrating bony and soft tissue landmarks of the posterior cruciate ligament (*PCL*)

stock, knee kinematics that better resemble the native, improved proprioception, femoral rollback on the tibia during extension, and better prosthesis stabilization, with the PCL preventing anterior translation of the femur on the tibia. In this regard, when performing the tibial cut, the surgeon should be extremely diligent not to damage the PCL attachment which may be spared in the majority of patients by performing a tibial bony cut of 4 mm or less when a posterior slope of 3–5° is used [44] (Fig. 1.2)

Biomechanically, the two bundles of the PCL provide codominant posterior translational stability [45, 46]. Secondarily the PCL resists rotational forces, particularly internal rotation between 90° and 120° [47, 48]. The individual bundles behave complementary at all flexion angles, demonstrating relative reciprocal changes in length, tension, and fiber orientation. At full extension, the PMB is taut and provides greater resistance to posterior tibial translational force [47, 49], becoming shorter and more horizontal with flexion [50]. Conversely, the ALB is longer and taut in 90° of flexion [51–54], but is also more vertical [50].

Understanding this relationship between tension, length, and orientation is the basis for codominant force resistance throughout knee motion [55] and helps elucidate the need for an anatomic double-bundle PCL when a reconstruction is needed. In cases where the cruciates are sacrificed in a TKA, the posterior cam-post-stabilization creates equivalent but nonanatomic medial and lateral femoral condyle posterior translation, which increases wear at the post and decreases internal tibial rotation [34]. A PCL-retaining TKA can lead to paradoxical anterior translation of the femoral condyles in flexion, which may be due to the vertical position the PCL adopts in the absence of the ACL [56]. Bicruciate-retaining TKA has shown good midterm results, and as acute injury reconstruction has shown, a shift toward more anatomic reconstruction leads to better results and improved kinematics.

1.4 Posterolateral Corner

The posterolateral corner (PLC) of the knee is comprised of three main primary lateral stabilizing structures: the fibular collateral ligament (FCL), popliteus tendon (PLT), and popliteofibular ligament (PFL) [57–61]. PLC injuries are present in nearly 16% of all knee ligament injuries [62]; however, the FCL, which is the primary varus stabilizer [52, 63, 64], is damaged in only 23% of PLC injuries [65] which may make identification difficult. The FCL attaches 1.4 mm proximal and 3.1 mm posterior to the lateral epicondyle [61]. It extends distally, with an average length of 7 cm [66], attaching 8.2 mm posterior to the anterior margin of the fibular head and 28.4 mm distal to the tip of the fibular styloid [61].

The popliteus muscle originates on the posteromedial tibia, becoming tendinous intra-articular as it courses superiorly, and runs deep to the FCL attaching 18.5 mm anterior to it with the knee flexed at 70°. In the lateral third of the popliteal fossa, the musculotendinous junction of the popliteus gives rise to the PFL which has two divisions. The larger posterior division attaches 1.6 mm distal to the posteromedial aspect of the tip of the fibular styloid process, and the smaller anterior division attaches 2.8 mm distal to the anteromedial aspect of the tip of the fibular styloid process [61].

In addition to the three main lateral knee stabilizers, a number of secondary structures provide static and dynamic resistance to the PLC. The mid-third lateral capsular ligament is a capsular thickening that attaches to the lateral epicondyle anterior to the popliteus and to the tibia just posterior to Gerdy's tubercle. It may function as a secondary varus stabilizer [61] and has a meniscofemoral and meniscotibial ligament component [67, 68]. The coronary ligament is also a component of the capsule found both medially and laterally attaching the menisci to their respective tibial plateau [69]. The lateral gastrocnemius tendon is the next important structure, because it is less frequently injured and can be used as a landmark during surgical reconstruction [70]. It is found posterior to the femoral FCL attachment along the supracondylar process and courses distally, fusing with the medial gastrocnemius and the soleus to form the sural triceps muscle. Additionally, there are two heads of the biceps femoris that attach to the fibula and enclose the distal attachment of the FCL. The short head of the biceps femoris has two arms that attach along the lateral aspect of the fibular styloid. The capsular arm has a distal thickening that extends vertically from the fabella to the fibular styloid to form the fabellofibular ligament. The fabella is a sesamoid bone (or cartilaginous analogue the rest of the time) that is found within the proximal lateral gastrocnemius tendon in approximately 30% of individuals [71]. The long head of the biceps also has two arms: a direct arm that inserts onto the posterolateral aspect of the fibular head and an anterior arm that is a crucial access point during FCL reconstruction as it fans out superficial to the FCL [70, 72].

The peroneal nerve, which can be damaged in up to one-third of PLC injuries [65, 73], runs deep to the biceps femoris and must be identified surgically where it emerges 1–2 cm proximal to the fibular head before coursing around the fibular neck and dividing into superficial and deep branches [70, 72]. After a biceps tendon avulsion off the

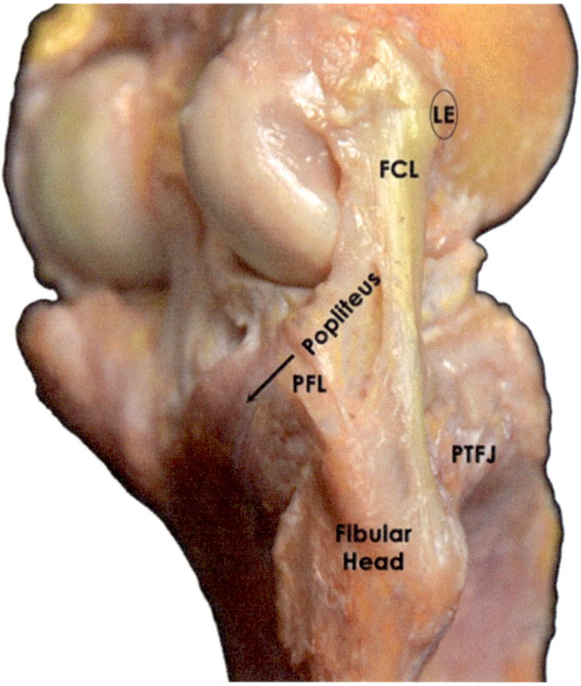

Fig. 1.3 Lateral view of a right cadaveric knee demonstrating isolated fibular collateral ligament (*FCL*) with attachments to the lateral femoral epicondyle (*LE*) and the fibular head, popliteus muscle and tendon, popliteofibular ligament (*PFL*), and proximal tibiofibular joint (*PTFJ*)

fibula, the nerve may migrate within the soft tissue of the posterolateral compartment, and additional care during dissection should be taken. Finally, the broad fascia of the iliotibial band (ITB) is the most superficial layer of the lateral aspect of the knee, covering all of the lateral femoral structures as it attaches from the anterior superior iliac spine onto Gerdy's tubercle on the anterolateral aspect of the tibia.

Opposing convex articular surfaces of the lateral femoral condyle and lateral tibial plateau create inherent bony instability in the lateral knee [74, 75]. Consequently, hyperextension and noncontact varus stress can cause injury, as well as a direct blow to the anteromedial knee [65]. Restraint to varus force is primarily accomplished by the FCL, particularly at 30° of flexion when there is less contribution from the other PLC structures that lend secondary support [65, 72]. The FCL also provides external rotational stability between 0° and 30° of flexion, along with the PLT in greater flexion and the PCL beyond 90° [76]. The PLT and the other PLC structures also provide secondary stabilization for anteroposterior tibial translation [52, 77, 78] and minor secondary restraint to internal rotation; however, those forces are controlled primarily by the ACL in low flexion angles and the anterolateral ligament in higher flexion [70, 79]. Although PLT release may be useful for lateral flexion gap tightness [80], resection can affect gap balancing and stability in TKA [81], and iatrogenic laceration results in decreased functional scores 2–3 years postoperatively following TKA [82]. Furthermore, overaggressive lateral structure releases have been implicated in TKA dislocations [83], and intraoperative injury to these structures can result in acute instability in flexion [84], warranting a preservation of the native anatomy (Fig. 1.3).

1.5 Medial/Posteromedial Structures

The medial collateral ligament (MCL) can be divided into a deep (dMCL) and superficial (sMCL) component. The two divisions of the MCL, along with the posterior oblique ligament (POL), provide the primary stability to the medial knee [85–88]. The MCL is a well-vascularized, extracapsular ligament, which grants it superior intrinsic healing capabilities compared to the anterior cruciate ligament [89–92]. Evidence of growth factor bioactivity and healing following injury has validated these early observations and provided a foundation for future treatment modalities [93–95].

The sMCL is recognized as the largest medial structure. It has a single femoral attachment 3.2 mm proximal and 4.8 mm posterior to the medial epicondyle and two distinct but synergistic tibial attachments [89]. The distal tibial division blends deep to the pes anserine bursa and has a bony attachment 61.2 mm distal to the joint line. The proximal attachment blends with the soft tissue of the anterior arm of the semimembranosus tendon 12.2 mm distal to the tibial joint line.

Additionally, fibrous extensions from the distal aspect of the semimembranosus tendon blend with the posteromedial aspect of the joint capsule to form three POL arms. The superficial and capsular arms are thin fascial expansions. The central (tibial) arm is the largest and thickest reinforcement of the posteromedial joint capsule, and it attaches on the femur 7.7 mm distal and 6.4 mm posterior to the adductor tubercle or 1.4 mm distal and 2.9 mm anterior to the gastrocnemius tubercle.

Finally, the medial aspect of the joint capsule thickens to form two components of the dMCL. The meniscofemoral component attaches 12.6 mm distal to the femoral attachment of the sMCL, and the shorter and thicker meniscotibial component attaches just distal to the edge of the articular cartilage of the medial tibial plateau [93]. In addition to the three primary medial structures (sMCL, POL, and dMCL), other major structures of the medial compartment include the adductor magnus tendon (AMT), medial patellofemoral ligament (MPFL), medial hamstring tendons, medial gastrocnemius tendon (MGT), and vastus medialis obliquus muscle.

Medial knee stability is provided by the sMCL, POL, and dMCL [85–88]. The sMCL and POL also contribute to anterior and posterior drawer loads in the intact knee [88]. The fixation differences between the proximal soft tissue attachment and the distal bony insertion of the sMCL provide biomechanical synergy [87, 96]. The proximal tibial division opposes valgus forces independently of flexion angle, whereas the more static distal division experiences the highest valgus load at 60° of flexion. Additionally, the sMCL provides resistance to external rotation, and to a lesser extent internal rotation, at increasing flexion angles [87, 88].

The POL functions reciprocally and complementarily to the sMCL, producing significantly higher load responses to internal torque at full extension. The POL also resists valgus forces, along with the meniscotibial attachments of the dMCL. The meniscotibial attachment resists valgus forces at 60° of flexion, and the meniscofemoral attachment resists valgus forces throughout flexion, though the dMCL mainly opposes external rotation between 30° and 90° [87].

In TKA with varus deformity, subperiosteal detachment of the medial soft tissue at the proximal tibia affects balancing relative to the function of the structures in the

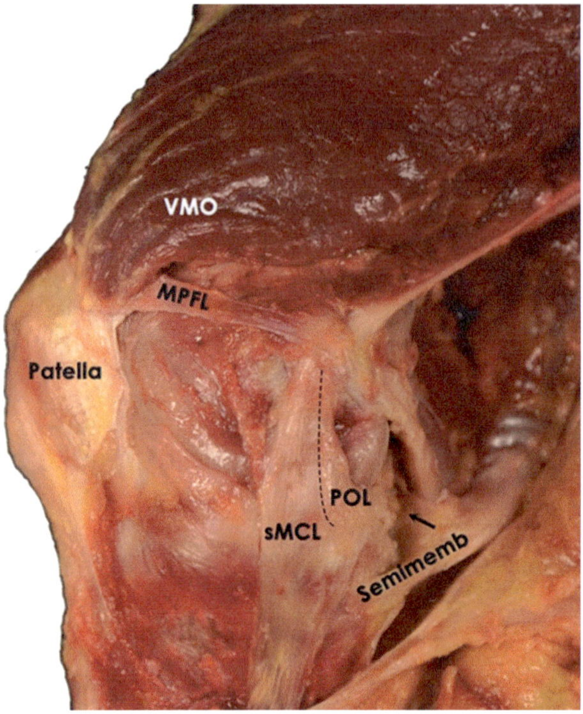

Fig. 1.4 Medial view of a right cadaveric knee demonstrating isolated superficial medial collateral ligament (sMCL), medial patellofemoral ligament (MPFL), posterior oblique ligament (POL), semimembranosus tendon (Semimemb), and vastus medialis oblique (VMO)

intact state. Flexion tightness requires anterior medial soft tissue release, whereas posterior release affects the extension gap [97]. Additionally, a sleeve of medial soft tissue is often tethered to osteophytes during removal, and greater bone removal may lead to increased gapping and early implant failure [98]. While soft tissue balancing is an important aspect of successful TKA, a preservation of the normal anatomy is important for implant longevity (Fig. 1.4).

1.6 Conclusions and Future Perspectives

Detailed anatomic knowledge is of outmost importance at the time of surgical procedures such as ligament reconstructions and joint arthroplasty. Oftentimes, ligament imbalances are present at the time of knee arthroplasties that may need to be addressed in conjunction with the bony work, and therefore a precise understanding of the anatomy and biomechanics is key. Furthermore, with the advent of cruciate-retaining prostheses, the awareness of the anatomy and the biomechanical consequences of the disruption of the structures can potentially yield better results. Further studies are needed to more thoroughly evaluate the long-term clinical effectiveness of various surgical techniques and prosthesis models, potentially with native ligamentous sparring methods to better preserve the anatomy and joint proprioception.

References

1. Nam D, Nunley RM, Barrack RL. Patient dissatisfaction following total knee replacement: a growing concern? Bone Joint J. 2014;96-B(11 Supple A):96–100.
2. Grazio S, Balen D. Obesity: risk factor and predictor of osteoarthritis. Lijec Vjesn. 2009;131(1–2) 22–26. PMID: 19348352.
3. Bourne RB, Chesworth BM, Davis AM, Mahomed NN, Charron KD. Patient satisfaction after total knee arthroplasty: who is satisfied and who is not? Clin Orthop Relat Res. 2010;468(1):57–63.
4. Baker PN, van der Meulen JH, Lewsey J, Gregg PJ. The role of pain and function in determining patient satisfaction after total knee replacement. Data from the National Joint Registry for England and Wales. J Bone Joint Surg Br. 2007;89(7):893–900.
5. D'Lima DD, Chen PC, Colwell Jr CW. Polyethylene contact stresses, articular congruity, and knee alignment. Clin Orthop Relat Res. 2001;392:232–8.
6. Berend ME, Ritter MA, Meding JB, Faris PM, Keating EM, Redelman R, et al. Tibial component failure mechanisms in total knee arthroplasty. Clin Orthop Relat Res. 2004;428:26–34.
7. Ensini A, Catani F, Leardini A, Romagnoli M, Giannini S. Alignments and clinical results in conventional and navigated total knee arthroplasty. Clin Orthop Relat Res. 2007;457:156–62.
8. Jeffery RS, Morris RW, Denham RA. Coronal alignment after total knee replacement. J Bone Joint Surg Br. 1991;73(5):709–14.
9. Oswald MH, Jakob RP, Schneider E, Hoogewoud HM. Radiological analysis of normal axial alignment of femur and tibia in view of total knee arthroplasty. J Arthroplasty. 1993;8(4):419–26.
10. Sikorski JM. Alignment in total knee replacement. J Bone Joint Surg Br. 2008;90(9):1121–7.
11. Giuliani JR. Anterior cruciate ligament anatomy a review of the anteromedial and posterolateral bundles. J Knee Surg. 2009;22(2):148–54.
12. Anderson CJ, Westerhaus BD, Pietrini SD, Ziegler CG, Wijdicks CA, Johansen S, Engebretsen L, LaPrade RF. Kinematic impact of anteromedial and posterolateral bundle graft fixation angles on double bundle anterior cruciate ligament reconstructions. Am J Sports Med. 2010;38(8):1575–83.
13. Ziegler CG, Pietrini SD, Westerhaus BD, Anderson CJ, Wijdicks CA, Johansen S, Engebretsen L, LaPrade RF. Arthroscopically pertinent landmarks for tunnel positioning in single-bundle and double-bundle anterior cruciate ligament reconstructions. Am J Sports Med. 2011;39(4):743–52.
14. Ellman MB, LaPrade CM, Smith SD, Rasmussen MT, Engebretsen L, Wijdicks CA, et al. Structural properties of the meniscal roots. Am J Sports Med. 2014;42(8):1881–7.
15. LaPrade CM, Ellman MB, Rasmussen MT, James EW, Wijdicks CA, Engebretsen L, et al. Anatomy of the anterior root attachments of the medial and lateral menisci: a quantitative analysis. Am J Sports Med. 2014;42(10):2386–92.
16. Girgis FG, Marshall JL, Monajem A. The cruciate ligaments of the knee joint. Anatomical, functional and experimental analysis. Clin Orthop Relat Res. 1975;106:216–31.
17. Goodfellow JW, Kershaw CJ, Benson MK, O'Connor JJ. The Oxford knee for unicompartmental osteoarthritis. The first 103 cases. J Bone Joint Surg Br. 1988;70(5):692–701.
18. Hernigou P, Deschamps G. Posterior slope of the tibial implant and the outcome of unicompartmental knee arthroplasty. J Bone Joint Surg Am. 2004;86-A(3):506–11.
19. Mancuso F, Dodd CA, Murray DW, Pandit H. Medial unicompartmental knee arthroplasty in the ACL-deficient knee. J Orthop Traumatol. 2016;17(3):267–75.

20. Weber E. Mechanik der menschlichen Gehwerkzeuge. Göttingen: Dieterichsche Buchhandlung; 1836.
21. Amis A, Dawkins GP. Functional anatomy of the anterior cruciate ligament. Fibre bundle actions related to ligament replacements and injuries. J Bone Joint Surg Br. 1991;73(2):260–7.
22. Butler DL, Noyes FR, Grood ES. Ligamentous restraints to anterior–posterior drawer in the human knee A biomechanical study. J Bone Joint Surg Am. 1980;62(2):259–70.
23. Gabriel MT, Wong EK, Woo SL, Yagi M, Debski RE. Distribution of in situ forces in the anterior cruciate ligament in response to rotatory loads. J Orthop Res. 2004;22(1):85–9.
24. Paessler HH, Michel D. How new is the lachman test? Am J Sports Med. 1992;20(1):95–8.
25. Markolf KL, Gorek JF, Kabo JM, Shapiro MS. Direct measurement of resultant forces in the anterior cruciate ligament An in vitro study performed with a new experimental technique. J Bone Joint Surg Am. 1990;72(4):557–67.
26. Sakane M, Fox RJ, Woo SL, Livesay GA, Li G, Fu FH. In situ forces in the anterior cruciate ligament and its bundles in response to anterior tibial loads. J Orthop Res. 1997;15(2):285–93.
27. Musahl V, Plakseychuk A, VanScyoc A, Sasaki T, Debski RE, McMahon PJ, Fu FH. Varying femoral tunnels between the anatomical footprint and isometric positions: effect on kinematics of the anterior cruciate ligament-reconstructed knee. Am J Sports Med. 2005;33(5):712–8.
28. Barrack RL. Proprioception in the anterior cruciate deficient knee. Am J Sports Med. 1989;17(1):1–6.
29. Georgoulis AD. The presence of proprioceptive mechanoreceptors in the remnants of the ruptured ACL as a possible source of re-innervation of the ACL autograft. Knee Surg Sports Traumatol Arthrosc. 2001;9(6):364–8.
30. Hollinghursta D, Stoneyb J, Warda T, Gilla HS, Newmanc JH, Murray DW, Bearda DJ. No deterioration of kinematics and cruciate function 10 years after medial unicompartmental arthroplasty. Knee. 2006;13(6):440–4
31. Miller RK, Goodfellow JW, Murray DW, O'Connor JJ. In vitro measurement of patellofemoral force after three types of knee replacement. J Bone Joint Surg Br. 1998;80(5):900–6.
32. Price AJ, Rees JL, Beard DL, Gill RH, Dodd CA, Murray DM. Sagittal plane kinematics of a mobile-bearing unicompartmental knee arthroplasty at 10 years: a comparative in vivo fluoroscopic analysis. J Arthroplasty. 2004;19(5):590–7.
33. Dennis D, Komistek R, Scuderi G, et al. In vivo three-dimensional determination of kinematics for subjects with a normal knee or a unicompartmental or total knee replacement. J Bone Joint Surg Am. 2001;83-A(Suppl 2 Pt 2):104–15.
34. Yoshiya S, Matsui N, Komistek RD, Dennis DA, Mahfouz M, Kurosaka M. In vivo kinematic comparison of posterior cruciate-retaining and posterior stabilized total knee arthroplasties under passive and weight-bearing conditions. J Arthroplasty. 2005;20(6):777–83.
35. Lee SH, Petersilge CA, Trudell DJ, Haghighi P, Resnick DL. Extrasynovial spaces of the cruciate ligaments: anatomy, MR imaging, and diagnostic implications. AJR Am J Roentgenol. 1996;166(6):1433–7.
36. Parolie JM, Bergfeld JA. Long-term results of nonoperative treatment of isolated posterior cruciate ligament injuries in the athlete. Am J Sports Med. 1986;14:35–8.
37. Makris CA, Georgoulis AD, Papageorgiou CD, Moebius UG, Soucacos PN. Posterior cruciate ligament architecture: evaluation under microsurgical dissection. Arthroscopy. 2000;16:627–32.
38. Lopes Jr OV, Ferretti M, Shen W, Ekdahl M, Smolinski P, Fu FH. Topography of the femoral attachment of the posterior cruciate ligament. J Bone Joint Surg Am. 2008;90:249–55.
39. Anderson CJ, Ziegler CG, Wijdicks CA, Engebretsen L, LaPrade RF. Arthroscopically pertinent anatomy of the anterolateral and posteromedial bundles of the posterior cruciate ligament. J Bone Joint Surg Am. 2012;94(21):1936–45.
40. Spiridonov SI, Slinkard NJ, LaPrade RF. Isolated and combined grade-III posterior cruciate ligament tears treated with double-bundle reconstruction with use of endoscopically placed femoral tunnels and grafts: operative technique and clinical outcomes. J Bone Joint Surg Am. 2011;93(19):1773–80.
41. Race A, Amis AA. The mechanical properties of the two bundles of the human posterior cruciate ligament. J Biomech. 1994;27:13–24.

42. Kennedy JC, Hawkins RJ, Willis RB, Danylchuck KD. Tension studies of human knee ligaments. Yield point, ultimate failure, and disruption of the cruciate and tibial collateral ligaments. J Bone Joint Surg Am. 1976;58:350–5.
43. Gupte CM, Bull AM, Thomas RD, Amis AA. A review of the function and biomechanics of the meniscofemoral ligaments. Arthroscopy. 2003;19:161–71.
44. Cinotti G, Sessa P, Amato M, Ripani FR, Giannicola G. Preserving the PCL during the tibial cut in total knee arthroplasty. Knee Surg Sports Traumatol Arthrosc. 2015. [Epub ahead of print].
45. Markolf KL, Zemanovic JR, McAllister DR. Cyclic loading of posterior cruciate ligament replacements fixed with tibial tunnel and tibial inlay methods. J Bone Joint Surg Am. 2002;84-A:518–24.
46. Kennedy NI, Wijdicks CA, Goldsmith MT, et al. Kinematic analysis of the posterior cruciate ligament, Part 1: the individual and collective function of the anterolateral and posteromedial bundles. Am J Sports Med. 2013;41:2828–38.
47. Sekiya JK, Whiddon DR, Zehms CT, Miller MD. A clinically relevant assessment of posterior cruciate ligament and posterolateral corner injuries. Evaluation of isolated and combined deficiency. J Bone Joint Surg Am. 2008;90:1621–7.
48. Wijdicks CA, Kennedy NI, Goldsmith MT, et al. Kinematic analysis of the posterior cruciate ligament, Part 2: a comparison of anatomic single- versus double-bundle reconstruction. Am J Sports Med. 2013;41:2839–48.
49. Markolf KL, Feeley BT, Tejwani SG, Martin DE, McAllister DR. Changes in knee laxity and ligament force after sectioning the posteromedial bundle of the posterior cruciate ligament. Arthroscopy. 2006;22:1100–6.
50. Ahmad CS, Cohen ZA, Levine WN, Gardner TR, Ateshian GA, Mow VC. Codominance of the individual posterior cruciate ligament bundles. An analysis of bundle lengths and orientation. Am J Sports Med. 2003;31:221–5.
51. Butler DL, Noyes FR, Grood ES. Ligamentous restraints to anterior-posterior drawer in the human knee. A biomechanical study. J Bone Joint Surg Am. 1980;62:259–70.
52. Gollehon DL, Torzilli PA, Warren RF. The role of the posterolateral and cruciate ligaments in the stability of the human knee. A biomechanical study. J Bone Joint Surg Am. 1987;69:233–42.
53. Markolf KL, Slauterbeck JR, Armstrong KL, Shapiro MS, Finerman GA. A biomechanical study of replacement of the posterior cruciate ligament with a graft. Part II: forces in the graft compared with forces in the intact ligament. J Bone Joint Surg Am. 1997;79:381–6.
54. Covey DC, Sapega AA, Riffenburgh RH. The effects of sequential sectioning of defined posterior cruciate ligament fiber regions on translational knee motion. Am J Sports Med. 2008;36:480–6.
55. Matava MJ, Ellis E, Gruber B. Surgical treatment of posterior cruciate ligament tears: an evolving technique. J Am Acad Orthop Surg. 2009;17:435–46.
56. Kleinbart FA, Bryk E, Evangelista J, Scott WN, Vigorita VJ. Histologic comparison of posterior cruciate ligaments from arthritic and age-matched knee specimens. J Arthroplasty. 1996;11(6):726–31.
57. Harner CDC, Mauro CSC, Lesniak BP, Romanowski JR. Biomechanical consequences of a tear of the posterior root of the medial meniscus. Surgical technique. J Bone Joint Surg Am. 2008;91(Suppl 2):257–70.
58. Seebacher J, Inglis A. The structure of the posterolateral aspect of the knee. J Bone Joint Surg Am. 1982;64(4):536–41.
59. Watanabe Y, Moriya H, Takahashi K. Functional anatomy of the posterolateral structures of the knee. Arthroscopy. 1993;9(1):57–62.
60. Veltri D, Deng X, Torzilli P, Maynard M, Warren R. The role of the popliteofibular ligament in stability of the human knee a biomechanical study. Am J Sports Med. 1996;24(1):19–27.
61. LaPrade RF, Ly TV, Wentorf FA, Engebretsen L. The posterolateral attachments of the knee: a qualitative and quantitative morphologic analysis of the fibular collateral ligament, popliteus tendon, popliteofibular ligament, and lateral gastrocnemius tendon. Am J Sports Med. 2003;31(6):854–60.

62. LaPrade RF, Wentorf FA, Fritts H, Gundry C, Hightower CD. A prospective magnetic resonance imaging study of the incidence of posterolateral and multiple ligament injuries in acute knee injuries presenting with a hemarthrosis. Arthroscopy. 2007;23(12):1341–7.
63. Grood ES, Stowers SF, Noyes FR. Limits of movement in the human knee. Effect of sectioning the posterior cruciate ligament and posterolateral structures. J Bone Joint Surg Am. 1988;70(1):88–97.
64. Gwathmey Jr FW, Tompkins MA, Gaskin CM, Miller MD. Can stress radiography of the knee help characterize posterolateral corner injury. Clin Orthop Relat Res. 2012;470(3):768–73.
65. LaPrade RF. Injuries to the posterolateral aspect of the knee: association of anatomic injury patterns with clinical instability. Am J Sports Med. 1997;25(4):433–8.
66. Sanchez AR, Sugalski MT, LaPrade RF. Anatomy and biomechanics of the lateral side of the knee. Sports Med Arthrosc Rev. 2006;14(1):2–11.
67. Terry GC, LaPrade RF. The posterolateral aspect of the knee: anatomy and surgical approach. Am J Sports Med. 1996;24:732–9.
68. LaPrade RF, Bollom TS, Gilbert TJ, Wentorf FA, Chaljub G. The MRI appearance of individual structures of the posterolateral knee: a prospective study of normal and surgically verified grade 3 injuries. Am J Sports Med. 2000;28:191–9.
69. Lougher L, Southgate CR, Holt MD. Coronary ligament rupture as a cause of medial knee pain (Lougher 2003). Arthroscopy. 2003;19(10):E19–20.
70. Chahla J, Moatshe G, Dean CS, LaPrade RF. Posterolateral corner of the knee: current concepts (Chahla 2016). Arch Bone Jt Surg. 2016 Apr;4(2):97–103.
71. Kawashima T, Takeishi H, Yoshitomi S, Ito M, Sasaki H. Anatomical study of the fabella, fabellar complex and its clinical implications. Surg Radiol Anat. 2007;29(8):611–6.
72. Crespo B, James EW, Metsavaht L, LaPrade RF. Injuries to posterolateral corner of the knee: a comprehensive review from anatomy to surgical treatment. Rev Bras Ortop. 2014;50(4):363–70. doi:10.1016/j.rboe.2014.12.008.
73. Veltri DM, Deng XH, Torzilli PA, Warren RF, Maynard MJ. The role of the cruciate and posterolateral ligaments in stability of the knee. A biomechanical study. Am J Sports Med. 1995;23(4):436–43.
74. LaPrade RF, Wentorf FA, Olson EJ, Carlson CS. An in vivo injury model of posterolateral knee instability. Am J Sports Med. 2006;34(8):1313–21.
75. LaPrade RF, Griffith CJ, Coobs BR, Geeslin AG, Johansen S, Engebretsen L. Improving outcomes for posterolateral knee injuries. J Orthop Res. 2014;32(4):485–91. doi:10.1002/jor.22572. Epub 2014 Jan 4.
76. LaPrade RF, Tso A, Wentorf F. Force measurements on the fibular collateral ligament, popliteofibular ligament, and popliteus tendon to applied loads. Am J Sports Med. 2004;32(7):1695–701.
77. LaPrade RF, Resig S, Wentorf F, Lewis JL. The effects of grade III posterolateral knee complex injuries on anterior cruciate ligament graft force. A biomechanical analysis. Am J Sports Med. 1999;27(4):469–75.
78. LaPrade RF, Wozniczka JK, Stellmaker MP, Wijdicks CA. Analysis of the static function of the popliteus tendon and evaluation of an anatomic reconstruction: the "fifth ligament" of the knee. Am J Sports Med. 2010;38(3):543–9.
79. Parsons EM, Gee AO, Spiekerman C, Cavanagh PR. The biomechanical function of the anterolateral ligament of the knee: response. Am J Sports Med. 2015;43(8):NP22. doi:10.1177/0363546515597218.
80. Laskin RS. Total knee replacement. London: Springer; 1991. p. 41–53.
81. Cottino U, Bruzzone M, Rosso F, Dettoni F, Bonasia DE, Rossi R. The role of the popliteus tendon in total knee arthroplasty: a cadaveric study. Joints. 2015;3(1):15–9.
82. de Simone V, Demey G, Magnussen RA, Lustig S, Servien E, Neyret P. Iatrogenic popliteus tendon injury during total knee arthroplasty results in decreased knee function two to three years postoperatively. Int Orthop. 2012;36(10):2061–5. doi:10.1007/s00264-012-1631-5. Epub 2012 Aug 1.

83. Schwab JH, Haidukewych GJ, Hanssen AD, Jacofsky DJ, Pagnano MW. Flexion instability without dislocation after posterior stabilized total knees. Clin Orthop Relat Res. 2005;440:96–100.
84. Sharkey PF, Hozack WJ, Booth Jr RE, Balderston RA, Rothman RH. Posterior dislocation of total knee arthroplasty. Clin Orthop Relat Res. 1992;278:128–33.
85. LaPrade RF, Engebretsen AH, Ly TV, Johansen S, Wentorf FA, Engebretsen L. The anatomy of the medial part of the knee. J Bone Joint Surg Am. 2007;89(9):2000–10.
86. Wijdicks CA, Ewart DT, Nuckley DJ, Johansen S, Engebretsen L, LaPrade RF. Structural properties of the primary medial knee ligaments. Am J Sports Med. 2010;38(8):1638–46. doi:10.1177/0363546510363465.
87. Griffith CJ, LaPrade RF, Johansen S, Armitage B, Wijdicks C, Engebretsen L. Medial knee injury: Part 1, static function of the individual components of the main medial knee structures. Am J Sports Med. 2009;37(9):1762–70. doi:10.1177/0363546509333852. Epub 2009 Jul 16.
88. Griffith CJ, Wijdicks CA, LaPrade RF, Armitage BM, Johansen S, Engebretsen L. Force measurements on the posterior oblique ligament and superficial medial collateral ligament proximal and distal divisions to applied loads. Am J Sports Med. 2009;37(1):140–8. doi:10.1177/0363546508322890. Epub 2008 Aug 25.
89. Palmer I. On the injuries to the ligaments of the knee joint: a clinical study. 1938. Clin Orthop Relat Res. 2007;454:17–22.
90. Frank CB. Ligament structure, physiology and function. J Musculoskelet Neuronal Interact. 2004;4(2):199–201.
91. Azar FM. Evaluation and treatment of chronic medial collateral ligament injuries of the knee. Sports Med Arthrosc. 2006;14(2):84–90.
92. Woo SL, Vogrin TM, Abramowitch SD. Healing and repair of ligament injuries in the knee. J Am Acad Orthop Surg. 2000;8(6):364–72.
93. Molloy T, Wang Y, Murrell G. The roles of growth factors in tendon and ligament healing. Sports Med. 2003;33:381–94.
94. Chamberlain CS, Crowley E, Vanderby R. The spatiotemporal dynamics of ligament healing. Wound Repair Regen. 2009;17:206–15.
95. Nishimori M, Matsumoto T, Ota S, Kopf S, Mifune Y, Harner C, Ochi M, Fu FH, Huard J. Role of angiogenesis after muscle derived stem cell transplantation in injured medial collateral ligament. J Orthop Res. 2012;30(4):627–33. doi:10.1002/jor.21551. Epub 2011 Sep 12.
96. Robinson JR, Bull AM, Thomas RR, Amis AA. The role of the medial collateral ligament and posteromedial capsule in controlling knee laxity. Am J Sports Med. 2006;34(11):1815–23.
97. Meloni MC, Hoedemaeker RW, Violante B, Mazzola C. Soft tissue balancing in total knee arthroplasty. Joints. 2014;2(1):37–40.
98. Russell N, Stitzlein MD, Alexander L, Neuwirth MD, Tyler R, Morris MD, Neil P, Sheth MD. A systematic approach to soft-tissue balancing in primary varus total knee arthroplasty. University of Pennsylvania Orthopaedic Journal. 2015;25:71–4.

Soft Tissue Balance of the Native Knee Provides Guidance for Balancing a Total Knee Arthroplasty

2

Joshua D. Roth and Stephen M. Howell

Contents

2.1 Definition of Soft Tissue Balance

Soft tissue balance is a frequently used term; however, it does not have a universally accepted definition. Soft tissue balance is a measure of the relative tensions in the soft tissue restraints over the full range of flexion [1, 2]. The soft tissues about the knee should be considered "balanced" when they are appropriately tensioned to provide stability to the knee without causing stiffness, limited motion, or pain.

Understanding the soft tissue balance in the native knee is a good starting point for developing a strategy for balancing a total knee arthroplasty (TKA).

J.D. Roth (✉)
Biomedical Engineering Graduate Group, University of California, Davis, Davis, CA 95616, USA

Mechanical Engineering Department, University of Wisconsin-Madison, Madison, WI 53706, USA
e-mail: jdroth@ucdavis.edu

S.M. Howell
Biomedical Engineering Graduate Group, University of California, Davis, Davis, CA 95616, USA

S. Matsuda et al. (eds.), *Soft Tissue Balancing in Total Knee Arthroplasty*,
DOI 10.1007/978-3-662-54082-4_2

In the native condition, the knee is inherently stable and has adequate mobility to enable individuals to perform a wide range of activities without pain, stiffness, or feelings of instability. Changes from the native state (e.g., due to ligamentous injury, degenerative joint disease, or TKA) will cause some level of soft tissue "imbalance." However, restoration of the soft tissue balance of the native knee is a reasonable goal when performing TKA to best restore native knee biomechanics.

Native knee biomechanics are determined by both active (i.e., muscles) and passive (i.e., articular surfaces and soft tissue restraints) components [3–7]. Unlike the active components that may be altered postoperatively through physical therapy [8–11], the passive components are set intraoperatively by the surgeon through the design of the components, alignment of the components, and soft tissue releases performed [12, 13]. The interaction between the articular surfaces and the soft tissue restraints determines passive knee biomechanics and is fundamental to the soft tissue balance of the knee [3–6]. This interaction sets the length of each restraint and thus the tension in each restraint based on the stiffness and the reference length of that particular structure.

There are numerous methods used in clinical practice to measure soft tissue balance. These range in complexity from spacer blocks [14] to intraoperative force sensors [15, 16]. Unfortunately, none of these technologies are able to directly measure the tension in an individual soft tissue restraint. Unlike most of these methods which are designed for intraoperative use, the laxities of the knee can be measured pre-, intra-, and postoperatively. This versatility enables the laxities to be measured in both native knees and TKAs. Hence, surgeons are able to use the laxities of the native knee to guide soft tissue balancing during TKA.

2.2 The Laxities of the Native Knee: A Measure of Soft Tissue Balance

The laxity of the knee in a particular anatomic direction is the relative displacement (either translation or rotation) of the tibia on the femur under an applied load (either force or torque) from the relative position of the tibia on the femur under no applied load (i.e., the neutral or resting position) (Fig. 2.1) [7, 17, 18]. Hence, the laxity in a particular anatomic direction is a measure of soft tissue balance because it is determined by the tension in the soft tissue restraints acting in parallel to stabilize the knee in that anatomic direction [7]. The laxities commonly used to describe soft tissue balance are the varus and valgus (V-V), internal and external rotation (I-E), anterior and posterior (A-P), and distraction (D) laxities.

These seven laxities in the native knee have been reported by numerous studies [3, 13, 17–28]. Each study differs in the experimental setup used and the loads

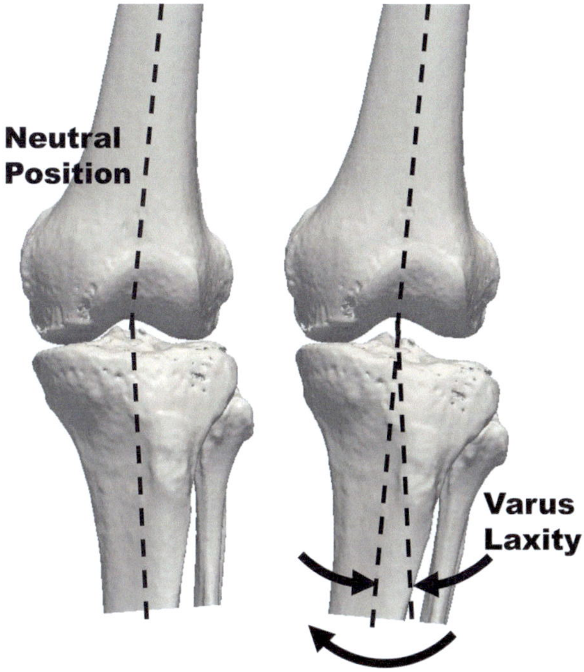

Fig. 2.1 Renderings of bone models of the femur, tibia, and fibula show how the varus laxity of the knee is determined. The other six laxities are determined in a similar way. In general, the laxity in a particular anatomic direction is the relative displacement (either translation or rotation) of the tibia on the femur under an applied load (either force or torque) from the relative position of the tibia on the femur under no applied load (i.e., the neutral or resting position) [7, 17, 18]

applied. While these differences lead to differences in the magnitude of the measured laxities, these studies generally agree that the laxities of the knee are negligible in extension and increase with knee flexion (Fig. 2.2).

To provide some quantitative results, the following paragraphs present a representative set of the seven laxities measured in vitro in native knees using a robotic load application system [17, 18]. The V-V, I-E, A-P, and D laxities were determined under applied loads of ±5 Nm [20], ±3 Nm [3], ±45 N [21], and 100 N [29], respectively. These loads were selected to just engage the soft tissue restraints [3, 20, 21].

In V-V, the knee has negligible laxity at 0° of flexion where the varus laxity (mean ± standard deviation) is 0.7° ± 0.3°, and the valgus laxity (mean ± standard deviation) is 0.4° ± 0.2° (Fig. 2.3a). Both V-V laxities increase with knee flexion, but the varus laxity increases more (five times greater on average at 90° of flexion than that at 0° of flexion) than the valgus laxity (three times greater on average at 90° of flexion than that at 0° of flexion).

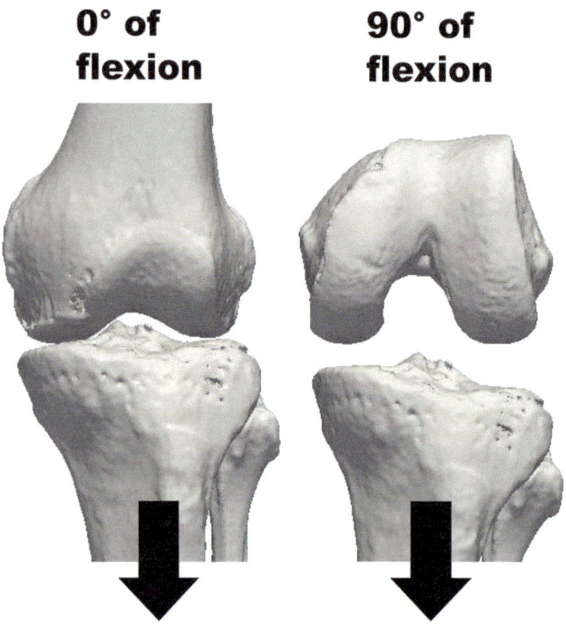

Fig. 2.2 Renderings of bone models of the femur, tibia, and fibula show the general pattern of the distraction laxity. In general, the V-V and I-E laxities follow this same general pattern where the laxity is negligible at 0° of flexion and is much greater at 90° of flexion

In I-E, the knee is also the least lax at 0° of flexion (Fig. 2.3b). At 0° of flexion, the internal rotation laxity (mean ± standard deviation) is 4.6° ± 1.4°, and the external rotation laxity (mean ± standard deviation) is 4.4° ± 1.7°. Both I-E laxities increase from 0° to 45° of flexion (three times greater on average at 45° of flexion than that at 0° of flexion) and stay relatively constant and symmetric from 45° of flexion to 90° of flexion.

In A-P, the knee is also least lax at 0° of flexion (Fig. 2.3c). At 0° of flexion, the anterior translation laxity (mean ± standard deviation) is 2.1 ± 0.5 mm, and the posterior translation laxity (mean ± standard deviation) is 2.4 ± 1.2 mm. Both A-P laxities are greatest around 45° of flexion where the anterior translation laxity is on average three times greater than that at 0° of flexion, but the posterior translation laxity is not significantly greater than that at 0° of flexion.

In distraction, the knee is also least lax at 0° of flexion (Fig. 2.3d). At 0° of flexion, the distraction laxity (mean ± standard deviation) is 0.6 ± 0.1 mm. Similar to the I-E laxities, the distraction laxity increases from 0° to 45° of flexion (three times greater on average at 45° of flexion than that at 0° of flexion) and then remains fairly constant throughout the rest of flexion.

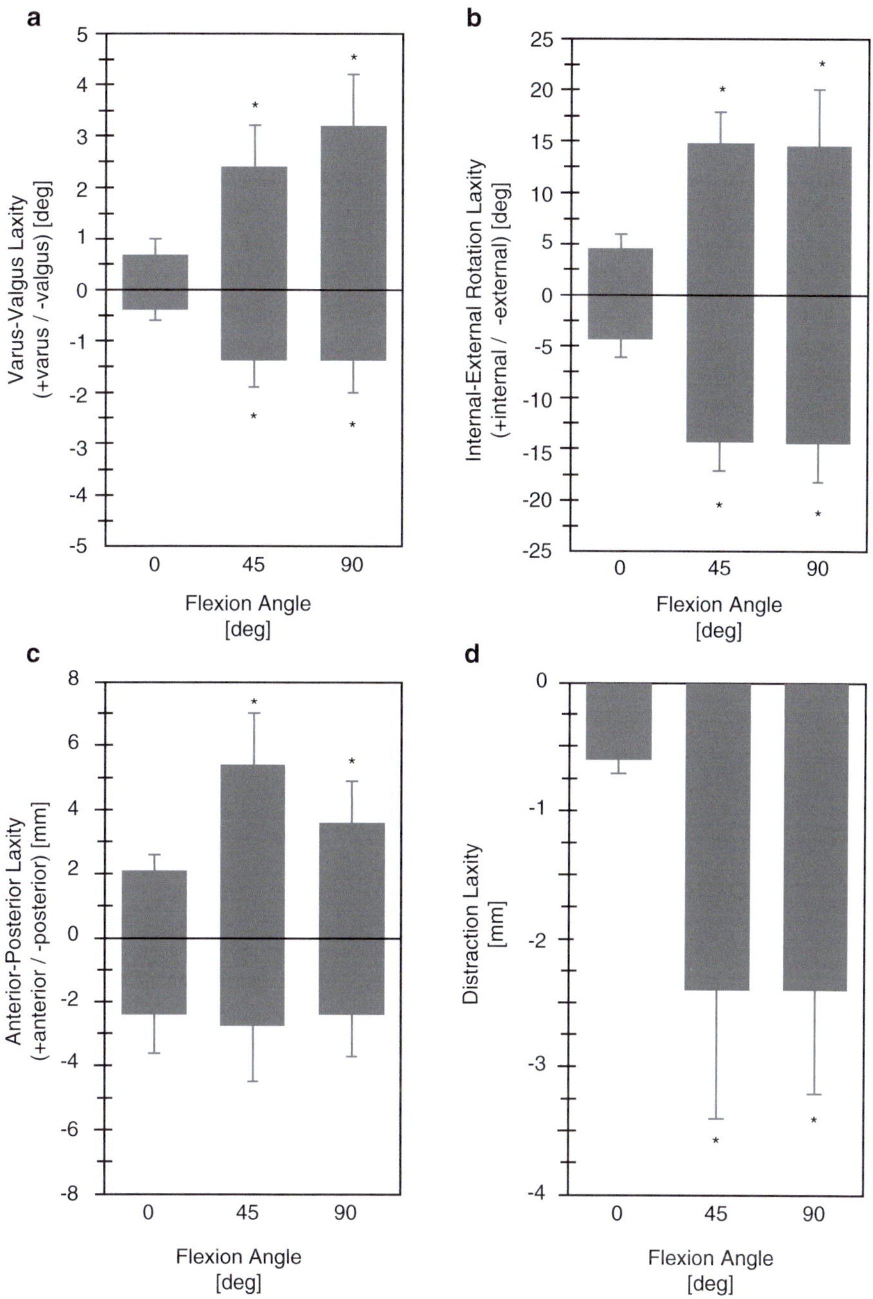

Fig. 2.3 The column graphs show the laxities of the native knee (columns are the means and error bars are the standard deviations) at 0°, 45°, and 90° of flexion in (**a**) V-V, (**b**) I-E, (**c**) A-P, and (**d**) D. An asterisk indicates that the laxity at either 45° or 90° of flexion is greater than that at 0° of flexion [17]

2.3 Using the Soft Tissue Balance of the Native Knee to Guide Balancing During TKA

If the preferred functional outcome after TKA is restoration of native biomechanics, then the soft tissue balance of the native knee is a reasonable choice to guide balancing during TKA. As previously mentioned, the native knee is inherently stable and has adequate mobility to enable individuals to perform a wide range of activities without pain, stiffness, or feelings of instability. Additionally, the laxities of the knee can be measured pre-, intra-, and postoperatively which allows the laxities of the native knee to be translated into clinical practice. There are two complexities that surgeons should be aware of when applying the previously described laxities in clinical practice. The first complexity is that at the time of surgery, the patient's soft tissue balance has changed from native due to the degenerative changes present in the joint [30–33]. Degradation of the articular surfaces increases the laxities of the knee by bringing together the origin and insertion of the soft tissue restraints (i.e., pseudo-ligamentous laxity) [34]. Growth of osteophytes often re-tensions the soft tissue restraints which in turn reduces the laxities of the knee [35]. Remodeling of the soft tissue restraints (e.g., either lengthening or contracture) may also change the laxities of the knee [30].

A second complexity is that soft tissue balance in the native knee has wide variability in terms of the laxities [18, 36]. This is likely caused by the variability in both the mechanical properties of the soft tissue restraints [37–40] and shapes of the articular surfaces [41]. This variability demonstrates that average laxities reported in the literature are unlikely to represent the native laxities of an individual patient. Hence, striving to achieve the same soft tissue balance in all patients during TKA is unlikely to restore the native soft tissue balance for a particular patient. It is important to note that the laxities do not vary widely at 0° of flexion [18], and therefore the average values at 0° of flexion are reasonable estimates of the native laxities of a particular patient at 0° of flexion.

The contralateral knee should be considered when determining how to approach these complexities. If the patient's contralateral knee has no to mild degenerative changes, then the laxities of the contralateral knee may be used to define the native soft tissue balance for that patient because side-to-side differences in the laxities are negligible [42]. However, if the contralateral knee also has moderate to severe degenerative changes, then the surgeon must assume that the previously reported average laxities at 0° of flexion are native for the patient. The soft tissue balance can then be checked in a relative sense based on the expected increases in the laxities with flexion relative to those at 0° of flexion (Fig. 2.3).

2.4 Potential Consequences of Not Restoring Native Soft Tissue Balance

Although complexities exist with striving to restore the native soft tissue balance, surgeons should be aware that there are at least three potential consequences for not striving to restore native soft tissue balance. The first consequence is that overly tight soft tissue restraints compared to native may cause abnormal kinematics. For example, studies have reported that patients following gap-balanced TKA exhibit abnormal kinematics in flexion [43, 44]. The goal of gap balancing in terms of soft tissue balance is to tighten the knee in flexion so that the laxities in flexion match those in extension [1, 45–47]. If the ideal balance is achieved in a gap-balanced TKA, then the knee will be overly tight in flexion especially in the lateral compartment [17]. One possible explanation for these abnormal kinematics is that the overly tight soft tissue restraints in flexion especially in the lateral compartment may limit the posterior translation of the femur on the tibia. This translation is present in the native knee and is necessary for achieving deep flexion [48–51]. This consequence is supported by a recent clinical study that showed patients preferred a more lax knee after TKA [52].

A second consequence is that soft tissue releases will frequently be required [53–57]. Soft tissue releases have several detrimental effects on the knee. First, soft tissue releases increase multiple laxities [58, 59]. Therefore, a release performed to achieve the desired change in one laxity may increase other laxities that do not need to be changed. Second, it is difficult to control the amount of release performed, and hence under- and over-release of the soft tissue restraints are possible [56, 60, 61].

The third consequence is that non-native tensions in the soft tissue restraints may feel abnormal to the patient because the soft tissue restraints are innervated with both proprioceptors and mechanoreceptors [27, 62–66]. Hence, even subtle changes in the soft tissue balance may be perceived as pain, stiffness, or instability by the patient [27, 67].

2.5 Summary

The soft tissues are "balanced" in the native knee because the joint is inherently stable and has adequate mobility for individuals to perform a wide range of activities. As such, restoration of the native soft tissue balance is a reasonable goal for soft tissue balancing in TKA to best restore native biomechanics and provide the patient with a knee that feels as close to normal as possible. Failing to restore native soft tissue balance may lead to instability, stiffness, limited motion, pain, or an abnormal feeling knee.

The benefits of striving to restore native soft tissue balance are evident in the positive clinical outcomes following kinematically aligned TKA. In kinematically aligned TKA, the components are aligned to best restore the native articular surfaces, and the surgeon strives to restore the native soft tissue balance without soft tissue releases [68]. A recent cadaveric study showed that kinematically aligned TKA does closely restore native soft tissue balance as judged by the laxities [69]. Patients after kinematically aligned TKA have better pain relief, have higher functional scores, achieve greater flexion, have more normal kinematics, and are three times more likely to report that their knee feels normal than patients after mechanically aligned TKA, in which surgeons most often strive to achieve balanced gaps [70–73].

References

1. Sikorski JM. Alignment in total knee replacement. J Bone Joint Surg Br. 2008;90(9):1121–7. doi:10.1302/0301-620X.90B9.20793.
2. Heesterbeek PJ, Haffner N, Wymenga AB, Stifter J, Ritschl P. Patient-related factors influence stiffness of the soft tissue complex during intraoperative gap balancing in cruciate-retaining total knee arthroplasty. Knee Surg Sports Traumatol Arthrosc. 2015:1–9. doi:10.1007/s00167-015-3694-5.
3. Blankevoort L, Huiskes R, de Lange A. The envelope of passive knee joint motion. J Biomech. 1988;21(9):705–20. doi: 10.1016/0021-9290(88)90280-1.
4. Schipplein OD, Andriacchi TP. Interaction between active and passive knee stabilizers during level walking. J Orthop Res. 1991;9(1):113–9. doi: 10.1002/jor.1100090114.
5. Dyrby CO, Andriacchi TP. Secondary motions of the knee during weight bearing and non-weight bearing activities. J Orthop Res. 2004;22(4):794–800. doi:10.1016/j.orthres.2003.11.003.
6. Wilson DR, Feikes JD, O'Connor JJ. Ligaments and articular contact guide passive knee flexion. J Biomech. 1998;31(12):1127–36. doi: 10.1016/S0021-9290(98)00119-5.
7. Halewood C, Amis AA. Clinically relevant biomechanics of the knee capsule and ligaments. Knee Surg Sports Traumatol Arthrosc. 2015;23(10):2789–96. doi:10.1007/s00167-015-3594-8.
8. Davidson BS, Judd DL, Thomas AC, Mizner RL, Eckhoff DG, Stevens-Lapsley JE. Muscle activation and coactivation during five-time-sit-to-stand movement in patients undergoing total knee arthroplasty. J Electromyogr Kinesiol. 2013;23(6):1485–93. doi:10.1016/j.jelekin.2013.06.008.
9. Meier W, Mizner RL, Marcus RL, Dibble LE, Peters C, Lastayo PC. Total knee arthroplasty: muscle impairments, functional limitations, and recommended rehabilitation approaches. J Orthop Sports Phys Ther. 2008;38(5):246–56. doi:10.2519/jospt.2008.2715.
10. Thomas AC, Judd DL, Davidson BS, Eckhoff DG, Stevens-Lapsley JE. Quadriceps/hamstrings co-activation increases early after total knee arthroplasty. Knee. 2014;21(6):1115–9. doi:10.1016/j.knee.2014.08.001.
11. Petterson SC, Mizner RL, Stevens JE, Raisis L, Bodenstab A, Newcomb W, Snyder-Mackler L. Improved function from progressive strengthening interventions after total knee arthroplasty: a randomized clinical trial with an imbedded prospective cohort. Arthritis Rheum. 2009;61(2):174–83. doi:10.1002/art.24167.
12. Athwal KK, Hunt NC, Davies AJ, Deehan DJ, Amis AA. Clinical biomechanics of instability related to total knee arthroplasty. Clin Biomech (Bristol, Avon). 2014;29(2):119–28. doi:10.1016/j.clinbiomech.2013.11.004.
13. Bull AM, Kessler O, Alam M, Amis AA. Changes in knee kinematics reflect the articular geometry after arthroplasty. Clin Orthop Relat Res. 2008;466(10):2491–9. doi:10.1007/s11999-008-0440-z.
14. Mihalko WM, Saleh KJ, Krackow KA, Whiteside LA. Soft-tissue balancing during total knee arthroplasty in the varus knee. J Am Acad Orthop Surg. 2009;17(12):766–74.
15. Camarata DA. Soft tissue balance in total knee arthroplasty with a force sensor. Orthop Clin North Am. 2014;45(2):175–84. doi:10.1016/j.ocl.2013.12.001.
16. Gustke K. Use of smart trials for soft-tissue balancing in total knee replacement surgery. J Bone Joint Surg Br. 2012;94(11 Suppl A):147–50. doi:10.1302/0301-620X.94B11.30621.
17. Roth JD, Howell SM, Hull ML. Native knee laxities at 0°, 45°, and 90° of flexion and their relationship to the goal of the gap-balancing alignment method of total knee arthroplasty. J Bone Joint Surg Am. 2015;97(20):1678–84. doi:10.2106/jbjs.n.01256.
18. Roth JD, Hull ML, Howell SM. The limits of passive motion are variable between and unrelated within normal tibiofemoral joints. J Orthop Res. 2015;33(11):1594–602. doi:10.1002/jor.22926.

19. Markolf KL, Graff-Radford A, Amstutz HC. In vivo knee stability. A quantitative assessment using an instrumented clinical testing apparatus. J Bone Joint Surg Am. 1978;60(5):664–74.
20. Markolf KL, Mensch JS, Amstutz HC. Stiffness and laxity of the knee–The contributions of the supporting structures. J Bone Joint Surg Am. 1976;58-A(5):583–94.
21. Eagar P, Hull ML, Howell SM. A method for quantifying the anterior load-displacement behavior of the human knee in both the low and high stiffness regions. J Biomech. 2001;34(12):1655–60. doi:10.1016/s0021-9290(01)00142-7.
22. Nowakowski AM, Majewski M, Müller-Gerbl M, Valderrabano V. Measurement of knee joint gaps without bone resection: "Physiologic" extension and flexion gaps in total knee arthroplasty are asymmetric and unequal and anterior and posterior cruciate ligament resections produce different gap changes. J Orthop Res. 2012;30(4):522–7. doi:10.1002/jor.21564.
23. Ghosh KM, Blain AP, Longstaff L, Rushton S, Amis AA, Deehan DJ. Can we define envelope of laxity during navigated knee arthroplasty? Knee Surg Sports Traumatol Arthrosc. 2014;22(8):1736–43. doi:10.1007/s00167-013-2574-0.
24. Wang X, Malik A, Bartel DL, Wickiewicz TL, Wright T. Asymmetric varus and valgus stability of the anatomic cadaver knee and the load sharing between collateral ligaments and bearing surfaces. J Biomech Eng. 2014;136(8) doi:10.1115/1.4027662.
25. Moewis P, Boeth H, Heller MO, Yntema C, Jung T, Doyscher R, Ehrig RM, Zhong Y, Taylor WR. Towards understanding knee joint laxity: errors in non-invasive assessment of joint rotation can be corrected. Med Eng Phys. 2014;36(7):889–95. doi:10.1016/j.medengphy.2014.03.017.
26. Haimes JL, Wroble RR, Grood ES, Noyes FR. Role of the medial structures in the intact and anterior cruciate ligament-deficient knee. Limits of motion in the human knee. Am J Sports Med. 1994;22(3):402–9. doi:10.1177/036354659402200317.
27. Delport P, Labey L, De Corte R, Innocenti B, Vander Sloten J, Bellemans J. Collateral ligament strains during knee joint laxity evaluation before and after TKA. Clin Biomech (Bristol, Avon). 2013;28(7):777–82. doi:10.1016/j.clinbiomech.2013.06.006.
28. Okazaki K, Miura H, Matsuda S, Takeuchi N, Mawatari T, Hashizume M, Iwamoto Y. Asymmetry of mediolateral laxity of the normal knee. J Orthop Sci. 2006;11(3):264–6. doi:10.1007/s00776-006-1009-x.
29. Mayman D, Plaskos C, Kendoff D, Wernecke G, Pearle AD, Laskin R. Ligament tension in the ACL-deficient knee: assessment of medial and lateral gaps. Clin Orthop Relat Res. 2009;467(6):1621–8. doi:10.1007/s11999-009-0748-3.
30. Bellemans J, Vandenneucker H, Vanlauwe J, Victor J. The influence of coronal plane deformity on mediolateral ligament status: an observational study in varus knees. Knee Surg Sports Traumatol Arthrosc. 2010;18(2):152–6. doi:10.1007/s00167-009-0903-0.
31. Rudolph KS, Schmitt LC, Lewek MD. Age-related changes in strength, joint laxity, and walking patterns: are they related to knee osteoarthritis? Phys Ther. 2007;87(11):1422–32. doi: 10.2522/ptj.20060137.
32. Brage ME, Draganich LF, Pottenger LA, Curran JJ. Knee laxity in symptomatic osteoarthritis. Clin Orthop Relat Res. 1994,304(7):181 9.
33. Sharma L, Lou C, Felson DT, Dunlop DD, Kirwan-Mellis G, Hayes KW, Weinrach D, Buchanan TS. Laxity in healthy and osteoarthritic knees. Arthritis Rheum. 1999;42(5):861–70. doi:10.1002/1529-0131(199905)42:5<861::AID-ANR4>3.0.CO;2-N.
34. Lewek MD, Rudolph KS, Snyder-Mackler L. Control of frontal plane knee laxity during gait in patients with medial compartment knee osteoarthritis. Osteoarthritis Cartilage. 2004;12(9):745–51. doi:10.1016/j.joca.2004.05.005.
35. Pottenger LA, Phillips FM, Draganich LF. The effect of marginal osteophytes on reduction of varus-valgus instability in osteoarthritic knees. Arthritis Rheum. 1990;33(6):853–8. doi:10.1002/art.1780330612.
36. Cyr AJ, Maletsky LP. Unified quantification of variation in passive knee joint constraint. Proc Inst Mech Eng H. 2014;228(5):494–500. doi:10.1177/0954411914530274.

37. Woo SL, Hollis JM, Adams DJ, Lyon RM, Takai S. Tensile properties of the human femur-anterior cruciate ligament-tibia complex. The effects of specimen age and orientation. Am J Sports Med. 1991;19(3):217–25. doi: 10.1177/036354659101900303.
38. Robinson JR, Bull AM, Amis AA. Structural properties of the medial collateral ligament complex of the human knee. J Biomech. 2005;38(5):1067–74. doi:10.1016/j.jbiomech.2004.05.034.
39. LaPrade RF, Bollom TS, Wentorf FA, Wills NJ, Meister K. Mechanical properties of the posterolateral structures of the knee. Am J Sports Med. 2005;33(9):1386–91. doi:10.1177/0363546504274143.
40. Race A, Amis AA. The mechanical properties of the two bundles of the human posterior cruciate ligament. J Biomech. 1994;27(1):13–24. doi:10.1016/0021-9290(94)90028-0.
41. Smoger LM, Fitzpatrick CK, Clary CW, Cyr AJ, Maletsky LP, Rullkoetter PJ, Laz PJ. Statistical modeling to characterize relationships between knee anatomy and kinematics. J Orthop Res. 2015;33(11):1620–30. doi:10.1002/jor.22948.
42. Shultz SJ, Shimokochi Y, Nguyen AD, Schmitz RJ, Beynnon BD, Perrin DH. Measurement of varus-valgus and internal-external rotational knee laxities in vivo–Part I: assessment of measurement reliability and bilateral asymmetry. J Orthop Res. 2007;25(8):981–8. doi:10.1002/jor.20397.
43. Dennis DA, Komistek RD, Colwell Jr CE, Ranawat CS, Scott RD, Thornhill TS, Lapp MA. In vivo anteroposterior femorotibial translation of total knee arthroplasty: a multicenter analysis. Clin Orthop Relat Res. 1998;356(11):47–57.
44. Dennis DA, Komistek RD, Mahfouz MR, Walker SA, Tucker A. A multicenter analysis of axial femorotibial rotation after total knee arthroplasty. Clin Orthop Relat Res. 2004;428(11):180–9.
45. Babazadeh S, Stoney JD, Lim K, Choong PFM. The relevance of ligament balancing in total knee arthroplasty: how important is it? A systematic review of the literature. Orthop Rev (Pavia). 2009;1(2)e26. doi: 10.4081/or.2009.e26.
46. Bottros J, Gad B, Krebs V, Barsoum WK. Gap balancing in total knee arthroplasty. J Arthroplasty. 2006;21(4 Suppl 1):11–5. doi:10.1016/j.arth.2006.02.084.
47. Griffin FM, Insall JN, Scuderi GR. Accuracy of soft tissue balancing in total knee arthroplasty. J Arthroplasty. 2000;15(8):970–3. doi:10.1054/arth.2000.6503.
48. Pinskerova V, Johal P, Nakagawa S, Sosna A, Williams A, Gedroyc W, Freeman MA. Does the femur roll-back with flexion? J Bone Joint Surg Br. 2004;86(6):925–31. doi: 10.1302/0301-620X.86B6.14589.
49. Dennis DA, Mahfouz MR, Komistek RD, Hoff W. In vivo determination of normal and anterior cruciate ligament-deficient knee kinematics. J Biomech. 2005;38(2):241–53. doi:10.1016/j.jbiomech.2004.02.042.
50. Freeman MA, Pinskerova V. The movement of the knee studied by magnetic resonance imaging. Clin Orthop Relat Res. 2003;410(5):35–43. doi:10.1097/01.blo.0000063598.67412.0d.
51. Freeman MA. Soft tissues: a question of balance. Orthopedics. 1997;20(9):827–31. doi: 10.3928/0147-7447-19970901-24.
52. Kuster MS, Bitschnau B, Votruba T. Influence of collateral ligament laxity on patient satisfaction after total knee arthroplasty: a comparative bilateral study. Arch Orthop Trauma Surg. 2004;124(6):415–7. doi:10.1007/s00402-004-0700-7.
53. Gu Y, Roth JD, Howell SM, Hull ML. How frequently do four methods for mechanically aligning a total knee arthroplasty cause collateral ligament imbalance and change alignment from normal in white patients? J Bone Joint Surg Am. 2014;96(12):e101. doi: 10.2106/JBJS.M.00306.
54. Hunt NC, Ghosh KM, Athwal KK, Longstaff LM, Amis AA, Deehan DJ. Lack of evidence to support present medial release methods in total knee arthroplasty. Knee Surg Sports Traumatol Arthrosc. 2014;22(12):3100–12. doi:10.1007/s00167-014-3148-5.
55. Peters CL, Jimenez C, Erickson J, Anderson MB, Pelt CE. Lessons learned from selective soft-tissue release for gap balancing in primary total knee arthroplasty: an analysis of 1216

consecutive total knee arthroplasties: AAOS exhibit selection. J Bone Joint Surg Am. 2013;95(20):e152. doi:10.2106/JBJS.L.01686.

56. Kwak DS, In Y, Kim TK, Cho HS, Koh IJ. The pie-crusting technique using a blade knife for medial collateral ligament release is unreliable in varus total knee arthroplasty. Knee Surg Sports Traumatol Arthrosc. 2016;24(1):188–94. doi:10.1007/s00167-014-3362-1.
57. Goudie S, Deep K. Collateral soft tissue release in primary total knee replacement. Comput Aided Surg. 2014;19(1–3):29–33. doi:10.3109/10929088.2014.889212.
58. Kanamiya T, Whiteside LA, Nakamura T, Mihalko WM, Steiger J, Naito M. Ranawat Award paper. Effect of selective lateral ligament release on stability in knee arthroplasty. Clin Orthop Relat Res. 2002;404(11):24–31.
59. Saeki K, Mihalko WM, Patel V, Conway J, Naito M, Thrum H, Vandenneuker H, Whiteside LA. Stability after medial collateral ligament release in total knee arthroplasty. Clin Orthop Relat Res. 2001;392(11):184–9.
60. Abdel MP, Haas SB. The unstable knee: wobble and buckle. Bone Joint J. 2014;96-B(11 Supple A):112–4. doi:10.1302/0301-620X.96B11.34325.
61. Parratte S, Pagnano MW. Instability after total knee arthroplasty. J Bone Joint Surg Am. 2008;90(1):184–94.
62. Zimny ML, Wink CS. Neuroreceptors in the tissues of the knee joint. J Electromyogr Kinesiol. 1991;1(3):148–57. doi:10.1016/1050-6411(91)90031-Y.
63. Yan J, Sasaki W, Hitomi J. Anatomical study of the lateral collateral ligament and its circumference structures in the human knee joint. Surg Radiol Anat. 2010;32(2):99–106. doi:10.1007/s00276-009-0547-2.
64. Johansson H. Role of knee ligaments in proprioception and regulation of muscle stiffness. J Electromyogr Kinesiol. 1991;1(3):158–79. doi:10.1016/1050-6411(91)90032-Z.
65. Sojka P, Sjolander P, Johansson H, Djupsjobacka M. Influence from stretch-sensitive receptors in the collateral ligaments of the knee joint on the gamma-muscle-spindle systems of flexor and extensor muscles. Neurosci Res. 1991;11(1):55–62. doi:10.1016/0168-0102(91)90066-8.
66. De Avila GA, O'Connor BL, Visco DM, Sisk TD. The mechanoreceptor innervation of the human fibular collateral ligament. J Anat. 1989;162:1–7.
67. Creaby M, Wrigley T, Lim B-W, Hinman R, Bryant A, Bennell K. Self-reported knee joint instability is related to passive mechanical stiffness in medial knee osteoarthritis. BMC Musculoskelet Disord. 2013;14(1):326. doi: 10.1186/1471-2474-14-326.
68. Nedopil AJ, Howell SM, Hull ML. Does malrotation of the tibial and femoral components compromise function in kinematically aligned total knee arthroplasty? Orthop Clin North Am. 2016;47(1):41–50. doi: 10.1016/j.ocl.2015.08.006.
69. Roth JD. How well does kinematically aligned total knee arthroplasty prevent clinically important changes in passive knee function? An in vitro biomechanical study of tibiofemoral laxities and contact. Dissertation, University of California, Davis; 2016. Publication No. 10124447.
70. Dossett HG, Estrada NA, Swartz GJ, LeFevre GW, Kwasman BG. A randomised controlled trial of kinematically and mechanically aligned total knee replacements: two-year clinical results. Bone Joint J. 2014;96-B(7):907–13. doi:10.1302/0301-620X.96B7.32812.
71. Dossett HG, Swartz GJ, Estrada NA, LeFevre GW, Kwasman BG. Kinematically versus mechanically aligned total knee arthroplasty. Orthopedics. 2012;35(2):e160–9. doi:10.3928/01477447-20120123-04.
72. Howell SM, Hodapp EE, Vernace JV, Hull ML, Meade TD. Are undesirable contact kinematics minimized after kinematically aligned total knee arthroplasty? An intersurgeon analysis of consecutive patients. Knee Surg Sports Traumatol Arthrosc. 2013;21(10):2281–7. doi:10.1007/s00167-012-2220-2.
73. Nam D, Nunley RM, Barrack RL. Patient dissatisfaction following total knee replacement: a growing concern? Bone Joint J. 2014;96-B(11 Supple A):96–100. doi:10.1302/0301-620X.96B11.34152.

Kinematics of the Normal Native Knee

3

Jan Victor

Contents

3.1 Introduction

'Kinematics' is a term often used in orthopaedics, unfortunately not always in the correct sense of the word. The term 'kinematics' is derived from mechanical engineering and refers to the relative motion of rigid bodies. In mechanical engineering the description has to be mathematically exact and correct. Tibiofemoral kinematics of the knee is hard to describe unequivocally and mathematically correct. The reason for this is twofold:

1. The native knee has a natural and intrinsic laxity, allowing it to follow several kinematic patterns.
2. The kinematic pattern of the native knee consists of rotation around different axes, in addition to translations.

J. Victor, MD, PhD
Ghent University, Ghent, Belgium

S. Matsuda et al. (eds.), *Soft Tissue Balancing in Total Knee Arthroplasty*,
DOI 10.1007/978-3-662-54082-4_3

3.2 Why Should We, Orthopaedic Surgeons, Bother with Kinematics?

As explained, the term kinematics refers to the relative motion of the femur and the tibia. In other words, it describes how the normal knee is moving. This understanding precedes all discussions on pathophysiology, diagnosis and treatment and forms the basis of our clinical work. Also, understanding normal kinematics is mandatory for improving our surgical techniques. A simplified example can make this very clear. Imagine a door with three hinges (Fig. 3.1). One of the hinges is broken (marked with a red star). It is clear that the door has a single axis of rotation, allowing us to open and close it. If we replace the broken hinge with a new hinge, but we put the new hinge outside of the axis of rotation, it is intuitively clear that the door will either not open anymore or, alternatively, the hinge will break. In orthopaedic terms one can translate this, respectively, into a stiff joint or a failed procedure. This example applies equally to ligament and joint replacement surgery.

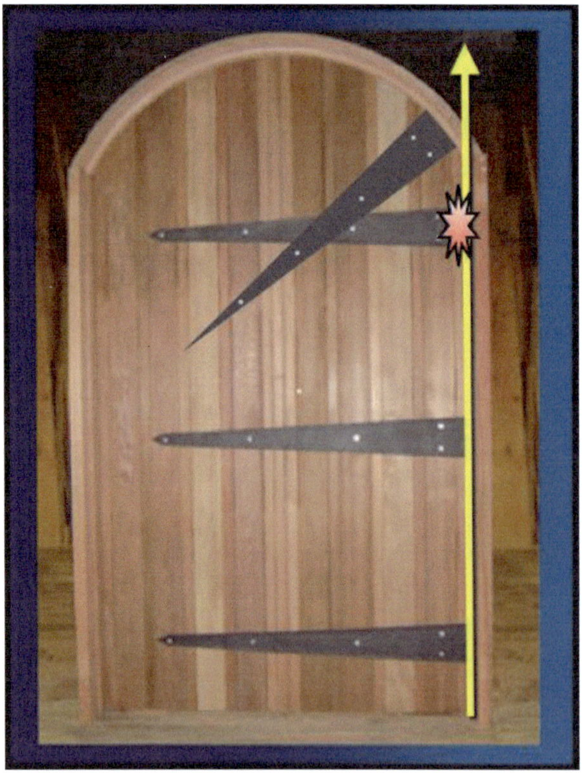

Fig. 3.1 Example of the door with axis of rotation (*yellow arrow*), broken (*red star*) and replaced hinge, outside of the axis of rotation

3.3 Historic Insights in Tibiofemoral Kinematics

The study of how the femur moves on the tibia has a long history. The first known description dates back to 1836 when Weber and Weber [1] described the movement on the medial side to be 'like a cradle'. Since that first description, based upon direct visual observation of a cadaveric specimen, several methods have been used to examine the kinematics of the human knee.

The first radiological study was performed by Zuppinger [2], who stated that the femur rolled back across the tibia during flexion as a result of the so-called rigid four-bar link mechanism provided by the two cruciate ligaments. In 1971, Frankel [3] introduced the concept of the instant centre of rotation to the orthopaedic community. He emphasized that as one link (rigid body) rotates around the other, there is at any given moment in time a point with zero velocity. That point is called the instant centre of rotation (Fig. 3.2).

He concluded that 'due to the shapes of the bones and the restraints on motion imposed by the ligaments, capsule, and muscles, the instantaneous centres for successive positions of the links of the knee move'.

The initial work by Frankel was carried out by taking 'true lateral' X-rays of the knee in patients lying on the side, at discrete intervals of 10–20° in the range of full extension to 90° of flexion. The knee was treated as if it were a 'planar mechanism'. In other words, the movement of the knee was reduced to a two-dimensional projection of a three-dimensional reality (Fig. 3.3). Menschik introduced in 1974 the concept of the four-bar linkage, representing the cruciate ligaments in two dimensions as two rigid bars and the lines connecting their insertion points on the femur and tibia as the two other rigid bars [4]. The instant centre of rotation is located at the point of intersection of the cruciate ligaments. This 'rigid four-bar linkage' was later widely popularized by Müller.

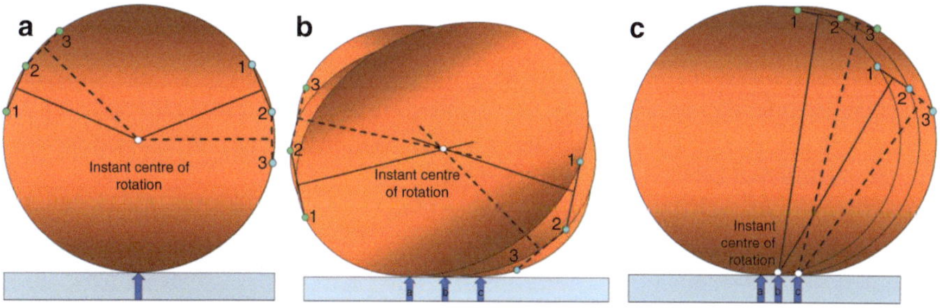

Fig. 3.2 The instant centre of rotation determined with the method of Reuleaux [3]. The points on the body move from position 1 to position 2 and from 2 to 3. The perpendicular bisector for a pair of displacement points is drawn. The intersection of the bisectors is the point with zero velocity, called the instant centre of rotation. The contact point is represented by the *blue arrow*. (**a**) For a circular body undergoing rotation with gliding, the instant centre of rotation and the contact point remain fixed. (**b**) For a non-circular body undergoing rotation with gliding, the instant centre of rotation remains fixed, but the contact point shifts. (**c**) For a circular body undergoing rotation with rolling, the instant centre of rotation coincides with the contact point and moves accordingly

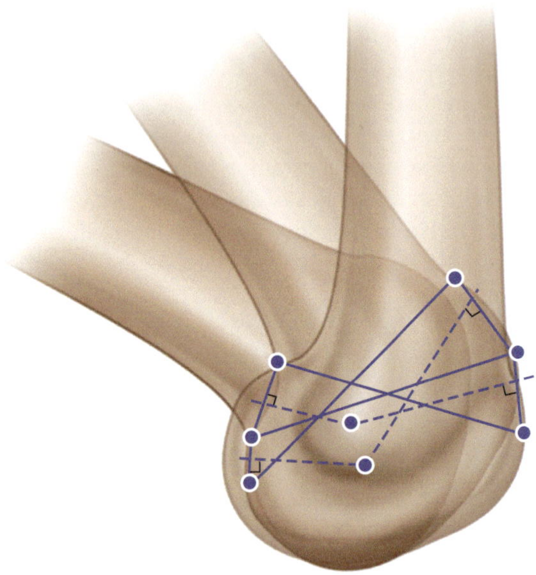

Fig. 3.3 The moving instant centre of rotation of the knee, as described by Frankel [3] in a two-dimensional model

In the years following, the limitations of this methodology became clear, with the major flaw being the inability to ascertain the location of the axes of rotation before performing kinematic analyses [5]. In 1983, Grood and Suntay presented a joint coordinate system providing a geometric description of the three-dimensional rotational and translational motion between two rigid bodies, applied to the knee joint. The main step forward was the definition of a 'floating axis'. With this model, the described joint displacements became independent of the order in which the component rotations and translations occur [6].

The new mathematical insights led to the concept of the helical axis and opened the door for a correct scientific description of the kinematics of the knee [7]. However, as the mathematical accuracy improved, the complexity increased and the model appeared to be impractical and difficult to apply to the clinical setting: the clinicians failed to understand the engineers.

Hollister, and later Churchill, tried to bridge the gap [8, 9]. Hollister's model essentially described knee motion as pure rotations occurring around two axes: the so-called flexion-extension axis and the so-called longitudinal rotation axis, with the understanding of the flexion-extension axis not being exactly located in the coronal plane and the longitudinal axis not being exactly located in the sagittal plane [8]. As a consequence, these mathematical 'simple rotations' meant in reality flexion-extension, varus-valgus and internal-external rotation of the knee joint, once again confusing the clinician trying to apply this knowledge to the practical setting. Churchill addressed this problem by allowing a mathematical error in the kinematic description, based on a loaded rig experiment with an ankle load of 100 N and a combined hamstrings load of 30 N [9]. They used an optimization technique to identify the locations of the so-called 'optimal flexion' and 'longitudinal rotation' axes. Knee motion was then described with the following formula:

$$K = \theta_{\mathrm{OF}} + \theta_{LR} + R_{\theta} + R_{\mathrm{X}} + R_{\mathrm{Y}} + R_{\mathrm{Z}},$$

where K = complete three-dimensional motion, θ_{OF} = rotation about the optimal flexion axis and θ_{LR} = rotation about the longitudinal rotation axis. He concluded that the optimal flexion axis coincided with the transepicondylar axis if one accepts the following errors and limitations: residual rotation ($R\theta$) = 2,9°, residual translations ($R_{\mathrm{X}} + R_{\mathrm{Y}} + R_{\mathrm{Z}}$) = 3.4 mm and applicable motion range 5–90° of flexion. Despite those limitations, the advantage of this approach was the link between the kinematic description and certain anatomic landmarks, allowing clinicians to apply this knowledge in practice.

In recent times, technological progress allowed more advanced tools to be used, including ex vivo studies with MRI on cadaveric specimens [10, 11]; in vivo analyses using 2D fluoroscopy with shape matching techniques, based on CT models [12–15]; roentgen stereo photogrammetric analysis [16]; and open dual coil MRIs [17–19]. These newer methods revealed a more complete, three-dimensional insight in the morphology and kinematic patterns of the normal knee in loaded and unloaded conditions.

3.4 Why Do Kinematic Descriptions of the Knee Vary So Much?

An interesting finding, derived from the study of historic publications on the subject, is worth describing. Hill and Nakagawa [17, 18] described tibiofemoral kinematics, respectively, from 5° to 90° of flexion, based on analysis of load-bearing flexion, and a few months later from 90° to full flexion, based on analysis of subjects performing a deep squat. One would expect the end position of the first study (90° flexion), to be identical to the starting position of the second study (90° flexion). In fact, it is not (Fig. 3.4)! Meticulous and dedicated researchers carried out

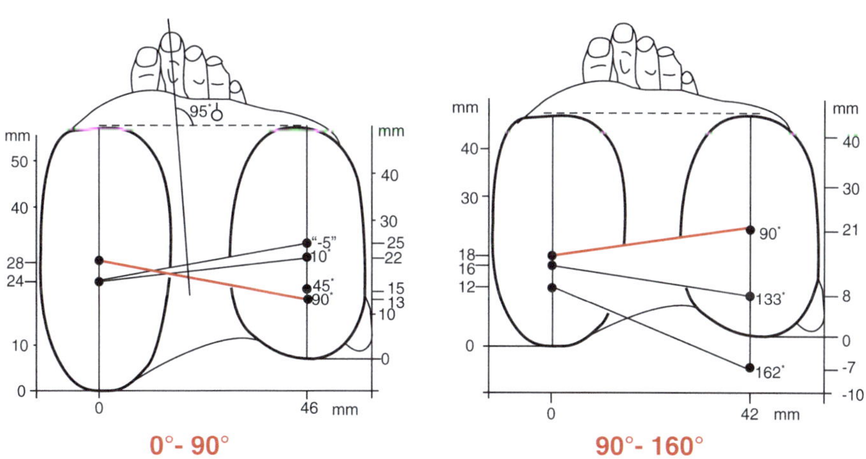

Fig. 3.4 Kinematic patterns found in the publications by Hill and Nakagawa [17, 18]. The end position of study 1 does not match the starting position of study 2 (represented by the *red line*)

both studies, so why is this discrepancy observed? The reason is that kinematics will vary with muscular action and imposed activity.

3.5 The Influence of Load on Tibiofemoral Kinematics

We measured passive kinematics of the human knee, using a cadaveric model [20]. In passive modus, the medial condyle is sliding slightly forwards (up to 35° of flexion), followed by some gradual posterior translation with increasing flexion. In contrast, the lateral condyle displays gradual posterior translation from full extension to full flexion. The excursion of the lateral condyle is greater than the excursion of the medial condyle and extends more posteriorly (Fig. 3.5).

When the quadriceps is loaded, the kinematics of the knee change significantly [21]. The translation of the femur relative to the tibia is significantly reduced (Fig. 3.6).

The forces acting on the tibia in the sagittal plane can explain this. Between full extension and 65° of flexion, the force vector acting on the tibia has an anterior directed component (Fig. 3.7). This force vector is reversed beyond 65° of flexion, pulling the tibia backwards and mitigating the traditional passive kinematics, especially on the lateral compartment. This kinetic analysis explains the observed differences.

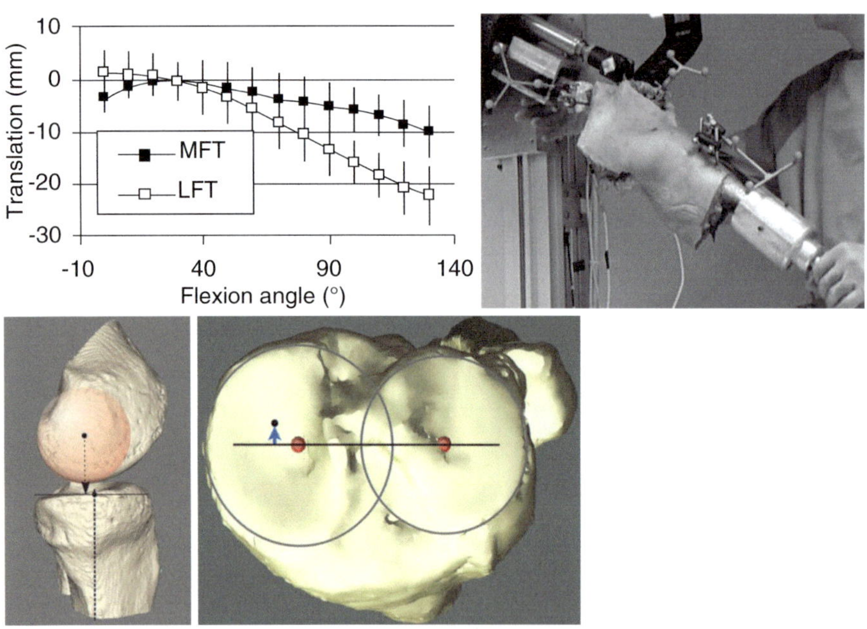

Fig. 3.5 Passive kinematics of the normal knee, based upon a cadaveric model [20]. The white boxes represent the relative position of the medial condyle on the anteroposterior axis, expressed as the distance from the projected centre of the condyle to the midline of the tibia, and the *black boxes* the relative position of the lateral condyle

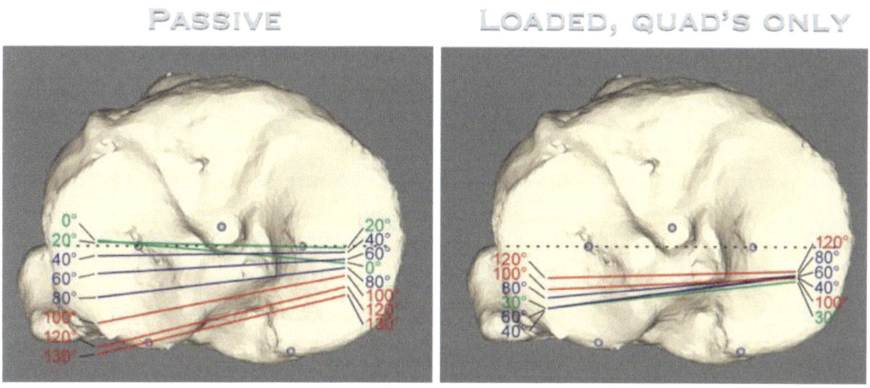

Fig. 3.6 Comparison of the passive and loaded tibiofemoral kinematics [21]

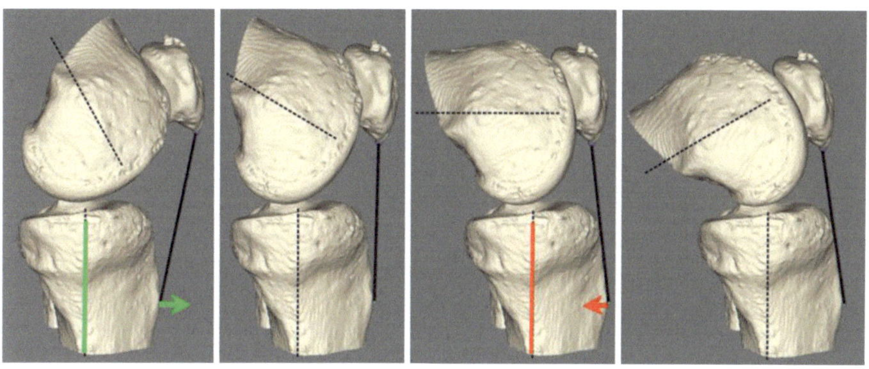

Fig. 3.7 Sagittal view of the knee with force vector analysis illustrating the effect of extensor mechanism forces on tibiofemoral kinematics [21]

Conclusion

Description of knee kinematics is complex. Correct mathematical methods are hard to understand intuitively and do not help the surgeon get a grip on knee function during diagnosis and surgical treatment. They are important however in accurately analysing the outcome of our procedures. More intuitive graphic descriptions offer the advantage of clarity and surgical value but fail to describe precisely the observed kinematics. Both ways of presenting deserve a place in the literature.

It is important to understand that tibiofemoral kinematics is not a static and dogmatic finding that repetitively happens in exactly the same way in any type of knee. In reality, kinematics depend on joint geometry, type of activity, knee alignment, body weight, muscle action and ligament laxity. The surgeon should look at this variability in terms of the 'boundaries of laxity'. Within the normal stress-strain curves of ligaments, the excursion of the femur relative to the tibia will encounter its limits in these ligaments that allow for a passive kinematic path that has been described in several studies. As the knee is loaded during body movement and muscular action, this kinematic path will vary, within the limits of natural laxity.

Every surgical procedure should respect this passive kinematic path as an optimum and refrain from pushing these boundaries of laxity. Failure to do so leads to stiffness, chronic pain, instability and/or failure of the surgical procedure.

References

1. Weber WE, Weber E. Mechanics of the human walking apparatus. Translated by Maquet P and Furlong R Berlin etc: Springer, 1992: 75 (original publication: Mechanik der menschelichen Gehwerkzeuge. Göttingen, 1836).
2. Zuppinger H. Die aktive flexion im unbelasten Kniegelenk: Züricher Habil Schr. Wiesbaden: Bergmann; 1904. p. 703–63.
3. Frankel VH, Burstein AH, Brooks DB. Biomechanics as determined by analysis of the instant centers of motion. J Bone Joint Surg Br. 1971;53-A:945–77.
4. Menschik A. Mechanik des Kniegelenks. Teil 1 Z Orthop. 1974;112:481–95.
5. Soudan K, Van Audekercke R, Martens M. Methods, difficulties and inaccuracies in the study of human joint kinematics and pathokinematics by the instant axis concept. Example: the knee joint. J Biomech. 1979;12:27–33.
6. Grood ES, Suntay WJ. A joint coordinate system for the clinical description of three-dimensional motions: application to the knee. J Biomech Eng. 1983;105:136–44.
7. Blankevoort L, Huiskes R, de Lange A. Helical axes of passive knee joint motions. J Biomech. 1990;23:1219–29.
8. Hollister AM, Jatana S, Singh AK, Sullivan WW, Lupichuk AG. The axes of rotation of the knee. Clin Orthop. 1993;290:259–68.
9. Churchill DL, Incavo SJ, Johnson CC, Beynnon BD. The transepicondylar axis approximates the optimal flexion axis of the knee. Clin Orthop. 1998;356:111–8.
10. Iwaki H, Pinskerova V, Freeman MAR. Tibiofemoral movement 1: the shapes and relative movements of the femur and the tibia in the unloaded cadaver knee. J Bone Joint Surg. 2000;82(8):1189–95.
11. Eckhoff DE, Hogan C, DiMatteo L, et al. Difference between the epicondylar and cylindrical axis of the knee. Clin Orthop. 2007;461:238–44.
12. Banks SA, Hodge WA. Accurate measurement of three-dimensional knee replacement kinematics using single-plane fluoroscopy. IEEE Trans Biomed Eng. 1996;43:638–49.
13. Komistek RD, Dennis DA, Mahfouz M. *In vivo* fluoroscopic analysis of the normal human knee. Clin Orthop. 2003;410:69–81.
14. Lu TW, Tsai TY, Kuo MY, Hsu HC, Chen HL. *In vivo* three dimensional kinematics of the normal knee during active extension under unloaded and loaded conditions using single-plane fluoroscopy. Med Eng Phys. 2008;30(8):1004–12. doi:10.1016/j.medengphy.2008.03.001.
15. Moro-oka T, Hamai S, Miura H, Shimoto T, Higaki H, Fregly BJ, Iwamoto Y, Banks SA. Dynamic activity dependence of *in vivo* normal knee kinematics. J Orthop Res. 2008;26:428–34.
16. Karrholm J, Brandsson S, Freeman MAR. Tibiofemoral movement 4: changes of axial rotation caused by forced rotation at the weight bearing knee studied by RSA. J Bone Joint Surg. 2000;82-B:1201–3.
17. Hill PF, Vedi V, Williams A, Iwaki H, Pinskerova V, Freeman MAR. Tibiofemoral movement 2: the loaded and unloaded living knee studied by MRI. J Bone Joint Surg Br. 2000;82-B:1196–8.

18. Nakagawa S, Kadoya Y, Todo S, Kobayashi A, Sakamoto H, Freeman MAR, Yamano Y. Tibiofemoral movement 3: full flexion in the living knee studied by MRI. J Bone Joint Surg Br. 2000;82-B:1199–200.
19. Johal P, Williams A, Wragg P, Hunt D, Gedroyc W. Tibio-femoral movement in the living knee. A study of weight bearing and non-weight bearing knee kinematics using 'interventional' MRI. J Biomech. 2005;38:269–76.
20. Victor J, Van Glabbeek F, Vander Sloten J, Parizel PM, Somville J, Bellemans J. An Experimental model for kinematic analysis of the knee. J Bone Joint Surg Am. 2009;91:150–63.
21. Victor J, Labey L, Wong P, Innocenti B, Bellemans J. The influence of muscle load on tibiofemoral kinematics. J Orthop Res. 2010;28(4):419–28.

Part II

Operative Procedure 1: Primary TKA

Primary Principles in Soft Tissue Balancing

4

Jacobus H. Müller and Willem van der Merwe

Contents

Soft tissue balance and alignment are integral to the success of a total knee arthroplasty (TKA). In 1985 it was already reported that most failures can be attributed to incorrect ligament balance or incorrect alignment [1]. Since 1985, numerous new and improved total knee replacement systems, surgical instruments, surgical methods, and computer-assisted surgery tools have seen the light. Ligament balancing and alignment however still remain the biggest considerations that impact the successful outcome of a total knee arthroplasty.

Once the anterior cruciate ligament (and posterior cruciate ligament in non-cruciate retaining TKA) is resected, knee stability relies on the interaction between the remaining ligamentous structures and articular surface geometries [2]. Patient satisfaction and clinical outcome scores are superior in balanced knees [3–5], whereas the restoration of joint space is also conducive to proprioception and balance [6]. Imbalance in TKA is linked to increased component wear, instability, decreased active range of motion, and increased risks of joint pain [3–5]. Up to 40% of early revisions are avoidable if optimal balance was achieved during the primary surgery [4]. It is thus important to appreciate what is meant by a soft tissue balanced joint.

J.H. Müller
Biomedical Engineering Research Group, Department of Mechanical and Mechatronic Engineering, Stellenbosch University, Stellenbosch, South Africa
e-mail: cobusmul@sun.ac.za

W. van der Merwe (✉)
Sports Science Institute of South Africa Orthopaedic Clinic, Cape Town, South Africa
e-mail: willem@ssoc.co.za

S. Matsuda et al. (eds.), *Soft Tissue Balancing in Total Knee Arthroplasty*,
DOI 10.1007/978-3-662-54082-4_4

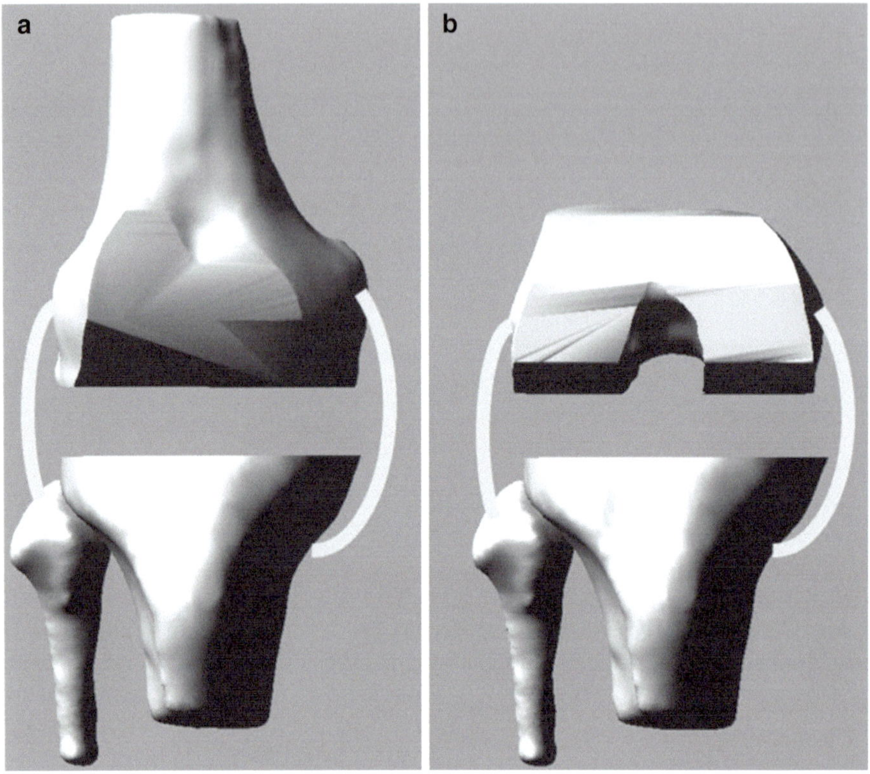

Fig. 4.1 Rectangular (**a**) extension gap and (**b**) flexion gap

A soft tissue balanced joint has been defined to have equal and rectangular gaps between the resected bone surfaces in extension and flexion to induce equal tension in the medial and lateral soft tissues [3] (Fig. 4.1). This is achieved through either or a combination of soft tissue release, modification to bone cuts, component size variation, and component rotation to ensure central tracking of the femoral component. This definition however only provides arbitrary criteria of what constitutes a balanced condition [5]. A better understanding may be established from the characteristics of a balanced knee [7]:

- A balanced knee will have a full range of movement.
- The flexion medial-lateral balance will be symmetrical to result in a rectangular tibiofemoral gap.
- The flexion-extension gap will be balanced with minimal to no medial-lateral tightness or laxity.
- The patella will track normal during the full range of motion due appropriate femoral rotation.
- Femoral roll back in deep flexion will be nonexcessive.
- There is proper rotational balance between the tibial and femoral components.

The resections of the tibia and femur during knee arthroplasty must result in rectangular flexion and extension gaps (equal medial and lateral soft tissue tensions) without changing the anatomical joint line [8].

Traditionally, resection of the femur and tibia can be done through three approaches, namely, the measured resection technique, the gap balancing technique, or a combination of the two techniques. The major difference between measured resection and gap balancing is the way in which femoral rotation is determined. During the measured resection technique, bony landmarks (Whiteside line, surgical epicondylar axis, posterior condylar axis, and the anterior-posterior axis) are used to set femoral component rotation, whereas the gap balancing technique relies on symmetrical tensioning of the medial and lateral soft tissues in flexion to set femoral rotation. The former technique may result in a wide range of soft tissue balance due to the difficulty of reproducibly identifying the bony landmarks intraoperatively [9]. This can lead to flexion gap asymmetry and condylar lift-off. To remedy the situation, the correct course of action depends on whether joint stiffness increase or decrease during flexion and the degree of asymmetry in the medial-lateral soft tissues and its variability with flexion [3]. Although the gap balancing technique provides better chances of achieving proper ligament balance in full extension and 90° flexion, midflexion stability is not guaranteed. This can be attributed to the risk of getting an incorrect tibial cut which serves as the platform from which the flexion gap is established [9]. Secondary to that is the uncertainty in the application and magnitude of the correct distraction force [9]. Since soft tissue balance can be manipulated by varying the medial-lateral extension and flexion gaps, incorrect resection may result in instability due to ligament imbalance.

Varus or valgus instability refers to a trapezoidal extension gap due to asymmetric contracture or laxity in the collateral ligaments (Fig. 4.2). This type of laxity can be either symmetric or asymmetric [8]. Symmetric instability may result due to excessive cartilage loss on the affected condyle. Alternatively, the patient might have had a varus or valgus alignment before the pathology set in. For these cases, a rectangular extension gap may then result in a pronounced varus or valgus alignment even though the ligaments might be balanced. On the other hand, asymmetric instability refers to contracture or excessive laxity of one of the collateral ligaments. Traditionally, surgeons employing gap balancing have relied on spacer blocks and distractors to achieve proper soft tissue balance [3]. Since these techniques rely solely on tactile feedback and subjective assessment [4, 10], success is strongly related to the skill level and experience of the surgeon. An attempt to circumvent this has seen the introduction of instrumented tibial trials and distractors with which the medial-lateral load components can be objectively measured [3]. Unfortunately, these new developments still shed little light on what the surgical steps should be to achieve a balanced condition [3].

Although there are no clear guidelines, e.g., it is still unclear what level of extension gap tightness is appropriate to avoid postoperative flexion contracture [2], some values have been found to produce good outcomes. The amount of laxity should be governed by the patient's perception of stability. A medial extension gap of 1–3 mm has been found to result in a stable feeling as well as not causing flexion contracture,

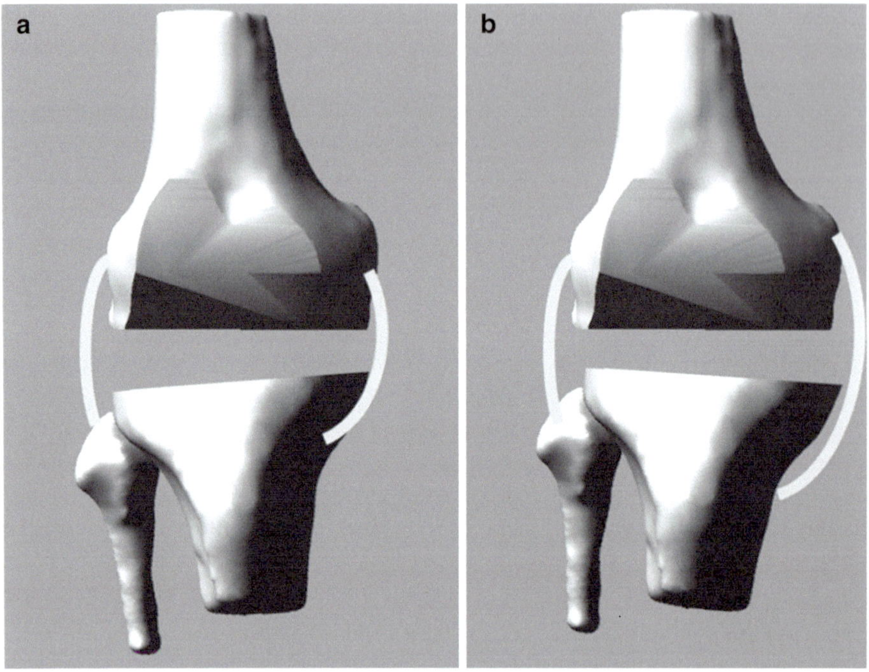

Fig. 4.2 Varus and valgus deformities after resection. (**a**) Varus deformity and (**b**) valgus deformity

whereas the lateral side should be 2.5° laxer than the medial side [2]. The medial flexion gap should be similar or close to the extension gap. This will achieve near-normal articulation, function, and patient satisfaction [2]. Unfortunately, there are no clear evidence on what constitutes a safe range for the lateral flexion gap other than some degree of laxity being acceptable [2]. Instrumented distractors and tibial trials have necessitated the need to quantify the flexion and extension gap balance in terms of force values.

Ideal force target values have not as of yet been validated; a medial-lateral ratio ranging between 0.5 and 0.55 is suggested [3, 4]. A case series ($n = 189$) has shown that a medial-lateral force differential less than 60 lb will result in good outcomes [4], whereas a more conservative ratio of less than 15 lb has also been ascribed [11]. It is however difficult to maintain this ratio throughout flexion [3] and furthermore unclear whether it is important to maintain the same ratio throughout flexion [10]. A recent case series ($n = 12$) measured the differential at 10°, 45°, and 90° [5]. The differentials (medial load min lateral load) were, respectively, 5.6, 9.8, and 4.3 lb. Laxities in the native knee are not uniform, and there is a need for more in depth analysis to determine appropriate target values [12]. Fortunately, there are qualitative measures and guidelines to address varus deformities, valgus deformities, flexion contracture, and genu recurvatum through soft tissue balancing.

A varus-deformed knee requires release of the deep medial collateral ligament and removal of osteophytes [8]. Persistent contracture may require release of the distal superficial medial collateral ligament in combination with the posterior-medial capsule and semimembranosus insertion [8]. Sacrifice of the posterior cruciate ligament will significantly increase the flexion gap on the medial side with little influence on the extension gap [13]. In cases with persistent deformity, it may be necessary to advance the lateral collateral ligament. It has been shown that lateral soft tissue laxity increased with increasing severity of knee deformities, while the medial side did not contract with increasing varus deformity [2]. This result suggests that release on the medial side may be unnecessary to make a space for implant replacement, even in severely deformed knees. Contrary to this, release of different parts of the medial collateral ligament will increase laxity at discrete ranges of flexion [14].

Valgus deformity is associated with tight lateral stabilizers and abnormal femoral lateral condylar anatomy. There is no consensus on what approach should be followed to address this type of deformity [8]. In general, the sequence of release starts off with the lateral collateral ligament followed by the posterior-lateral capsule, iliotibial band, posterior cruciate ligament, popliteus tendon, and biceps femoris. It should be noted that in one study ($n = 37$), valgus deformity was addressed solely through over resection of the distal femur and a constrained total knee arthroplasty system with no reported cases of loosening or instability at a 7.8-year follow-up [15]. This approach has merit, since it has been shown that lateral tissue release to address valgus deformities frequently produces asymmetric flexion-extension gaps and ligament instability [16]. The lateral flexion gap is affected most by the lateral collateral ligament, whereas the iliotibial band influences the extension gap size the most [16]. In the same study, a release sequence starting with the posterior cruciate ligament, posterior-lateral capsule, iliotibial band, popliteus tendon, and lateral collateral ligament resulted in a symmetric flexion-extension gap. The best approach however is to examine the flexion and extension gap after each step in a release sequence regardless of what sequence is used [8].

Flexion contracture arises due to the soft tissue contracture of the posterior capsule [8] (Fig. 4.3). The approach to address contracture typically entails release of the posterior capsule from the distal femur and then the proximal tibia after bone resection and removal of osteophytes. Genu recurvatum (Fig. 4.3) is generally a symptom of weak quadriceps structures since these patients rely on recurvatum during gait to compensate for their weaker quadriceps muscles [8]. This can be dealt with during surgery by reducing the extension gap. Care should be exercised when correcting recurvatum in patients with weak quadriceps muscles, since complete correction may result in their inability to lock their knees.

Perfect soft tissue balance during surgery remains elusive even with careful application of the surgical methods described above and in the remainder of this book. Reasons can be attributed to slight inequalities in the normal knee [17]. Stress relaxation occurs during surgery, which directly influences soft tissue balancing. Medial-lateral laxity has been shown to increase by 1 mm, whereas passive maximum extension can increase up to three degrees intrasurgery [18]. The lateral gap tends to be larger than the medial gap, whereas the extension gap is normally larger than the flexion gap [17]. On the upside, a larger extension gap aids in the prevention of flexion contracture and flexion instability. It may therefore be beneficial to

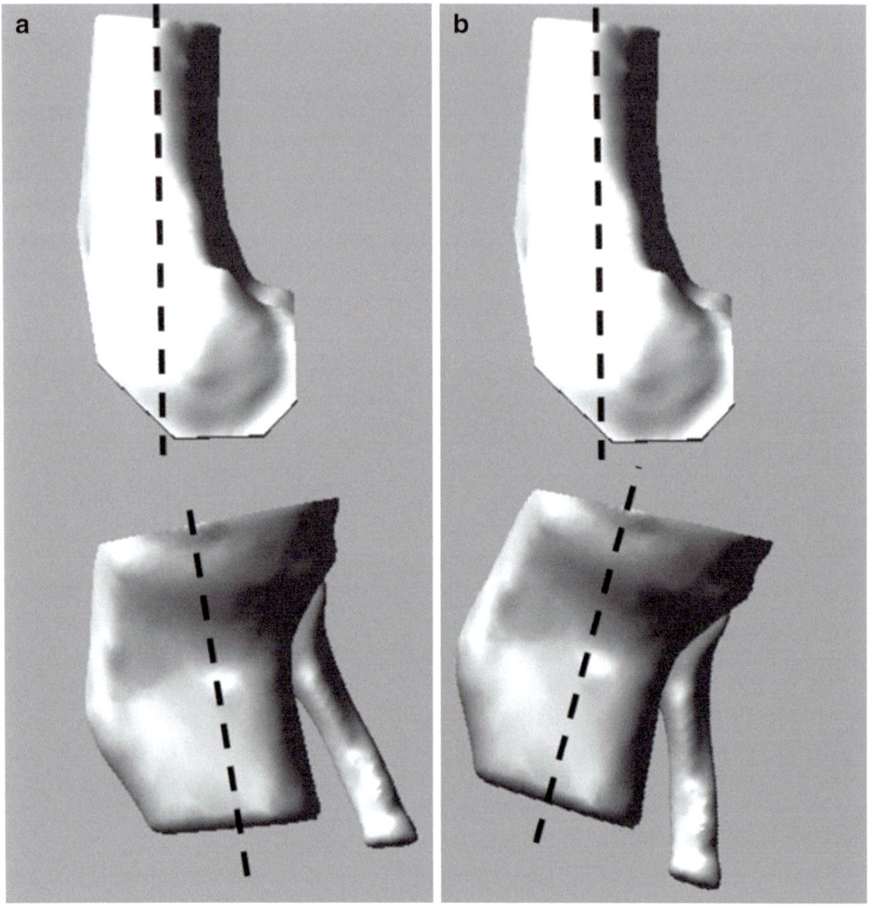

Fig. 4.3 (**a**) Flexion contracture and (**b**) genu recurvatum

have the extension gap somewhat larger than the flexion gap if it is not possible to achieve equal gap distances [17]. One remaining consideration is the impact of soft tissue balancing on proprioception. Proprioception significantly improves in knees that are balanced in both flexion and extension [19].

Insall et al. [1] in 1985 stated that "new methods will have to prove themselves against the standard already established for cemented prostheses." The same can be said of the ligament balancing technique. Reported results on the use of kinematic alignment are still inconclusive on whether it is truly better in comparison to the more traditional soft tissue balancing techniques. Although kinematic aligned knees tend to produce good functional outcomes (2-year follow-up, [20]), it remains to be seen whether this holds for longer periods. Of concern is the resistance to wear by the tibial insert which now also sees an increased shear load due to the oblique anatomic joint line. On the other hand, "a fresh look at soft tissue balancing is required" [21]. Too many times patients are still dissatisfied with the outcome after total knee arthroplasty. Soft tissue balancing techniques only require consideration of the flexion and extension gap, with little attention or tools available to objectively assess midflexion stability. Further work is therefore necessary to incorporate findings from studies such as [12] that compared laxities between full extension, 45° flexion, and 90° flexion into the surgical methods to establish proper ligament laxity throughout the entire range of knee flexion.

References

1. Insall JN, Binazzi R, Soudry M, Mestriner LA. Total knee arthroplasty. Clin Orthop Relat Res. 1985;192:13–22.
2. Matsuda S, Ito H. Ligament balancing in total knee arthroplasty—medial stabilizing technique. Asia Pac J Sports Med Arthrosc Rehabil Technol. 2015;2(4):108–13.
3. Meere PA, Schneider SM, Walker PS. Accuracy of balancing at total knee surgery using an instrumented tibial trial. J Arthroplasty. 2016;31(9):1938–42.
4. Meneghini RM, Ziemba-Davis MM, Lovro LR, Ireland PH, Damer BM. Can intraoperative sensors determine the "Target" ligament balance? Early outcomes in total knee arthroplasty. J Arthroplasty. 2016;31(10):2181–7.
5. Elmallah RK, et al. Can we really "Feel" a balanced total knee arthroplasty? J Arthroplasty. 2016;31(9 Suppl):102–5.
6. Wodowski AJ, Swigler CW, Liu H, Nord KM, Toy PC, Mihalko WM. Proprioception and knee arthroplasty: a literature review. Orthop Clin North Am. 2016;47(2):301–9.
7. Babazadeh S, Stoney JD, Lim K, Choong PF. The relevance of ligament balancing in total knee arthroplasty: how important is it? A systematic review of the literature. Orthop Rev. 2009;1(2):e26.
8. Gorab RS, Barnett SL. Ligamentous balancing in primary total knee replacement. Curr Opin Orthop. 2002;13(1):14–22.
9. Abdel MP. Measured resection versus gap balancing for total knee arthroplasty. Clin Orthop Relat Res. 2014;472(7):2016.
10. Nodzo SR, Franceschini V, Della Valle AG. Intraoperative load-sensing variability during cemented, posterior-stabilized total knee arthroplasty. J Arthroplasty. 2016;32(1):66–70.
11. Gustke KA, Golladay GJ, Roche MW, Elson LC, Anderson CR. A new method for defining balance: promising short-term clinical outcomes of sensor-guided TKA. J Arthroplasty. 2014;29(5):955–60.
12. Roth JD, Howell SM, Hull ML. Native knee laxities at 0°, 45°, and 90° of flexion and their relationship to the goal of the gap-balancing alignment method of total knee arthroplasty. J Bone Joint Surg Am. 2015;97(20):1678–84.
13. Mihalko W, Miller C, Krackow K. Total knee arthroplasty ligament balancing and gap kinematics with posterior cruciate ligament retention and sacrifice. Am J Orthop (Belle Mead NJ). 2000;29(8):610–6.
14. Whiteside LA, Saeki K, Mihalko WM. Functional medial ligament balancing in total knee arthroplasty. Clin Orthop Relat Res. 2000;380:45–57.
15. Easley ME, Insall JN, Scuderi GR, Bullek DD. Primary constrained condylar knee arthroplasty for the arthritic valgus knee. Clin Orthop Relat Res. 2000;380:58–64.
16. Peters CL, Mohr RA, Bachus KN. Primary total knee arthroplasty in the valgus knee: creating a balanced soft tissue envelope. J Arthroplasty. 2001;16(6):721–9.
17. Griffin FM, Insall JN, Scuderi GR. Accuracy of soft tissue balancing in total knee arthroplasty. J Arthroplasty. 2000;15(8):970–3.
18. Bellemans J, D'Hooghe P, Vandenneucker H, Van Damme G, Victor J. Soft tissue balance in total knee arthroplasty: does stress relaxation occur perioperatively? Clin Orthop Relat Res. 2006;452:49–52.

19. Attfield S, Wilton T, Pratt D, Sambatakakis A. Soft-tissue balance and recovery of proprioception after total knee replacement. Bone Joint J. 1996;78(4):540–5.
20. Dossett H, Estrada N, Swartz G, LeFevre G, Kwasman B. A randomised controlled trial of kinematically and mechanically aligned total knee replacements. Bone Joint J. 2014;96(7):907–13.
21. Delanois RE, Elmallah RK. A fresh look at soft-tissue balancing. J Bone Joint Surg Am. 2015;97(20):e69.

Measured (Anatomical Reference) Resection Technique for Cruciate-Retaining Total Knee Arthroplasty

5

Shaw Akizuki and Hiroshi Horiuchi

Contents

5.1 Introduction

The PCL is the thickest and strongest ligament in the knee joint. It is recognized as the first stabilizer in the sagittal and vertical planes and as the second stabilizer in the frontal plane. After cruciate-retaining total knee arthroplasty (CR-TKA), knee motion similar to that of the intact knee joint is obtained. The concept underlying this type of prosthesis may be called as soft tissue-guided motion in contrast with implant-guided motion with the posterior stabilized (PS) type of prosthesis [1].

S. Akizuki, MD, PhD (✉) • H. Horiuchi, MD, PhD
Center for Adult Joint Reconstruction, Nagano-Matsushiro General Hospital,
183 Matsushiro, Matsushiro Town, Nagano City 381-1231, Japan
e-mail: sakizuki@hosp.nagano-matsushiro.or.jp; hhoriuchi@hosp.nagano-matsushiro.or.jp

S. Matsuda et al. (eds.), *Soft Tissue Balancing in Total Knee Arthroplasty*,
DOI 10.1007/978-3-662-54082-4_5

The following points are very important for effective functioning of a cruciate-retaining (CR) prosthesis characterized by soft tissue-guided motion and reproduction of similar motion to the intact knee joint. First, the component must be positioned according to the anatomical landmarks of the patient while avoiding rotational error by the anterior reference method [2]. Second, soft tissue dissection must be minimized. Third, when PCL release is required, V-shaped osteotomy with cancellous bone graft (VOCG) is done at the tibial PCL attachment site, and tension on the ligament is adjusted with a cancellous bone graft. The anterior reference method has the advantage of avoiding formation of anterior notches that may cause fractures and allows sizing of femoral component in consideration of rotation but has the problem of the flexion gap wound being slightly larger than the extension gap. If TKA is performed with a PS-type prosthesis, flexion instability due to a large flexion gap may lead to dislocation when the joint is in deep flexion, and post breakage can also occur. On the other hand, CR-TKA avoids these problems because the PCL is preserved. The measured (anatomical reference) resection technique is not only applicable to varus and valgus knees but also to revision arthroplasty. We use a CR prosthesis for patients with an intact PCL, and this type has been applied to more than 95% of our TKA patients. This chapter reveals the rationale and key points of our measured (anatomical reference) resection technique for CR-TKA.

5.2 Exposure and Resection of Osteophytes

We manage primary knees with a straight skin incision and the trivector approach. The distal femur is always completely exposed as far as the tibial tubercle, and all osteophytes are resected up to the inner part of the medial collateral ligament (MCL). Dissection at the medial aspect of the tibia should be minimized and only osteophytes are resected (Fig. 5.1).

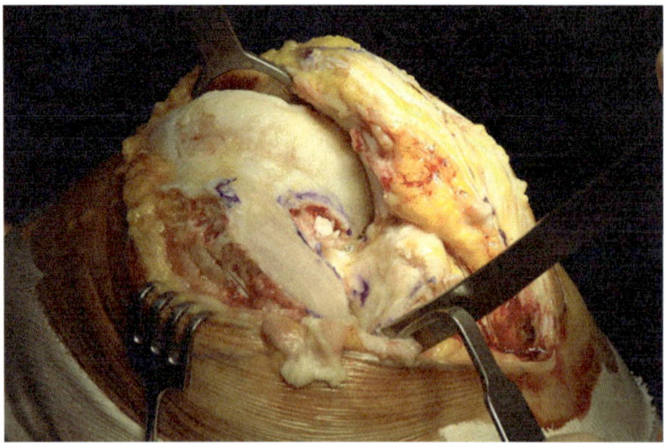

Fig. 5.1 Resection of medial femoral osteophytes that placed the MCL under tension. Medial dissection of the tibia is minimized because only osteophytes need to be resected

5.3 Preparation of the Femur

5.3.1 Determining the Rotational Alignment of the Femoral Component

Rotational alignment of the femoral component has a major influence on the outcome of TKA. Incorrect rotational alignment leads to mediolateral imbalance in extension and flexion, resulting in problems such as postoperative restriction of motion and patellofemoral joint incompatibility [3, 4]. It may also lead to excessive soft tissue release in an attempt to achieve adequate soft tissue balance. There are several methods for determining the rotational alignment of the femoral component [2, 5, 6]. Among them, the use of the surgical epicondylar axis (SEA) has the advantage of not being influenced by deformity of the articular surface and condyles. In addition, because it crosses the femoral and tibial axes at right angles in both flexion and extension, the correct balance between the tibial osteotomy surface and soft tissues can be achieved more easily [2]. Various methods of identifying the SEA have been proposed, such as estimation from preoperative images. While intraoperative identification of the SEA has been reported to be difficult [7, 8], we consider that identification by palpation during surgery is the most practical method. In fact, postoperative measurement of the difference of rotation between the SEA and the femoral component on CT scans reveals a difference within ±1° in approximately 80% of our patients. The medial epicondyle can be identified by inspection and palpation as the site of attachment of the medial collateral ligament or as a sulcus at the center of the horseshoe-shaped bony protrusion (Fig. 5.2a). On the other hand, it is difficult to visually identify the lateral epicondyle, because it is the site of attachment of the lateral collateral ligament, and the soft tissues are thicker than at the medial epicondyle. To perform palpation, the patella is retracted, and the top of the bony elevation is identified as the lateral epicondyle (Fig. 5.2b). After identification of the medial and lateral epicondyles, the SEA jig (SA original) is fixed to the epicondyles by pins (Fig. 5.3a). Then the anterior surface of the femur is resected in parallel with the SEA by the anterior reference method (Fig. 5.3b). This surface is used as the reference for every subsequent osteotomy and also for determining the appropriate size of the femoral component by anterior reference.

5.3.2 Sizing the Femoral Component by Anterior Reference

The anteroposterior (AP) size of the medial condyle is different from that of the lateral condyle when measured at the anterior osteotomy surface of the femur parallel to the SEA (reference osteotomy surface). Thus, sizing of the medial and lateral condyles is done individually, and the component is selected for CR-TKA with smaller AP size between that of the medial and lateral condyles (Fig. 5.4).

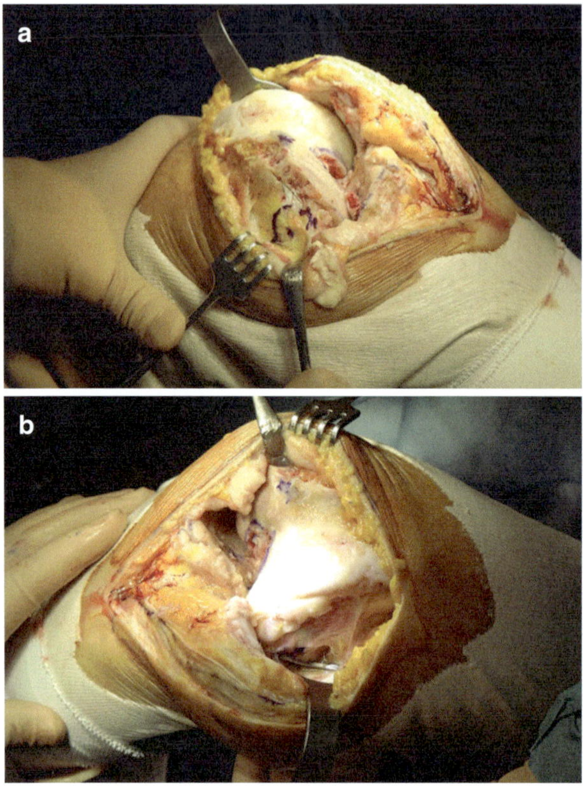

Fig. 5.2 (**a**) The medial epicondyle is palpated as a sulcus at the center of the horseshoe-shaped bony protrusion (*blue dot* in the center). (**b**) The patella is retracted and the lateral epicondyle is palpated as the top of the bony elevation (*blue dot*)

5.4 Preparation of the Tibia

5.4.1 Posterior Tibial Slope and PCL Preservation

In CR-TKA, a sagittal posterior slope is added during osteotomy because this increases flexion after surgery. As a result, the bone defect at the posterior part of the tibia can become smaller, and the PCL must be preserved together with the protecting bone in a manner mentioned later. The anteroposterior axis of the tibia must be determined carefully, because the posterior tibial slope influences varus and valgus tilt of the osteotomy surface. Several reports have been published concerning determination of the anteroposterior axis of the tibia, but this issue is still controversial [9, 10]. To maintain patellofemoral tracking, it is essential to avoid positioning the tibial component in internal rotation. We determine the AP axis of the tibia by adjusting the line that connects the center of the PCL attachment site to a point slightly lateral to the inner margin of the tibial tubercle depending on the degree of rotational freedom of the implant. Final rotational position is determined so that the

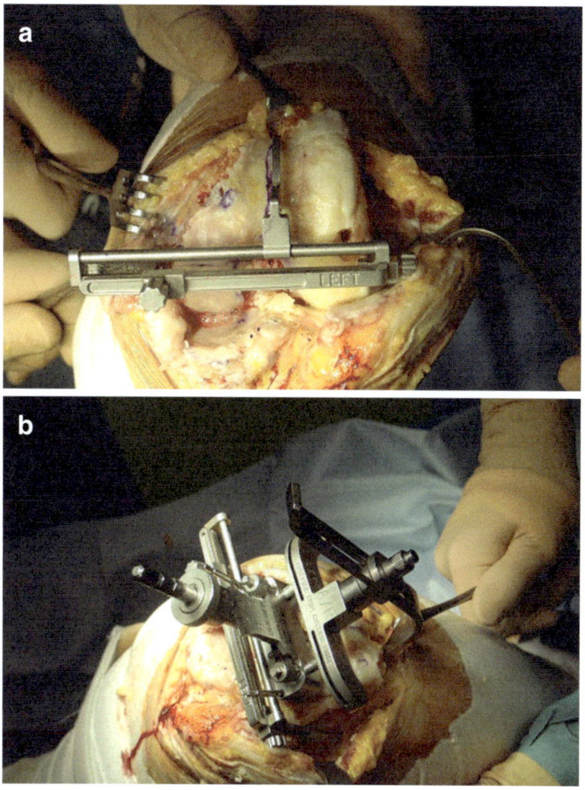

Fig. 5.3 (**a**) The SEA jig (SA original) is attached to both epicondyles and the Whiteside line is confirmed. (**b**) The intramedullary rod is combined with the SEA jig, and the anterior femoral surface parallel to the SEA is resected by the anterior reference method

trial component remains within the acceptable range in knee extension. Osteotomy of the proximal tibia is performed with an angel fin-shaped jig as close to the damaged surface as possible and within 8 mm of the normal articular surface (Fig. 5.5). If there is a residual defect after resection within 8 mm, autologous bone grafting is performed.

Prior to tibial osteotomy, to avoid cutting into the insertion of the PCL at its attachment site, a V-shaped bone fragment is formed around the PCL, and a bone chisel is used to protect it. At this time, the bone to which the anterior fibers of PCL are attached may be pulled away from the tibial surface by the tension of the PCL, but this can be overcome by implanting a cancellous bone graft in the space between the tibial component and the PCL attachment site. The angle of the posterior slope is made as close as possible to the original posterior slope angle in each patient. It has been a concern that the posterior tibial slope may influence long-term postoperative implant fixation, because it causes excess extension between the components when the knee joint is in full extension. Although the acceptable degree of hyperextension between the components differs with each implant, we have not found any such influence on the long-term outcome in our cementless CR-TKA series [11].

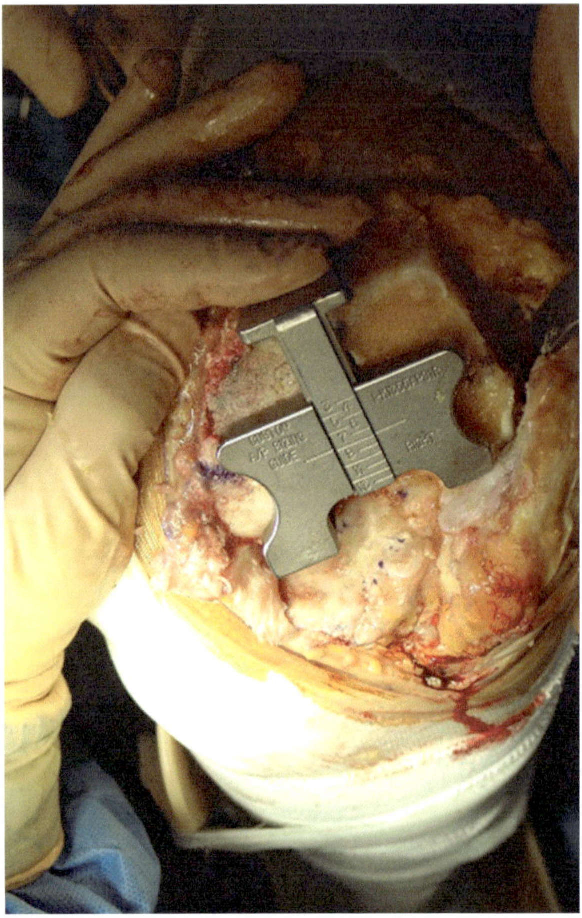

Fig. 5.4 Measuring the anteroposterior dimension of the medial condyle from the anterior femoral osteotomy surface (reference osteotomy surface) parallel to the SEA. The anteroposterior dimensions of both condyles are usually different

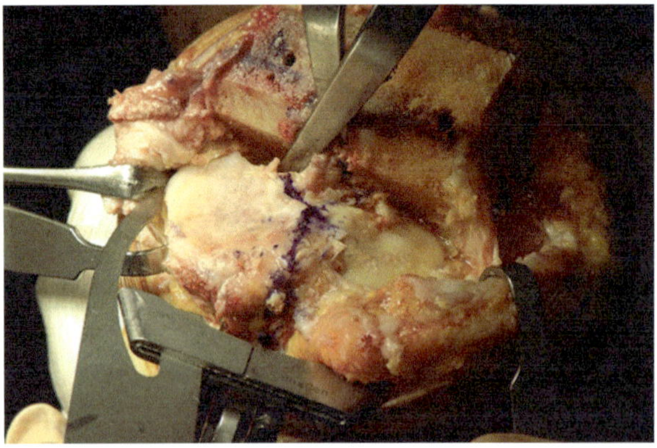

Fig. 5.5 The anteroposterior axis of the tibia is identified as a line connecting the center of the PCL attachment site to the point slightly lateral to the inner margin of the tibial tubercle and corresponds to the tibial axis (*blue line*). After the axis has been identified, the proximal tibial osteotomy line is set as close to the defect surface as possible and within 8 mm of the normal articular surface

5.4.2 Adjusting the Flexion-Extension and Medial-Lateral Gaps

The central parts of the femoral and tibial osteotomy surfaces are apposed to confirm that they are on the Mikulicz line. Regarding the soft tissue balance, slight medial tightness (within 3°) is acceptable when confirmed at 0° of extension and at 90° of flexion using a tension device with a force of approximately 40 pounds (Fig. 5.6). Slight medial tightness is considered to induce medial pivot after surgery [1]. In contrast, medial laxity is unacceptable because it leads to postoperative instability. However, it is acceptable for the flexion gap to be 2–3 mm larger than the extension gap.

If the femoral component is parallel to the SEA, medial laxity usually does not occur other than in patients with valgus deformity. Even in patients with slight medial tightness on extension, if the projecting portion of the posterior condyle is resected after trial component insertion, the posterior articular capsule will become looser, and an appropriate soft tissue balance is often acquired. If medial tightness is excessive, release of the pes anserine region or semimembranosus tendon may be indicated but is rarely performed.

PCL release is necessary if the flexion gap is too small, or PCL contracture and overstress are detected by the pull-out/lift-off (POLO) test, even though the posterior slope is appropriate.

5.4.3 V-Shaped Osteotomy with Cancellous Bone Graft (VOCG) for PCL Release

VOCG is performed to release PCL contracture because the bone is the only tissue that can undergo primary healing without scar formation. While we use a CR prosthesis in 95% of TKA patients, VOCG is only required for approximately 10%. This technique is employed to adjust PCL tension appropriately, and then bone union is

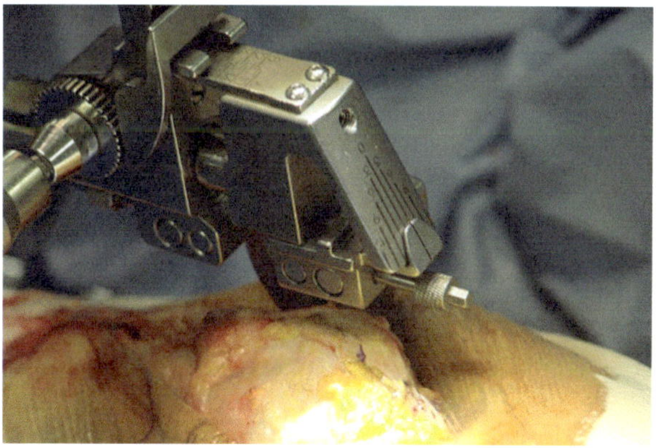

Fig. 5.6 The soft tissue balance and gap are confirmed using a tension device at 0° of extension and 90° of flexion

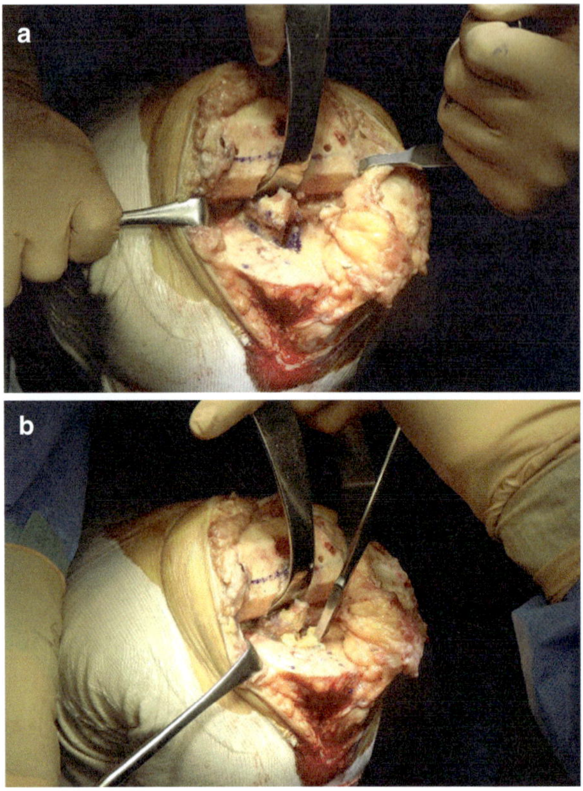

Fig. 5.7 (**a**) While maintaining periosteal continuity, V-shaped osteotomy is done from the tibial PCL attachment site to the posterior tibial cortex, allowing the PCL to float up together with the tibial fragment. (**b**) Cancellous bone grafting is done to fill gaps (VOCG)

obtained while maintaining the new position. First, V-shaped osteotomy is performed from the tibial PCL attachment site to the periosteum of the posterior tibial cortex, and the PCL is freed together with the attached tibial fragment (Fig. 5.7a). It is important to preserve the posterior periosteum for postoperative bone union. When reduction is performed with trial component insertion, the bone fragment floats up with attached PCL while maintaining continuity of the periosteum, resulting in decreasing tension of the PCL. The soft tissue balance should be confirmed again with a tension device.

Then cancellous bone grafts are placed to fill gaps and promote early bone union (Fig. 5.7b).

5.5 Fixation of the Components

After the tibial tray and polyethylene insert are fixed to the tibia, extension to flexion offset can be acquired accurately if the femoral component is inserted in a sliding manner with the knee in flexion. This can be done more easily with cementless fixation, which we perform in almost all patients. We have obtained excellent results with cementless CR-TKA by using hydroxyapatite-coated products to improve early fixation [12, 13]. This procedure can be used in cemented fixation, but care should be taken so that a thin film of cement is applied to the back surface of the posterior condyle of the femoral component.

5.6 Drain and Wound Closure

After fixation of all of the components (including the patellar component), we leave one drain inside the knee and use tranexamic acid with fibrin glue for hemostasis to suppress postoperative hemorrhage [14]. Then the incision (including the fat pad) is closed in the usual manner.

References

1. Horiuchi H, Akizuki S, Tomita T, Sugamoto K, Yamazaki T, Shimiz N. In vivo kinematics of cruciate-retaining total knee arthroplasty during weight-bearing and non-weight bearing deep knee bending. J Arthroplasty. 2013;27:1196–202.
2. Berger RA, Rubash HE, Seel MJ, Thompson WH, Crossett LS. Determining the rotational alignment of the femoral component in total knee arthroplasty using the epicondylar axis. Clin Orthop Relat Res. 1993;286:40–7.
3. Berger RA, Crossett LS, Jacobs JJ, Rubash HE. Malrotation causing patellofemoral complications after total knee arthroplasty. Clin Orthop Relat Res. 1998;356:144–53.
4. Insall JN, Scuderi GR, Komistek RD, Math K, Dennis DA, Anderson DT. Correlation between condylar lift-off and femoral component alignment. Clin Orthop Relat Res. 2002;403:143–52.
5. Stiehl JB, Abbott BD. Morphology of the transepicondylar axis and its application in primary and revision total knee arthroplasty. J Arthroplasty. 1995;10:785–9.
6. Olcott CW, Scott RD. The Ranawat Award. Femoral component rotation during total knee arthroplasty. Clin Orthop Relat Res. 1999;367:39–42.
7. Jenny JY, Boeri C. Low reproducibility of the intra-operative measurement of the transepicondylar axis during total knee replacement. Acta Orthop Scand. 2004;75:74–7.
8. Kinzel V, Ledger M, Shakespeare D. Can the epicondylar axis be defined accurately in total knee arthroplasty? Knee. 2005;12:293–6.
9. Dalury DF. Observations of the proximal tibia in total knee arthroplasty. Clin Orthop Relat Res. 2001;389:150–5.
10. Akagi M, Oh M, Nonaka T, Tsujimoto H, Asano T, Hamanishi C. An anteroposterior axis of the tibia for total knee arthroplasty. Clin Orthop Relat Res. 2004;420:213–9.
11. Watanabe H, Akizuki S, Takizawa T. Survival analysis of a cementless, cruciate-retaining total knee arthroplasty. Clinical and radiographic assessment 10 to 13 years after surgery. J Bone Joint Surg Br. 2004;86:824–9.
12. Akizuki S, Takizawa T, Horiuchi H. Fixation of a hydroxyapatite-tricalcium phosphate-coated cementless knee prosthesis. Clinical and radiographic evaluation seven years after surgery. J Bone Joint Surg Br. 2003;85:1123–7.
13. Gejo R, Akizuki S, Takizawa T. Fixation of the NexGen HA-TCP-coated cementless, screwless total knee arthroplasty: comparison with conventional cementless total knee arthroplasty of the same type. J Arthroplasty. 2002;17:449–56.
14. Akizuki S, Yasukawa Y, Takizawa T. A new method for hemostasis for cementless total knee arthroplasty. Bull Hosp Jt Dis. 1997;56:222–4.

PS: Gap Technique

6

Myung Chul Lee

Contents

Total knee arthroplasty (TKA) is the qualified surgical technique for the treatment of osteoarthritis of the knee joint [1]. The success of the TKA is dependent upon restoration of limb alignment, accurate implant position, and optimal gap balancing [2].

Malposition of the femoral or tibial component of the total knee arthroplasty can lead to early loosening, increased polyethylene wear, and poor patellar tracking [3–7]. Gap balancing affects the final knee kinematics and functional outcome. Balanced extension and flexion gaps are also highly essential [2, 8–10].

The gap balancing technique relies on ligament releases prior to performing bone cuts. These ligament releases correct fixed deformities and improve lower limb alignment prior to assessing femoral component rotation [11]. The concept of the gap technique was first suggested by Freeman et al. [12] more than 30 years ago. In its origin, the gap balancing technique began with a variable resection of the tibia, followed by resection of the posterior condyles in order to produce the flexion gap. The knee was then extended, and a resection of the distal femoral condyles was performed to produce an equal extension gap. In general, extension is dependent on ligament releases, and flexion is dependent on appropriate femoral sizing and rotation [7].

There are basically two gap balancing sequences, which rely on gap balancing first. First is the initial preparation of the flexion gap which is followed by matching

M.C. Lee
Department of Orthopaedic Surgery, Seoul National University Hospital, Seoul, South Korea
e-mail: leemc@snu.ac.kr

S. Matsuda et al. (eds.), *Soft Tissue Balancing in Total Knee Arthroplasty*,
DOI 10.1007/978-3-662-54082-4_6

the width of the extension gap to the width of the flexion gap. This is called the "gap technique" [12–14]. Second is the initial preparation of the extension gap followed by matching the width of the flexion gap to the width of the extension gap. This is called the "modified gap technique" [15–18].

6.1 Operative Procedure: Flexion Gap First (Gap Technique)

A skin incision is made with the knee in flexion, followed by exposure of the medial side of the knee by subperiosteal elevation of the anteromedial capsule and deep medial collateral ligament (MCL) off the tibia to the posteromedial corner of the knee.

Flexion of the knee allows for removal of the anterior cruciate ligament (ACL) and the anterior horns of the medial and lateral meniscus, along with any osteophytes that may lead to component malposition or soft tissue imbalance. The posterior horns of the meniscus can be excised after the femoral and tibial cuts have been made. The posterior cruciate ligament (PCL) can be resected at this time, or it can be removed later in the procedure along with the box cut that is made in the distal femur [19].

The tibia is cut perpendicular to its mechanical axis with the cutting block oriented using an intramedullary or extramedullary cutting guide. The amount of posterior slope present is dependent on the individual implant system being used or the preference of surgeon. An accurate proximal tibial cut is crucial because the tibial resection will serve as a reference for the femoral bone resections [20]. Before any soft tissue release is made, remove any medial or lateral osteophytes associated with the tibia and the femur. Remove posterior condylar osteophytes because they can inhibit flexion and tent the posterior soft tissue structures in extension, causing a flexion contracture [21].

When the joint is accurately tensioned in flexion, the tibial cut should be parallel in alignment to the transepicondylar axis (TEA) of the femur, and it will be perpendicular to the anterior-posterior (AP) axis of the tibia. Corrective soft tissue releases can then be performed if these axes do not align appropriately. Varus deformities can be corrected through a medial release, and valgus deformities can be corrected through a lateral release. (Detailed soft tissue management is discussed in Chap. 3.) Once the joint is accurately tensioned in flexion, anterior and posterior femoral condylar resections are made using an AP cutting block (Fig. 6.1). Spacer blocks or a tensioner can be inserted into the flexion gap to confirm that a proper flexion gap symmetry has been achieved (Fig. 6.2).

After precisely balancing the knee in flexion, the extension gap will be appropriately balanced. With the knee in extension, the extension gap is checked through placement of spacer blocks set to a similar tension level as the flexion gap (Fig. 6.3). An intramedullary or extramedullary guide is attached to the tensioning jig, and the lower extremity alignment is compared to the mechanical axis. Additional soft tissue balancing can be done to ensure precise alignment.

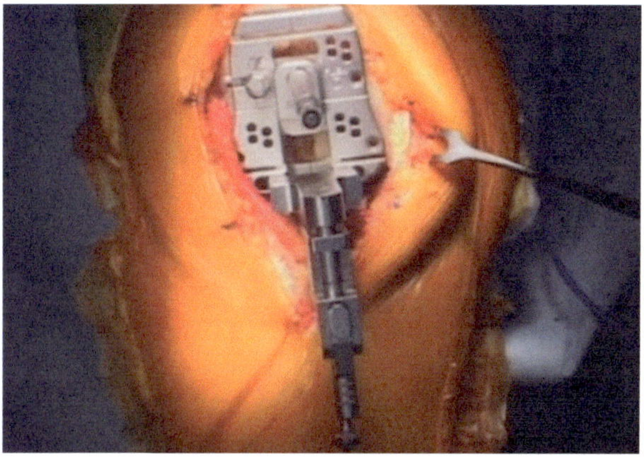

Fig. 6.1 If the knee joint is well tensioned in flexion, anterior and posterior femoral resections are made by using an AP cutting block

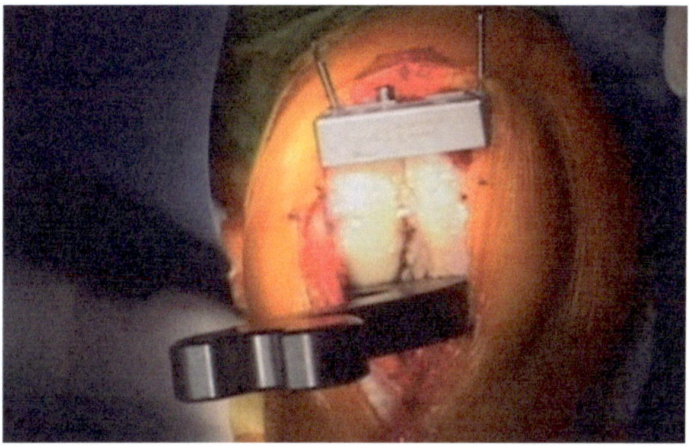

Fig. 6.2 Spacer blocks can be inserted into the flexion gap to confirm proper flexion gap symmetry

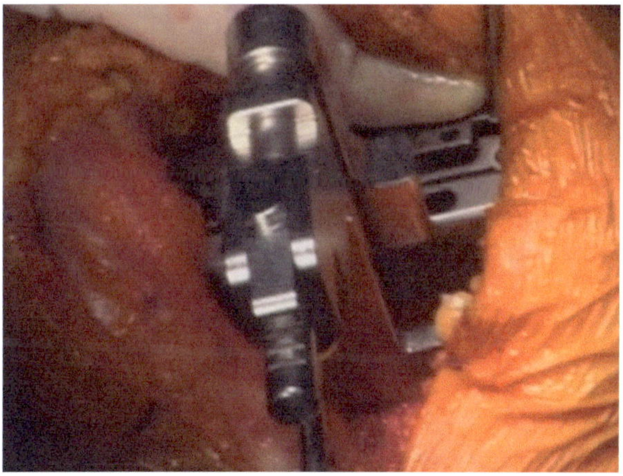

Fig. 6.3 With the knee in extension, extension gap is checked by spacer blocks that are set at a similar tension level to flexion gap

Once a symmetric flexion and extension gap is obtained, the distal femoral cutting guide is positioned, and the distal femoral cut is made. The spacer block or tensioner is inserted into the extension gap to check the symmetry between the extension gap and flexion gap.

6.2 Operative Procedure: Extension Gap First (Modified Gap Technique)

Alternatively, surgeons can balance the extension gap before the flexion gap. Using this technique, the distal femur is resected using an intramedullary guide followed by proximal tibial resection perpendicular to the longitudinal tibial axis. All osteophytes, including those on the femoral and tibial sides, are removed at this point, before any soft tissue release is performed because of their tensioning effect on adjacent ligamentous structures [21].

After the extension gap resection and osteophyte removal, gap symmetry, soft tissue balance, and lower extremity alignment are assessed. This assessment is achieved by placing a spacer block or tensioner into the extension gap (Fig. 6.4). Once ligament imbalance is checked, tight ligamentous structures are released until the extension gap is symmetric.

Once the knee is balanced symmetrically in extension, the goal is to balance the flexion gap and the extension gap. Spacer blocks can be used to apply equal tension to the collateral ligaments with the knee at 90 degrees of flexion. The transepicondylar and AP axis are constructed and used as a secondary indicator of femoral component rotation. When the knee is well balanced in extension and the tibial resection is precise, the resected proximal tibia should be parallel to the TEA and perpendicular to the AP axis (Fig. 6.5).

The appropriately sized AP femoral cutting block is then applied and inserted until it is parallel with the resected proximal tibia (Fig. 6.6). By adjusting the AP

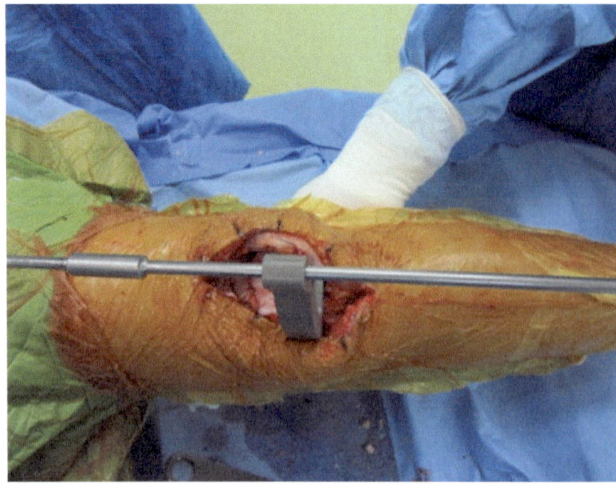

Fig. 6.4 After tibial resection, extension gap symmetry and lower extremity alignment are assessed by inserting spacer block into the extension gap

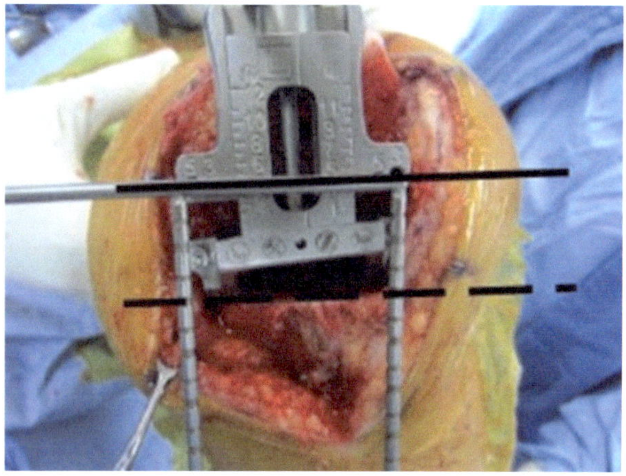

Fig. 6.5 When the knee is well balanced in extension and the tibial resection is precise, the resected proximal tibia (*dotted line*) should be parallel to the TEA and perpendicular to the AP axis (*straight line*)

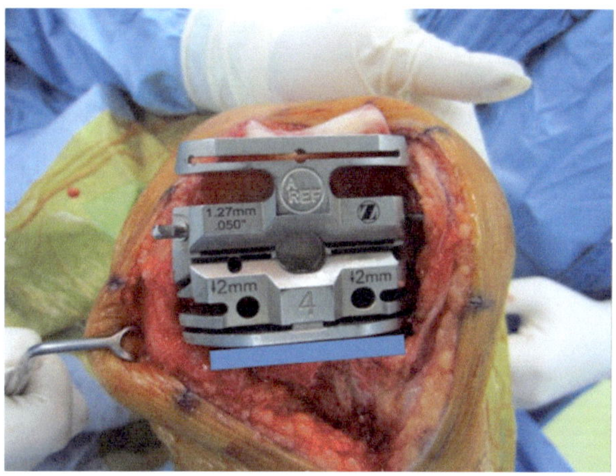

Fig. 6.6 Placement of the AP femoral cutting block parallel to the resected proximal tibia showing that the collateral ligaments are tensioned to create a rectangular flexion gap

cutting block anteriorly or posteriorly, a flexion gap width is created as to be the same as the extension gap. In order to confirm the flexion-extension gap symmetry, the same spacer block used to check the extension gap is placed under the AP cutting block and above the resected proximal tibia, and flexion gap tension is again assessed before resection of the posterior femoral condyles.

References

1. Laskin RS. The Genesis total knee prosthesis: a 10-year followup study. Clin Orthop Relat Res. 2001;388:95–102.
2. Insall JN. Presidential address to The Knee Society. choices and compromises in total knee arthroplasty. Clin Orthop Relat Res. 1988;226:43–8.
3. Berger RA, Rubash HE, Seel MJ, Thompson WH, Crossett LS. Determining the rotational alignment of the femoral component in total knee arthroplasty using the epicondylar axis. Clin Orthop Relat Res. 1993;286:40–7.

4. Boldt JG, Stiehl JB, Hodler J, Zanetti M, Munzinger U. Femoral component rotation and arthrofibrosis following mobile-bearing total knee arthroplasty. Int Orthop. 2006;30(5):420–5. doi:10.1007/s00264-006-0085-z.
5. Berger RA, Crossett LS, Jacobs JJ, Rubash HE. Malrotation causing patellofemoral complications after total knee arthroplasty. Clin Orthop Relat Res. 1998;356:144–53.
6. Romero J, Stahelin T, Binkert C, Pfirrmann C, Hodler J, Kessler O. The clinical consequences of flexion gap asymmetry in total knee arthroplasty. J Arthroplasty. 2007;22(2):235–40. doi:10.1016/j.arth.2006.04.024.
7. Fehring TK. Rotational malalignment of the femoral component in total knee arthroplasty. Clin Orthop Relat Res. 2000;380:72–9.
8. Hananouchi T, Yamamoto K, Ando W, Fudo K, Ohzono K. The intraoperative gap difference (flexion gap minus extension gap) is altered by insertion of the trial femoral component. Knee. 2012;19(5):601–5. doi:10.1016/j.knee.2011.08.001.
9. Katz MA, Beck TD, Silber JS, Seldes RM, Lotke PA. Determining femoral rotational alignment in total knee arthroplasty: reliability of techniques. J Arthroplasty. 2001;16(3):301–5.
10. Baldini A, Scuderi GR, Aglietti P, Chalnick D, Insall JN. Flexion-extension gap changes during total knee arthroplasty: effect of posterior cruciate ligament and posterior osteophytes removal. J Knee Surg. 2004;17(2):69–72.
11. Insall J, W Norman Scott. Insall & Scott surgery of the knee. Elsevier, The Netherlands. 4th ed. 2006.
12. Freeman MA, Samuelson KM, Levack B, de Alencar PG. Knee arthroplasty at the London Hospital. 1975-1984. Clin Orthop Relat Res. 1986;205:12–20.
13. Scott RD, Thornhill TS. Posterior cruciate supplementing total knee replacement using conforming inserts and cruciate recession. effect on range of motion and radiolucent lines. Clin Orthop Relat Res. 1994;309:146–9.
14. Daines BK, Dennis DA. Gap balancing vs. measured resection technique in total knee arthroplasty. Clin Orthop Surg. 2014;6(1):1–8. doi:10.4055/cios.2014.6.1.1.
15. Dennis DA, Komistek RD, Kim RH, Sharma A. Gap balancing versus measured resection technique for total knee arthroplasty. Clin Orthop Relat Res. 2010;468(1):102–7. doi:10.1007/s11999-009-1112-3.
16. Minoda Y, Iwaki H, Ikebuchi M, Yoshida T, Nakamura H. The flexion gap preparation does not disturb the modified gap technique in posterior stabilized total knee arthroplasty. Knee. 2012;19(6):832–5. doi:10.1016/j.knee.2012.03.007.
17. Minoda Y, Sakawa A, Aihara M, Tada K, Kadoya Y, Kobayashi A. Flexion gap preparation opens the extension gap in posterior cruciate ligament-retaining TKA. Knee Surg Sports Traumatol Arthrosc. 2007;15(11):1321–5. doi:10.1007/s00167-007-0394-9.
18. Moro-oka TA, Shiraishi H, Iwamoto Y, Banks SA. Modified gap-balancing technique in total knee arthroplasty: evaluation of the post-operative coronal laxity. Knee Surg Sports Traumatol Arthrosc. 2010;18(3):375–80. doi:10.1007/s00167-009-0977-8.
19. Canale ST, Beaty JH. Campbell's operative orthopaedics. 12th ed. Philadelphia: Elsevier Mosby; 2013.
20. Bottros J, Gad B, Krebs V, Barsoum WK. Gap balancing in total knee arthroplasty. J Arthroplasty. 2006;21(4 Suppl 1):11–5. doi:10.1016/j.arth.2006.02.084.
21. Sugama R, Kadoya Y, Kobayashi A, Takaoka K. Preparation of the flexion gap affects the extension gap in total knee arthroplasty. J Arthroplasty. 2005;20(5):602–7. doi:10.1016/j.arth.2003.12.085.

7 Bicruciate-Retaining TKA: How to Achieve Near-Normal Kinematics

Rob Middleton and Andrew Price

Contents

7.1 Theory of Joint Reconstruction

Total knee arthroplasty (TKA) is widely accepted as a successful treatment for end-stage knee osteoarthritis (OA), relieving pain and improving function, with long-lasting implants. The success of TKR is reflected in the increasing demand for the procedure. In the UK approximately 85,000 primary TKRs were performed in 2015 and more than 620,000 in the USA in 2009 [1, 2]. These numbers are on the rise as shown by temporal trends in multiple countries, with US TKR numbers projected to rise to 3.48 million by 2030 alone [3–6].

Of concern however is that approximately 10–20% of patients remain unsatisfied following primary TKR, often associated with pain, stiffness or that the knee does not feel 'normal' [7–10]. The causes for this are unclear, and likely multifactorial, but result in an increasingly large number of unsatisfied patients globally. The last 40 years of total knee arthroplasty component design and development have yet to close the gap with total hip arthroplasty patient satisfaction [11, 12].

R. Middleton • A. Price (✉)
Nuffield Orthopaedic Centre, Nuffield Department of Orthopaedics Rheumatology and Musculoskeletal Science, University of Oxford, Oxford, UK
e-mail: andrew.price@ndorms.ox.ac.uk

S. Matsuda et al. (eds.), *Soft Tissue Balancing in Total Knee Arthroplasty*,
DOI 10.1007/978-3-662-54082-4_7

When discussing prosthesis design, it is vital to understand the mechanics of the knee and the requirements of implants. Goodfellow and O'Connor classically described these features and highlighted that implant designs should allow the sliding and rolling movements of the knee, whilst applying only compressive forces to the underlying bone. The soft tissues, in particular the ligaments responsible for controlling joint movement and distraction, should be retained at their natural tensions [13]. Such principles are exemplified in their design of the Oxford unicompartmental knee arthroplasty (UKA), which retains all ligaments under physiological tension and restores knee kinematics to near normal [14–16]. Alongside this is the recognition that the ligaments of the knee themselves provide more than simple mechanical restraints to the knee and have a role in proprioception of the knee [17–19].

Two critical TKA design features are prosthesis constraint and prosthesis congruency. Congruency is the degree to which the femoral and tibial components match one another geometrically and can most simply be appreciated as the degree to which the concavity of the tibial tray matches the convexity of the femoral condyle. The proposed benefit of highly congruent femoral and tibial components is reduced wear given the greater surface area for force transmission. Constraint refers to the stability provided by the design of the prosthesis. Less constrained prostheses (e.g. cruciate-retaining TKA) rely on the soft tissue envelope and ligaments for stability, whereas highly constrained prostheses (e.g. rotating hinge) are inherently stable and can be used in those with global ligamentous deficiency. Highly constrained designs however transfer sheer stresses to the bone-cement interface, with resulting issues with loosening.

The ideal primary total knee arthroplasty would combine highly congruent surfaces to minimise polyethylene wear, but be unconstrained so as to allow the patients' ligaments to control natural knee motion, and prevent transmission of sheer stresses across the knee. This balance falls back to the understanding of knee anatomy as discussed above. However, the multitude of TKA prostheses available attests to the difficulty in perfecting this balance and the differing design mentalities to get there. Such a balance has been achieved in unicompartmental designs with a mobile bearing. For example, in the Oxford UKA, perfect congruency is achieved by way of two interfaces. The femoral component is spherical and is received by a matching radius spherical depression in the superior surface of the bearing. The inferior surface of the bearing is flat and articulates with a flat tibial tray. The design is also unconstrained, with movement of the bearing and knee dictated by the muscles and ligaments.

The value of retaining all ligaments of the knee during TKA has been recognised since the 1960s, even if the specific biomechanical reasons were unclear. The critical feature was of course to not violate the ACL attachments, which is a particular issue on the tibial side. This was achieved by either resurfacing the medial and lateral tibial plateaus individually, or by cutting a bony bridge anterior to the ACL, allowing for a single tibial tray. Modern bicruciate-retaining prostheses are the result of evolution of these original prosthesis designs.

Despite the availability of BCR TKAs, the vast majority of knee replacements today do not retain the ACL. The commonest TKA systems are either 'cruciate-retaining' (CR) or 'posterior-stabilised' (PS) designs, in relation to the posterior cruciate ligament (PCL). The ACL is sacrificed in both CR and PS designs. This is despite the finding that the ACL is intact in approximately 80% of knees at the time of TKA [20, 21]. There is thus a conflict between the principle of retention of ligaments during TKA and modern TKA practice. To understand this conflict, one needs to review the history of BCR TKA development and early prosthesis results.

7.2 History of Bicruciate-Retaining TKA

Bicruciate-retaining knee arthroplasty has existed as a concept since the 1940s, with a number of implants developed between the 1960s and 1980s. The first example is that of the polycentric knee (Fig. 7.1), designed by Frank Gunston in the late 1960s, following his fellowship with Sir John Charnley. Gunston recognised the variable radius of the femoral condyles, the composite movements of the knee and the 'polycentric' nature of the flexion axis. His design retained the collateral and cruciate ligaments, recognised the importance of cement fixation of components and replaced both articular surfaces. The polycentric knee itself consisted of semi-circular stainless steel femoral runners cemented into each condyle, with a corresponding high-density polyethylene track cemented into slots in the tibial plateau. Due to difficulty with manufacture, the femoral components were semi-circular rather than replicating femoral geometry exactly, with a diameter designed to best replicate natural flexion. As part of the operative technique, the level of the articulating surfaces was chosen to tension the collateral ligaments [22].

The 1970s saw the introduction of several BCR TKAs. The Coventry Geomedic knee consisted of a single femoral component with a bridge connecting the medial and lateral condylar replacements and did not resurface the trochlea (Fig. 7.2a). The

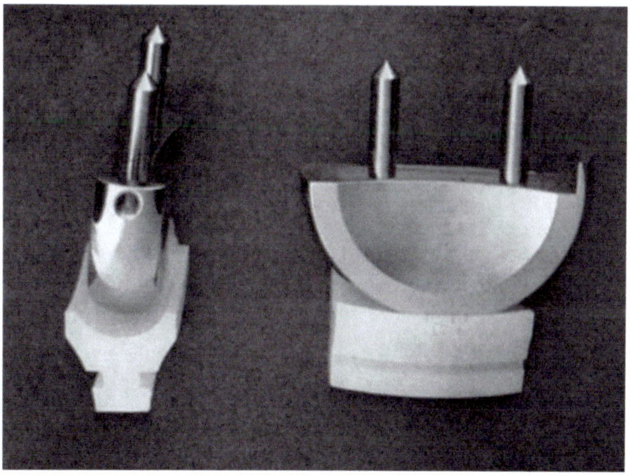

Fig. 7.1 The Gunston polycentric knee (From Gunston [22])

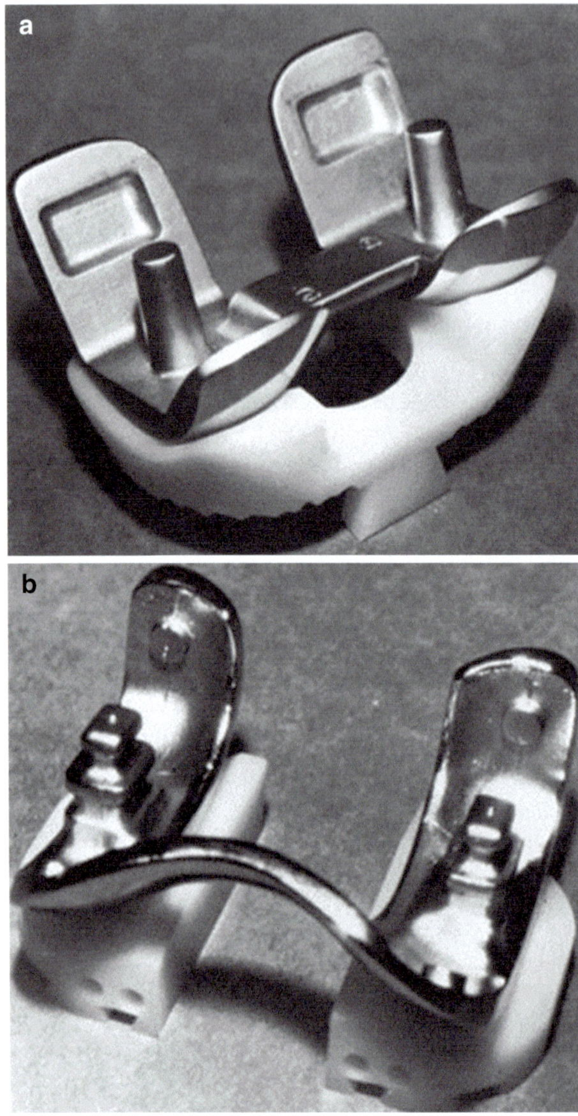

Fig. 7.2 (a) The Geomedic knee. (b) The duocondylar (From http://musculoskeletalkey.com/historic-development-classification-and-characteristics-of-knee-prostheses-2/)

tibial component was also a single component, made from high-density polyethylene, with concave surfaces to accept the femoral condyles resulting in a semi-constrained design. To allow retention of the ACL, the tibia component was U-shaped, requiring an anterior tibial bone bridge to be removed to allow seating [23]. The duocondylar from the Hospital for Special Surgery had a similar one-piece femoral component, without trochlear resurfacing (Fig. 7.2b). However, the tibial surfaces were replaced with two separate high-density polyethylene components, rather than a single component. These were concave in the coronal plane to

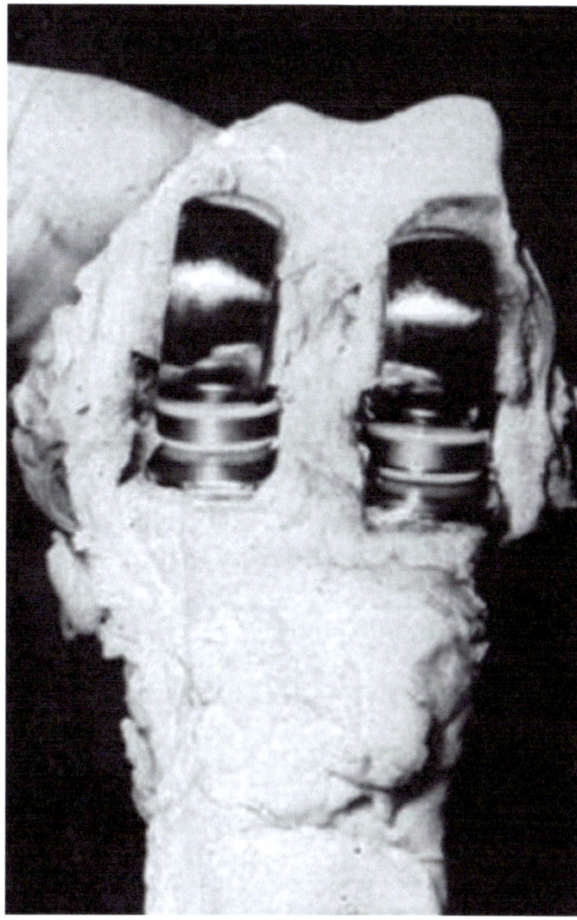

Fig. 7.3 The Oxford prosthesis implanted bi-compartmentally in a cadaveric knee as originally described by Goodfellow & O'Connor [13]

provide medio-lateral stability, with no restriction to movement in the sagittal plane [24]. The Townley anatomic total knee was the first bicruciate-retaining, tricompartmental knee arthroplasty system and was an unconstrained system. The introduction of additional bicruciate-retaining systems can trace their development back to these early designs. An excellent history of these developments is provided by Robinson [25].

Alongside the development of these total condylar replacements was the original development of the 'Oxford knee'. The components were highly similar to those used today, but were implanted bi-compartmentally (Fig. 7.3). This allowed for fully congruent yet fully unconstrained prostheses, in a procedure with no ligamentous releases. The transition to use of the Oxford knee as a unicompartmental prosthesis came from the recognition of poor results in ACL-deficient knees and that when the ACL is present, disease is often limited to the medial compartment [26–28].

BCR TKA was rapidly overtaken by the popularity of CR and PS TKA designs due to BCR TKA's greater technical difficulty, concerns regard its longevity and equivocal clinical benefits over these alternative designs [29].

7.3 Results

Gunston's original report of the polycentric knee included follow-up of between 1 and 2.5 years for 22 patients. All 22 patients reported improvements in pain, with an average range of motion of 8.4–101°. All but one patient were recorded having increased levels of mobility. Three knees required manipulation under anaesthesia for 'delayed healing'. One knee was arthrodesed due to lack of functional improvement (this was on a background of previous knee surgery, with suboptimal prosthesis placement, resulting in an unstable knee) [22]. 10-year follow-up of polycentric knees was reported by Lewallen et al. in 1984, for 209 knees. At 10 years only 42% were assessed as being 'successful' – defined as an ability to mobilise without aids, with mild discomfort, and did not require medical attention. A further 24% were reported as successful before 10 years, due to death or loss to follow-up. Thirty-four percent of the knees were classified as failures, with causes reported as instability in 13%, loosening in 7%, infection in 3%, patellofemoral pain in 4% and ankyloses in 2%. At time of revision surgery, loosening was found to be present in an additional 5%. Of note, failure rates were doubled in patients with components implanted in any degree of varus alignment or greater than 8° valgus alignment [30].

Skolnick et al. reported the 2-year outcomes after 119 geometric TKAs (with eight lost to follow up). As with the polycentric knee, pain relief was reported in the majority of patients (92%), an increased walking distance and a reduced requirement for walking aids with a 93% satisfaction rate. Range of motion in patients clinically reviewed was 7–87°. Post-operative flexion was reported as not significantly different to preoperatively, although there was a significantly different increase in extension achieved post-operatively. A deep infection rate of 1.8% was reported. 11.8% demonstrated radiographic tibial component loosening, with 9.1% requiring reoperation because of this. Approximately 80% demonstrated lucent lines at the cement-bone interface [31]. A 2–3.5-year follow-up of several TKA designs was reported by Insall et al. For the Geomedic (50 knees), the average range of motion was 90°, and an average increase in the Hospital for Special Surgery knee rating score of 69% and 85% was reported for osteoarthritis and rheumatoid arthritis patients, respectively. Eleven cases (nine of which were rheumatoid arthritis patients) were considered as failures due to one dislocation, two late infections, two patients with patellofemoral pain, two cases of tibial loosening and two with restricted range of motion. Of note, the authors report a radiolucent line in 80% of the geometric knees, although only 8% as loose, similar to Skolnick et al. [32]. A failure rate of 18.3% at 8.5-year follow-up was reported by Riley & Woodyard, on a cohort of 71 Geomedic TKAs, in which failure was defined as severe pain or need for reoperation [33]. Van Loon et al. reported 70% of knees remained painless at an average of 11-year follow-up and an average range of motion of 100°. A failure rate of 18%, most commonly due to tibial loosening, was similar to that of Riley & Woodyard. A survival rate (with an endpoint of implant removal) of 78% was given at 13 years; however this dropped to 58% if radiographically loose prostheses were included [34].

Ranawat et al. reported their experience of the duocondylar knee with a 2–4-year follow-up in 94 knees. Pain relief of 88.7% was achieved, although only 40.2% were considered excellent or complete pain relief. Average range of motion was 102°. Radiographic lucencies were found in 76% at 3 years, with 26% demonstrating progression. Five to seven patients required revision surgery for loose tibial components [35].

Townley reported his experience of 532 anatomic total knees, with a follow-up period of 2–11 years. An excellent or good outcome was found in 89%, in which the range of motion was beyond 90° and pain or activity restriction was mild to none, and there was no requirement for walking aids. A 2% rate of tibial loosening was reported [36]. A 23-year follow-up of the Townley Anatomic Knee by Pritchett demonstrated an 89% survivorship at 23 years, with revision for any reason as the endpoint. Goniometer measured flexion increased from a pre-operative mean of 104° to 117° post-operatively. Knee Society Scores increased from a pre-operative mean of 42 to a post-operative mean of 91. 5.6% required revision, with polyethylene wear being the most common cause. Tibial loosening was reported as rare [37].

Cloutier et al. has reported the 9–11-year follow-up of 107 Hermes 2C knee. This demonstrated a good or excellent outcome in 97%. The average range of motion was 107 ± 12.6°, normal anteroposterior stability in 89%, average knee score of 91 ± 8.4 and average functional score of 82 ± 21. With an endpoint of revision, the survival rate was 95 ± 2% at 10 years. No radiolucent lines were seen in 91%. Four percent of the knees (from the original cohort of 163) were revised, 3 for deep infection, one for instability after ACL rupture in a rheumatoid arthritis patient, one for a loose femoral component and two revisions for polyethylene wear [20]. The 22-year results for this same group have also been reported, although this constituted only 20% of the original cohort of 163. This demonstrated an average flexion of 103°, knee society score of 87 and function score of 68. With revision for any reason as an endpoint, survival at 22 years was 82.1%. This increased to 96.1% when aseptic loosening was chosen as the endpoint [38].

Such results highlight the difficulties with the earliest designs of BCR TKA with regard to implant loosening, particularly of the tibial components. The 10–20-year follow-up studies of more recent designs have much improved on these, however, and are more comparable to the widespread CR and PS TKAs. Patient satisfaction however, rather than survivorship, is another important factor to consider. A prospective randomised trial, in which patients underwent stage bilateral TKA, with different prostheses, supports BCR TKA. In 440 patients, with a minimum of 2-year follow-up, 89.1% preferred a BCR TKA in one knee to a PS TKA in the other. Also implanted in this study was a medial-pivot knee design, and this was preferred equally to the BCR TKA [39]. The reasons for the preference of a BCR TKA to a

CR or PS TKA may be due to the more normal kinematics achieved with a BCR TKA. This has been demonstrated with in vivo fluoroscopic kinematic analysis. The BCR TKA group on deep knee bend demonstrated more normal posterior femoral roll back, compared to a CR TKA, which demonstrated anterior femoral movement on flexion [40]. Anteroposterior laxity has also been shown to be more near normal in BCR TKA than CR TKA in a separate study [41].

Encouraging long-term results from more recently designed BCR TKAs, coupled with patient preference, and evidence of more normal knee kinematics argue that BCR TKA is a viable treatment option. With modern developments, BCR TKA may prove to be the superior option in appropriately selected patients and may help to reduce 10–20% of unsatisfied patients.

However there remain both technical and design challenges to be addressed in BCR TKA. Implantation of the prosthesis is technically demanding and has a notable learning curve in our experience. The inability to sublux the tibia anteriorly with an intact ACL reduces visualisation of the proximal tibia, potentially making resection, templating and implantation more difficult. Concerns remain regarding tibial island fracture or ACL avulsion; however, in experienced hands, rates of tibial island fracture are below 2% [37, 42]. On a similar theme is the issue of knee stiffness, where inadequate bony resection can result in a stiff knee with a reduced range of movement. Minimisation of tibial island fracture and stiffness requires a clear understanding of soft tissue balancing of the knee and the impact of femoral and tibial resection.

The femoral component in BCR TKA is very similar, or identical in some cases, to manufacturers' existing CR or PS systems. This is in contrast to the tibial component, which to retain the ACL insertion necessitates a cut-out in the plate to produce a U-shape to fit around the tibial island. This results in a narrow connecting beam anteriorly, with resulting concerns regarding fatigue failure. In response to this some manufacturers have used alternative manufacturing techniques or alloys with higher resistance to fatigue failure. More significantly concerns exist regarding tibial tray fixation and loosening. As discussed above several of the early designs suffered from early loosening, and newer designs often demonstrate radiolucent lines in short-term follow-up of unclear significance [32, 42]. The challenges arise again from the inability to sublux the tibia. This reduces the space available to insert the tibial component and so constrains the size of fixation pegs, or keels, that can be used. In comparison to standard TKA designs, BCR TKA tibial trays have significantly smaller fixation features or have required screw fixation. This is coupled with reduced access during application of cement and component impaction. Whilst progressive radiolucent lines are clearly a cause for concern, the implications of 'stable' radiolucent lines in the short-term are unclear. It may be that similarly to the Oxford unicompartmental knee, these radiolucent lines are common and do not herald failure [43]. The rates of radiolucent lines also differ between designs, for example, Cloutier et al. reported a rate of 9% at 9–11 years, versus 30% by Christensen et al. at an average of 18-month follow-up [20, 42]. This suggests that tibial tray designs can have a significant influence on the formation of these radiolucent lines. The question remains as to whether the presence of radiolucent lines has an impact on outcome or if such outcomes are similarly design specific. Only long-term follow-up studies can answer these questions for the emerging designs. Finally, with the tibial tray consisting of often two separate polyethylene components, the question remains as to whether different sized bearings can be used to allow for additional soft tissue balancing.

7.4 Contemporary Bicruciate Retaining TKA

With an increasing recognition of the unsatisfied 20% of patients following total knee replacement, and increasing patient expectations for return to function, it is not surprising that interest in BCR TKA has increased. Whilst some may suggest that BCR TKA has been tried before, with limited if any benefits over CR or PS TKA designs, we feel it would be premature to abandon the concept altogether. It is over 50 years since the first designs for BCR TKA emerged, and our understanding of the knee, implants and manufacturing have come a long way. Manufacturers have collaborated with a number of groups, and as such there are several BCR TKAs available. These include designs such as the Zimmer Biomet Vanguard XP, the BioPro Total Knee Original, the Ceraver Hermes 2C and the Smith & Nephew Journey II XR. These designs incorporate features of those designs that have come before them, with incremental changes to geometry as well as new materials.

Using the Vanguard XP as an example, one can see these design steps. The femoral component is based upon the established Vanguard CR knee system with a trochlear groove design to reduce patellar shear stress. The posterior condyle geometry has been altered with the aim of increased flexion without edge loading. Asymmetric condyles also feature, with a larger lateral condyle to allow greater roll back laterally. The tibial tray consists of the typical U-shaped tray of forged cobalt-chromium-molybdenum, with two pegs and two keels. This appears to be an approach recognising the survivorship reported of four pegged tibial components (although not in an ACL-retaining knee) and their experience of the Oxford knee which uses a keel [44]. Another example of modern technologies being incorporated is the use of vitamin E-infused bearings as a potential means to reduce revision due to polyethylene wear (as seen in the longer term follow-ups in previous prosthesis). These bearings also incorporate compartment-specific geometries, recognising the difference in kinematics between the medial and lateral sides (Fig. 7.4).

However, new prostheses, whilst attempting to address issues of prior designs, are not guaranteed to succeed. Christensen et al. have reported a higher reoperation with a new BCR TKA design in a retrospective review of 78 BCR TKAs compared to 294 CR TKAs at early follow-up [42]. Radiolucent lines were also seen in 30% as previously discussed.

There is no doubt that BCR TKAs will continue to evolve in response to ongoing research both in the lab and in the clinical setting.

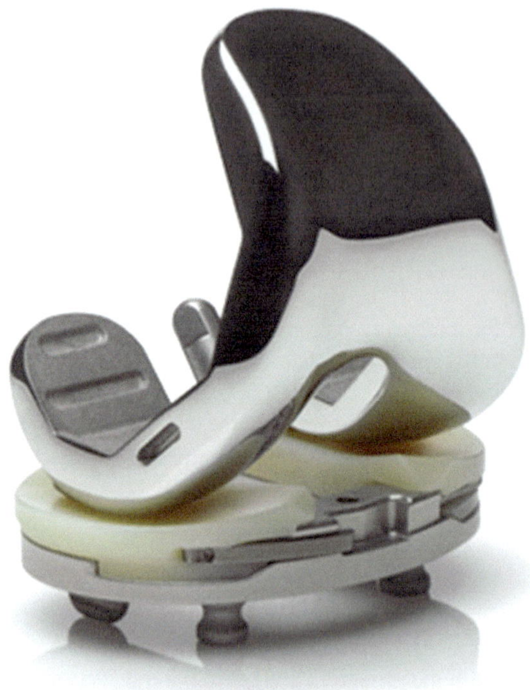

Fig. 7.4 The Vanguard XP BCR TKA

7.5 How Would BCR TKA Be Used?

With the increasing rates of total knee arthroplasty, and falling age at first surgery, it is essential that strategies are in place to optimise outcomes. We believe that retention of the knee ligaments, including the ACL, should be the aim wherever possible. We propose a stepwise approach to the surgical treatment of knee osteoarthritis with arthroplasty as below.

For patients with isolated medial compartment osteoarthritis and an intact ACL, a unicompartmental arthroplasty is our preferred solution. Such a condition is met in up to 50% of patients presenting for joint replacement surgery, if the Oxford criteria for selection are employed. Such surgery minimises surgical trauma, has a reduced mortality and provides patients with better functional outcomes compared to ACL-sacrificing TKA.

However an alternative approach is to use bicruciate-retaining TKA, when damage to other surfaces in the knee may prevent the use of a partial knee replacement, but the ACL is still intact. This combines the benefit of resurfacing multiple diseased articular surfaces whilst retaining the ACL. We estimate this constitutes a further 25% of patients for a partial knee replacement surgeon, but many higher numbers if they do not wish to use partial knee replacement. This provides the patient with pain relief whilst also maximising the potential for normal kinematics and superior functional outcome.

In the remaining 25% of patients with ACL-deficient knees and multicompartmental disease, a traditional CR or PS TKA can be implanted, as retaining the ACL is not an option.

The proportions above are estimates and will depend on the indications for the Oxford medial UKA used by the treating surgeon. Taking the Oxford indications for the Oxford UKA, approximately 50% of cases would be eligible for unicompartmental arthroplasty [45], with 25% being suitable for a BCR TKA and the remaining 25% receiving a CR or PS TKA. With more restrictive indications for medial UKA, these proportions may fall to approximately a third each.

7.6 Summary

BCR TKA is one potential avenue to address patient dissatisfaction after total knee replacement. The recognition of the soft tissue envelope and the importance of the ligaments in controlling movement of the knee have been present since the 1940s. The potential benefits of retaining the ACL include improve kinematics, proprioception and reduced prosthesis wear. Long-term follow-up data is available for select BCR TKAs demonstrating good outcomes, although with variable reports regarding functional outcome. Modern designs aim to build on the foundation laid down by the original innovators of knee prosthesis design, but further research is required to determine if these implants can deliver clinical improvements in outcome.

References

1. National Joint Registry for England and Wales. No Title. National Joint Reports - Knees - Primary procedures types by type of provider. http://www.njrreports.org.uk/knees-all-procedures-activity/K02v2NJR?reportid=B5FEC459-C763-4354-A5CD-1F2FCAE75C1B&defaults=DC__Reporting_Period__Date_Range="MAX",JYS__Filter__Calendar_Year__From__To="max-max",R__Filter__Country="All",H__Filter__Joint="Kne. Published 2015. Accessed 28 Oct 2016.
2. Weinstein AM, Rome BN, Reichmann WM, et al. Estimating the burden of total knee replacement in the United States. J Bone Joint Surg Am. 2013;95(5):385–92. doi:10.2106/JBJS.L.00206.
3. Kurtz S, Ong K, Lau E, Mowat F, Halpern M. Projections of primary and revision hip and knee arthroplasty in the United States from 2005 to 2030. J Bone Joint Surg Am. 2007;89(4):780–5. doi:10.2106/JBJS.F.00222.
4. Kurtz SM, Ong KL, Lau E, et al. International survey of primary and revision total knee replacement. Int Orthop. 2011;35(12):1783–9. doi:10.1007/s00264-011-1235-5.
5. Singh JA, Vessely MB, Harmsen WS, et al. A population-based study of trends in the use of total hip and total knee arthroplasty, 1969-2008. Mayo Clin Proc. 2010;85(10):898–904. doi:10.4065/mcp.2010.0115.
6. Culliford DJ, Maskell J, Beard DJ, Murray DW, Price AJ, Arden NK. Temporal trends in hip and knee replacement in the United Kingdom: 1991 to 2006. J Bone Joint Surg Br. 2010;92(1):130–5. doi:10.1302/0301-620X.92B1.22654.

7. Baker PN, van der Meulen JH, Lewsey J, Gregg PJ. National Joint Registry for England and Wales. The role of pain and function in determining patient satisfaction after total knee replacement. Data from the National Joint Registry for England and Wales. J Bone Joint Surg Br. 2007;89(7):893–900. doi:10.1302/0301-620X.89B7.19091.
8. Bourne RB, Chesworth BM, Davis AM, Mahomed NN, Charron KDJ. Patient satisfaction after total knee arthroplasty: who is satisfied and who is not? Clin Orthop Relat Res. 2010;468(1):57–63. doi:10.1007/s11999-009-1119-9.
9. PROMs Team (Health and Social Care Information Centre). Finalised Patient Reported Outcome Measures (PROMs) in England April 2013 to March 2014. 2015.
10. Nam D, Nunley RM, Barrack RL. Patient dissatisfaction following total knee replacement: a growing concern? Bone Joint J. 2014;96-B(11 Supple A):96–100. doi:10.1302/0301-620X.96B11.34152.
11. Anakwe RE, Jenkins PJ, Moran M. Predicting dissatisfaction after total hip arthroplasty: a study of 850 patients. J Arthroplasty. 2011;26(2):209–13. doi:10.1016/j.arth.2010.03.013.
12. Bourne RB, Chesworth B, Davis A, Mahomed N, Charron K. Comparing patient outcomes after THA and TKA: is there a difference? Clin Orthop Relat Res. 2010;468(2):542–6. doi:10.1007/s11999-009-1046-9.
13. Goodfellow J, O'Connor J. The mechanics of the knee and prosthesis design. J Bone Joint Surg Br. 1978;60-B(3):358–69. http://www.ncbi.nlm.nih.gov/pubmed/581081.
14. Jefferson RJ, Whittle MW. Biomechanical assessment of unicompartmental knee arthroplasty, total condylar arthroplasty and tibial osteotomy. Clin Biomech. 1989;4(4):232–42. doi:10.1016/0268-0033(89)90008-9.
15. Price AJ, Rees JL, Beard DJ, Gill HS, CAF D, Murray DW. Sagittal plane kinematics of a mobile-bearing unicompartmental knee arthroplasty at 10 years: a comparative in vivo fluoroscopic analysis. J Arthroplasty. 2004;19(5):590–7. http://www.ncbi.nlm.nih.gov/pubmed/15284980.
16. Jones GG, Kotti M, Wiik AV, et al. Gait comparison of unicompartmental and total knee arthroplasties with healthy controls. Bone Joint J. 2016;98-B(10 Supple B):16–21. doi:10.1302/0301-620X.98B10.BJJ.2016.0473.R1.
17. Johansson H. Role of knee ligaments in proprioception and regulation of muscle stiffness. J Electromyogr Kinesiol. 1991;1(3):158–79. doi:10.1016/1050-6411(91)90032-Z.
18. Bali K, Prabhakar S, Dhillon M. Proprioception in anterior cruciate ligament deficient knees and its relevance in anterior cruciate ligament reconstruction. Indian J Orthop. 2011;45(4):294. doi:10.4103/0019-5413.80320.
19. Katayama M, Higuchi H, Kimura M, et al. Proprioception and performance after anterior cruciate ligament rupture. Int Orthop. 2004;28(5):278–81. doi:10.1007/s00264-004-0583-9.
20. Cloutier JM, Sabouret P, Deghrar A. Total knee arthroplasty with retention of both cruciate ligaments. A nine to eleven-year follow-up study. J Bone Joint Surg Am. 1999;81(5):697–702. http://www.ncbi.nlm.nih.gov/pubmed/10360698.
21. Johnson AJ, Howell SM, Costa CR, Mont MA. The ACL in the arthritic knee: how often is it present and can preoperative tests predict its presence? Clin Orthop Relat Res. 2013;471(1):181–8. doi:10.1007/s11999-012-2505-2.
22. Gunston FH. Polycentric knee arthroplasty. Prosthetic simulation of normal knee movement. J Bone Joint Surg Br. 1971;53(2):272–7. http://www.ncbi.nlm.nih.gov/pubmed/5578223.
23. Coventry MB, Finerman GA, Riley LH, Turner RH, Upshaw JE. A new geometric knee for total knee arthroplasty. Clin Orthop Relat Res. 1972;83:157–62. http://www.ncbi.nlm.nih.gov/pubmed/5014807.
24. Ranawat CS, Shine JJ. Duo-condylar total knee arthroplasty. Clin Orthop Relat Res. 1973;(94):185–95. http://www.ncbi.nlm.nih.gov/pubmed/4743449.
25. Robinson RP. The early innovators of today's resurfacing condylar knees. J Arthroplasty. 2005;20(1 Suppl 1):2–26. doi:10.1016/j.arth.2004.11.002.
26. Goodfellow J, O'Connor J. The anterior cruciate ligament in knee arthroplasty. A risk-factor with unconstrained meniscal prostheses. Clin Orthop Relat Res. 1992;276:245–52. http://www.ncbi.nlm.nih.gov/pubmed/1537161.

27. White SH, Ludkowski PF, Goodfellow JW. Anteromedial osteoarthritis of the knee. J Bone Joint Surg Br. 1991;73(4):582–6. http://www.ncbi.nlm.nih.gov/pubmed/2071640.
28. Goodfellow J, O'Connor J, Pandit H, Dodd C, Murray D. Unicompartmental arthroplasty with the oxford knee. 2nd ed. Goodfellow Publishers Ltd, Oxford, United Kingdom; 2015.
29. Scuderi GR, Insall JN, Windsor RE, Moran MC. Survivorship of cemented knee replacements. J Bone Joint Surg Br. 1989;71(5):798–803. http://www.ncbi.nlm.nih.gov/pubmed/2584250.
30. Lewallen DG, Bryan RS, Peterson LF. Polycentric total knee arthroplasty. A ten-year follow-up study. J Bone Joint Surg Am. 1984;66(8):1211–8. http://www.ncbi.nlm.nih.gov/pubmed/6490696.
31. Skolnick MD, Coventry MB, Ilstrup DM. Geometric total knee arthroplasty. A two-year follow-up study. J Bone Joint Surg Am. 1976;58(6):749–53. http://www.ncbi.nlm.nih.gov/pubmed/956218.
32. Insall JN, Ranawat CS, Aglietti P, Shine J. A comparison of four models of total knee-replacement prostheses. J Bone Joint Surg Am. 1976;58(6):754–65. http://www.ncbi.nlm.nih.gov/pubmed/956219.
33. Riley D, Woodyard JE. Long-term results of Geomedic total knee replacement. J Bone Joint Surg Br. 1985;67(4):548–50. http://www.ncbi.nlm.nih.gov/pubmed/4030848.
34. van Loon CJ, Hu HP, Van Horn JR, De Waal Malefijt MC. The Geomedic knee prosthesis. A long-term follow-up study. Acta Orthop Belg. 1993;59(1):40–4. http://www.ncbi.nlm.nih.gov/pubmed/8484320.
35. Ranawat CS, Insall J, Shine J. Duo-condylar knee arthroplasty: hospital for special surgery design. Clin Orthop Relat Res. 1976;120:76–82. doi:10.1097/00003086-197307000-00023.
36. Townley CO. The anatomic total knee resurfacing arthroplasty. Clin Orthop Relat Res. 1985;(192):82–96. http://www.ncbi.nlm.nih.gov/pubmed/3967443.
37. Pritchett JW. Bicruciate-retaining total knee replacement provides satisfactory function and implant survivorship at 23 years. Clin Orthop Relat Res. 2015;473(7):2327–33. doi:10.1007/s11999-015-4219-8.
38. Sabouret P, Lavoie F, Cloutier J-M. Total knee replacement with retention of both cruciate ligaments: a 22-year follow-up study. Bone Joint J. 2013;95-B(7):917–22. doi:10.1302/0301-620X.95B7.30904.
39. Pritchett JW. Patients prefer a bicruciate-retaining or the medial pivot total knee prosthesis. J Arthroplasty. 2011;26(2):224–8. doi:10.1016/j.arth.2010.02.012.
40. Stiehl JB, Komistek RD, Cloutier JM, Dennis DA. The cruciate ligaments in total knee arthroplasty: a kinematic analysis of 2 total knee arthroplasties. J Arthroplasty. 2000;15(5):545–50. http://www.ncbi.nlm.nih.gov/pubmed/10959990.
41. Halewood C, Traynor A, Bellemans J, Victor J, Amis AA. Anteroposterior laxity after bicruciate-retaining total knee arthroplasty is closer to the native knee than ACL-resecting TKA: a biomechanical cadaver study. J Arthroplasty. 2015;30(12):2315–9. doi:10.1016/j.arth.2015.06.021.
42. Christensen JC, Brothers J, Stoddard GJ, et al. Higher Frequency of Reoperation With a New Bicruciate retaining Total Knee Arthroplasty. Clin Orthop Relat Res. 2017;475(1):62–69. doi:10.1007/s11999-016-4812-5.
43. Gulati A, Chau R, Pandit HG, et al. The incidence of physiological radiolucency following Oxford unicompartmental knee replacement and its relationship to outcome. J Bone Joint Surg Br. 2009;91(7):896–902. doi:10.1302/0301-620X.91B7.21914.
44. Schwartz AJ, Della Valle CJ, Rosenberg AG, Jacobs JJ, Berger RA, Galante JO. Cruciate-retaining TKA using a third-generation system with a four-pegged tibial component: a minimum 10-year followup note. Clin Orthop Relat Res. 2010;468(8):2160–7. doi:10.1007/s11999-010-1360-2.
45. Beard DJ, Holt MD, Mullins MM, Malek S, Massa E, Price AJ. Decision making for knee replacement: variation in treatment choice for late stage medial compartment osteoarthritis. Knee. 2012;19(6):886–9. doi:10.1016/j.knee.2012.05.005.

Five Quality Assurance Steps for Balancing a Kinematically Aligned Total Knee Arthroplasty

8

Stephen M. Howell and Alexander J. Nedopil

Contents

8.1 Overview

Kinematically aligned total knee arthroplasty (TKA) has gained interest because two randomized trials and a national multicenter study showed that patients treated with kinematic alignment reported significantly better pain relief, function, flexion, a more normal-feeling knee than mechanical alignment with a similar implant survivorship at 2, 3, and 6 years [1–5]. This chapter introduces the three goals of

S.M. Howell
Biomedical Engineering Graduate Group, University of California, Davis, Davis, CA 95616, USA

A.J. Nedopil (✉)
Department of Orthopaedics, University of California, Davis, 4860 Y Street, Suite 3800, Sacramento, CA 95817, USA
e-mail: nedopil@ucdavis.edu

S. Matsuda et al. (eds.), *Soft Tissue Balancing in Total Knee Arthroplasty*,
DOI 10.1007/978-3-662-54082-4_8

kinematically aligned TKA, which are to restore (1) the native tibial-femoral articular surfaces, (2) the native knee and limb alignments, and (3) the native laxities of the knee. Because kinematically aligned TKA is relatively new and not as well understood as mechanically aligned TKA, we present five Quality Assurance Steps that are used intraoperatively to verify both kinematic alignment of the femoral and tibial components to the native joint lines and correct balancing of the knee. Examples of patients with severe varus and valgus deformity and flexion contractures treated with kinematically aligned TKA are shown.

8.2 Goal One: Restore the Native Tibial-Femoral Articular Surfaces

One goal of kinematically aligned total knee arthroplasty (TKA) is to set the anterior-posterior, proximal-distal, and medial-lateral translation and flexion-extension, varus-valgus, internal-external rotation (6 degrees of freedom) of the femoral and tibial components to restore the native tibial-femoral articular surface of the knee. Setting the femoral and tibial components on the native tibial-femoral articular surface coaligns the axes of the components as close as possible with the three kinematic axes of the normal knee [2, 3, 6] (Fig. 8.1). One kinematic axis is the flexion axis of the tibia that penetrates the two centers of the circular portion of the posterior femoral condyles from about 20° to 120° like an axle passing through two wheels, which determines the native arc of flexion and extension of the tibia on the femur [6–10]. The second kinematic axis is the flexion axis of the patella that

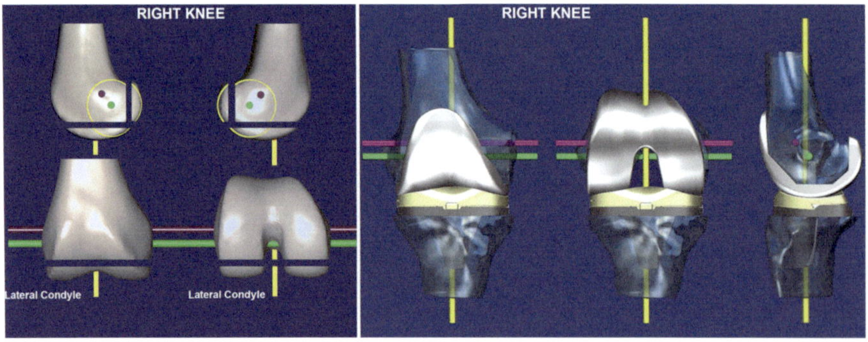

Fig. 8.1 A right femur (*left*) and kinematically aligned TKA (*right*) shows the relationships between the three kinematic axes of the knee and the joint lines of the distal and posterior femoral resections and the 6 degree-of-freedom position of the components [3]. The flexion axis of the tibia is the *green line*, the flexion axis of the patella is the *magenta line*, and the longitudinal rotational axis of the tibia is the *yellow line*. All three axes are closely parallel or perpendicular to the joint lines. The flexion-extension plane of the extended knee lies perpendicular to the flexion axes of the tibia and patella and centered in the knee. Compensating for wear and kerf and resecting bone from the distal and posterior femur condyles equal in thickness to the condyles of the femoral component kinematically aligns the femoral component by co-aligning the axis of the femoral component with the flexion axis of the tibia assuming that the condyles of the femoral component are symmetric in the flexion-extension plane of the tibia

lies parallel and averages 10 mm anterior and 12 mm proximal to the flexion axis of the tibia, which determines the native arc of flexion and extension of the patella on the femur [11, 12]. The flexion-extension plane of the extended knee lies perpendicular to these two kinematic axes in the center of the knee. The third kinematic axis is the longitudinal rotational axis of the tibia that lies approximately perpendicular to the flexion axes of the tibia and patella and determines the native arc of internal and external rotation of the tibia on the femur [10, 11]. These kinematic axes are closely parallel or perpendicular to the native tibial-femoral articular surface [6, 10–14]. Therefore, a change in the position of either component in one or more of the 6 degrees of freedom changes the native tibial-femoral articular surfaces. A change in the native articular surface malaligns the rotational axes of the components with the three kinematic axes of the knee, which changes the native resting length of the collateral, retinacular, and posterior cruciate ligaments. Changing the native resting length of these ligaments causes unnatural tightening and/or slackening of the ligaments and unnatural tibial-femoral and patella-femoral motions that patients may perceive as pain, binding, stiffness, or instability [6, 10, 15, 16].

8.3 Goal Two: Restore the Native Knee and Limb Alignments

The second goal of kinematically aligned TKA is to restore the native knee and limb alignments [3, 4, 15, 17]. Several studies support correction to the native or "constitutional" alignment when performing TKA as opposed to creating mechanical alignment to neutral (Fig. 8.2) [15, 18–20]. Creating mechanical alignment in patients with constitutional varus and valgus alignment is unnatural and causes greater strain deviations in the medial and lateral collateral ligaments from the native knee [15, 18, 21, 22]. Patients with preoperative varus have better clinical and functional outcome scores and the same implant survivorship at 7 years when the alignment is left in the native varus, as compared with patients overcorrected to neutral [19]. At a mean of 6 years after kinematically aligned TKA, restoration of the native alignments of the knee, limb, and tibia did not adversely affect implant survival and resulted in high function, which supports the consideration of kinematic alignment as an alternative to mechanical alignment when performing primary TKA [4].

Current evidence suggests that the native alignment of the limb does not cause osteoarthritis of the knee. The clinical findings of bilateral osteoarthritis with a varus deformity in one knee and a valgus deformity in the other ("wind swept"), and the lack of osteoarthritis in the majority of elderly Asian patients with severe constitutional varus suggest that native alignment plays little role in the development of osteoarthritis. Instead, the onset of osteoarthritis is associated with known changes in cartilage metabolism that occur with aging. Articular cartilage is a mechanosensitive tissue that, when healthy, increases anabolic activity and thickens when loaded. Chondrocytes experience age-related declines in their anabolic activity and thickening response which causes osteoarthritis as the ability to respond and compensate for high loads from activity and obesity is gradually lost [23].

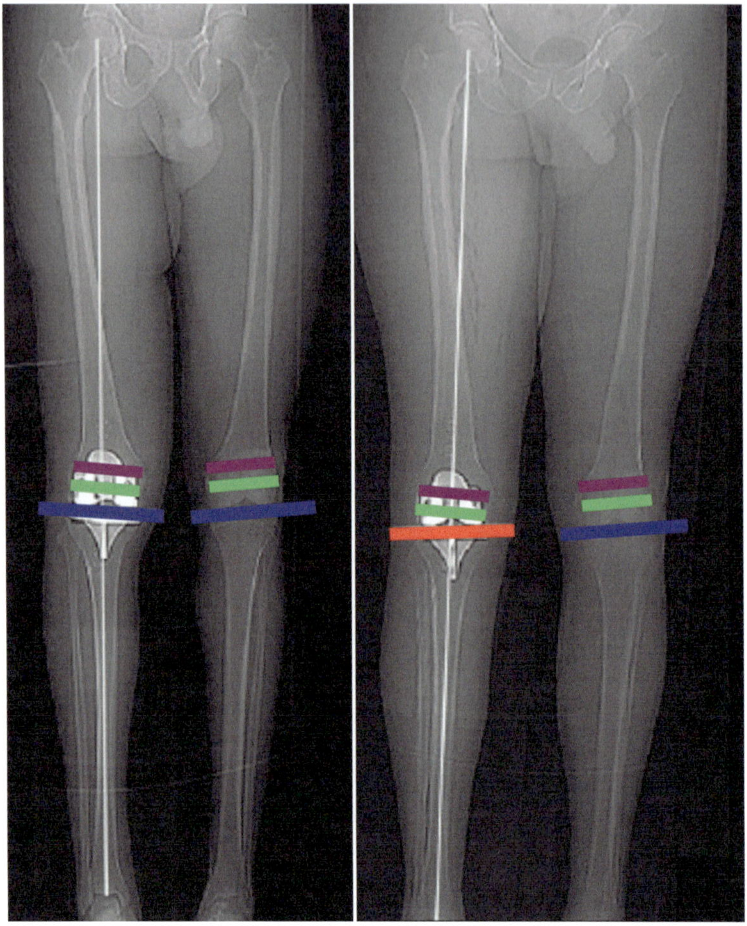

Fig. 8.2 Composite shows (1) the kinematically aligned TKA (*left patient*) restores the natural tibial-femoral joint surface (*blue line*) and the natural limb alignment (*white line*) and coaligns the axes of the femoral component with the flexion axes of the tibia (*green line*) and patella (*magenta line*), and (2) the mechanically aligned TKA (*right patient*) changes the natural tibial-femoral joint surface (*red line*), the natural limb alignment, and malaligns the axes of the femoral component oblique to the flexion axes of the tibia and patella. Studies have shown that kinematic alignment has less varus limb and varus knee outliers and has the same average limb and knee alignment as mechanical alignment [2, 34, 35]

8.4 Goal Three: Restore the Native Laxities of the Knee

The third goal of kinematically aligned TKA is to restore the native laxities of the knee, which are tighter at 0° of flexion than at 45° and 90° of flexion [16, 24] (Fig. 8.3). At 0° of flexion the native tibia-femoral joint behaves as a rigid body since the average varus (0.7°), valgus (0.5°), internal (4.6°), and external (4.4°) rotations

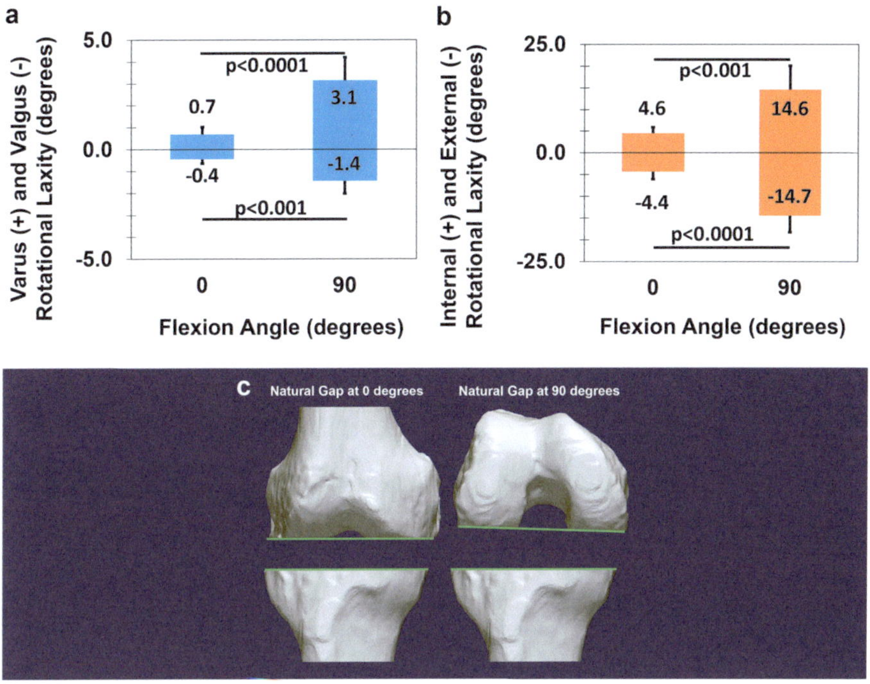

Fig. 8.3 A composite shows column graphs of the natural varus (+), valgus (−), internal (+), and external (−) rotational laxities of the normal knee at 0° and 90° of flexion (**a** and **b**) and the natural gaps of a right knee at 0° and 90° of flexion after making the resections using kinematic alignment (**c**) [24, 36]. Those paired columns connected by a p-value less than 0.05 indicate the laxity at 90° is greater than at 0° of flexion. The resected right knee shows a symmetrically shaped gap that is equal medially and laterally at 0° of flexion and an asymmetrically shaped gap lesser medially than laterally at 90° of flexion. Therefore, the surgical goal of gap balancing a TKA over-tightens the flexion gap. Error bars show ±1 standard deviation

of the tibia on the femur are negligible under applied loads that just engage the soft tissue restraints [16, 24, 25]. At 45° and 90° of flexion, the mean laxity is fivefold greater in varus (3.1°) rotation; fourfold greater in distraction; threefold greater in valgus (1.4°), internal (14.6°), and external (14.7°) rotation; and twofold greater in anterior translation than at 0° of flexion [16, 24]. The maintenance of these native differences in laxities between positions of knee flexion requires the maintenance of the native resting lengths of the collateral ligaments, posterior cruciate ligament, and retinacular ligaments. The alignment goal of gap balancing a TKA overtightens the laxities of the flexion gaps at 45° and 90° of flexion to match those at 0° of flexion, which patients may perceive as pain, stiffness, and/or limited flexion [6, 16].

Restoring the native laxities of knee at 0° of flexion requires removal of all osteophytes, extending the knee to 0°, and adjusting the varus-valgus angle and thickness of the tibial component until the varus, valgus, internal, and external rotational laxities are negligible [3]. Flexing the knee to 90° and adjusting the anterior-posterior slope and thickness of the tibial component until the offset of the anterior tibia from

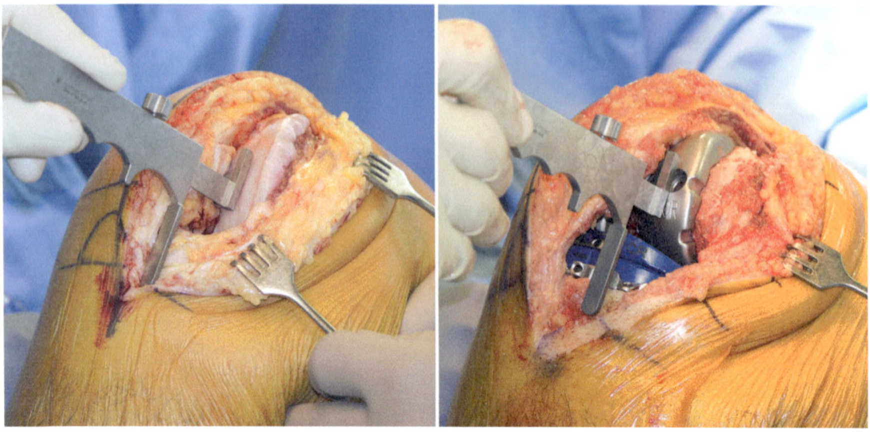

Fig. 8.4 Intraoperative photographs of a right knee with a varus deformity in 90° of flexion shows the measurement of the natural anterior offset of the tibia from the worn distal medial articular surface of the femur in a knee at the time of exposure (*left*) and at the time of reduction with the trial components (*right*). Compensating 2 mm for cartilage wear on the distal medial femur, adjusting the anterior-posterior slope and the thickness of the tibial component until the offset of the anterior tibia from the distal medial femoral condyle with the trial components matches that of the knee at the time of exposure, and setting the internal and external rotations of the tibia approximately 14° restores the laxities of the knee in 90° of flexion

the distal medial femoral condyle measured at the time of exposure matches the knee with the trial components, and the internal and external rotation of the tibia approximately 14° restores the native laxities of knee at 90° of flexion (Fig. 8.4) [3]. The ability of kinematically aligned TKA to restore the native knee and limb alignments and the laxities of the knee may explain the reports from a randomized clinical trial and a national, multicenter study that showed patients with a kinematically aligned TKA reported better pain relief, better function, better flexion, and a more normal-feeling knee than patients with a mechanically aligned TKA [2, 5].

8.5 Technique for Kinematically Aligning the Femoral Component to the Native Articular Surface

Kinematic alignment sets the femoral component at the native angle and level of the distal (0°) and posterior (90°) joint line. The surgical technique begins by using an offset caliper to measure the anterior-posterior offset of the anterior tibia from the distal medial femur with the knee in 90° of flexion (Fig. 8.4). Two millimeters is subtracted from the offset measurement if cartilage is missing on the distal medial femoral condyle. The measured offset is subsequently used as the reference for completing Quality Assurance Step 5 to restore the native F-E angle or slope of the tibial joint line. Once the knee is fully exposed, the locations of cartilage wear are assessed on the distal femur. A ring curette is used to remove any partially worn cartilage. The flexion-extension position of the femoral component is set by the

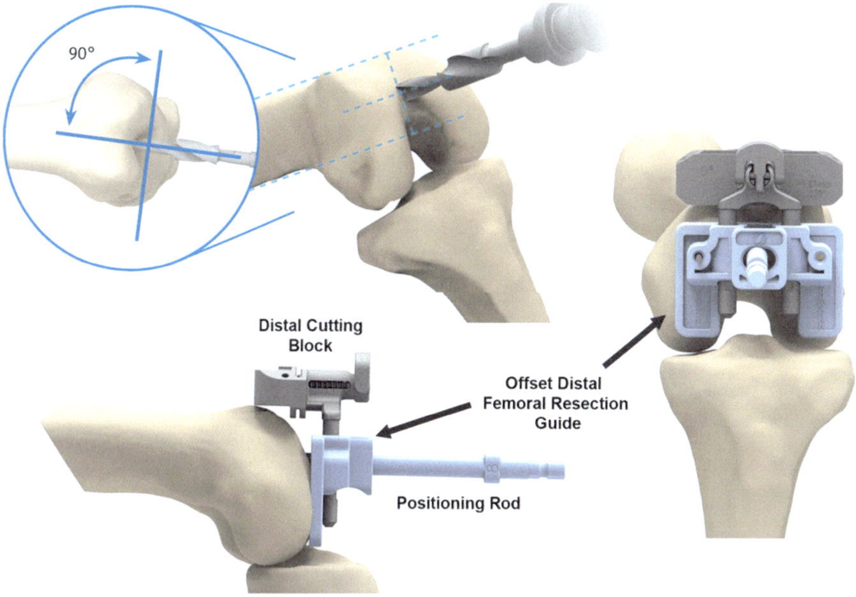

Fig. 8.5 Composite shows the method of setting the flexion extension and varus-valgus rotations and the proximal-distal translation of the kinematically aligned femoral component with disposable instruments (*blue*). The insertion of a positioning rod 8–10 cm through a hole drilled parallel to the anterior surface and perpendicular to the distal articular surface of the distal femur sets flexion-extension rotation of the femoral component. An assembly of the distal cutting block inserted into the offset distal femoral resection guide that compensates for 2 mm of cartilage wear on the worn condyle(s) is placed over the positioning rod in contact with the distal femur and sets varus-valgus rotation and proximal-distal translation of the femoral component

insertion of a positioning rod 8–10 cm through a drill hole placed parallel to the anterior surface of the distal femur and perpendicular to the distal articular surface (Fig. 8.5). The use of a starting hole midway between the top of the intercondylar notch and the anterior cortex reduces the risk of flexing the femoral component more than 5° from the anatomic axis of the femur, which is associated with patellofemoral instability [26]. Minimizing flexion of the femoral component completes Quality Assurance Step 1.

The varus-valgus rotation and proximal-distal translation of the femoral component are set by using a disposable distal referencing guide that compensates 2 mm when there is cartilage wear on the distal medial femoral condyle in the varus knee and 2 mm when there is cartilage wear on the distal lateral femoral condyle in the valgus knee. The distal resections are measured with a caliper. The anterior-posterior translation and internal-external rotation of the femoral component are set by placing a 0° rotation posterior referencing guide in contact with the posterior femoral condyles (Fig. 8.6). The positioning of the posterior referencing guide infrequently requires correction because complete cartilage loss on the posterior medial and posterior lateral femoral condyles is rare in most varus and valgus osteoarthritic knees [27]. The posterior resections are measured with a caliper. Correction for bone wear is rarely needed at 0° and 90° of flexion even in the most arthritic knees [3, 27]. Adjusting the thickness of the distal and posterior resections to match the thickness of the femoral component after compensating for cartilage wear and the kerf of the saw blade completes Quality Assurance Step 2.

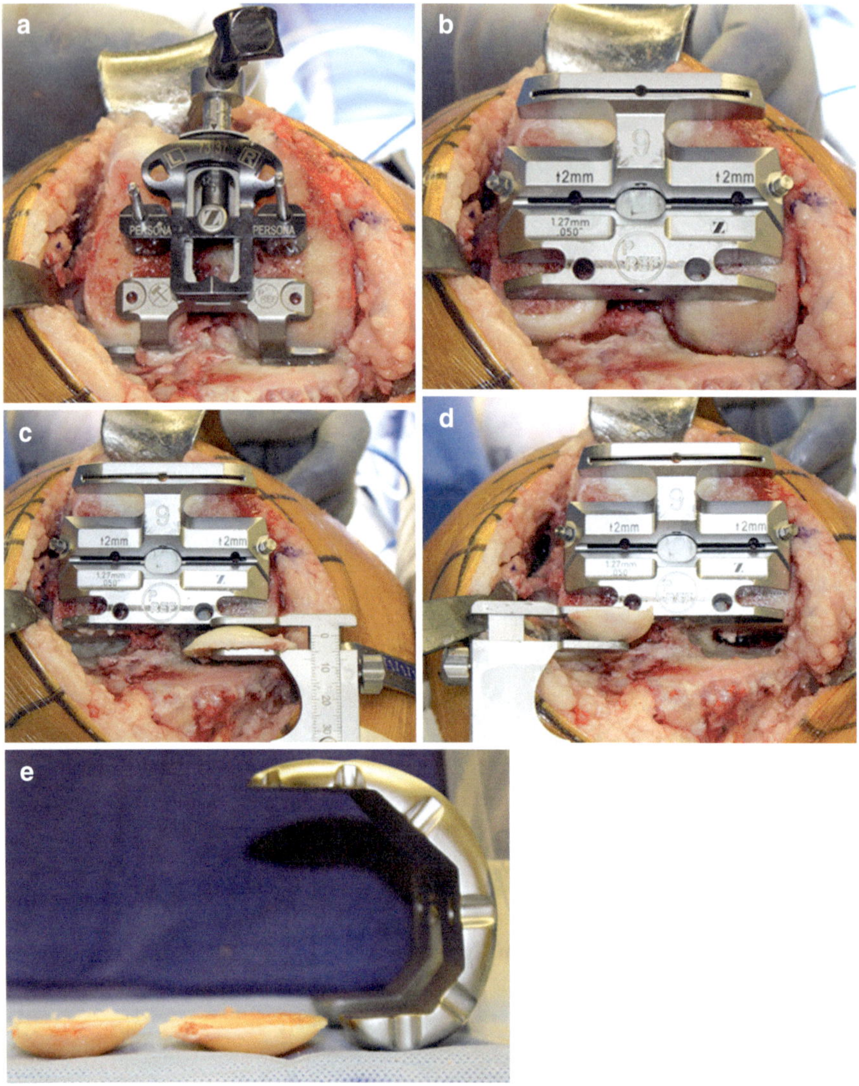

Fig. 8.6 Composite of a right varus osteoarthritic knee shows the steps for kinematically aligning the femoral component at 90° of flexion. A 0° rotation posterior referencing guide is inserted in contact with the posterior femoral condyles and pinned (**a**). The correct size chamfer guide is inserted into the pin holes (**b**). A caliper measures the thickness of the posterior medial femoral condyle (**c**) and posterior lateral femoral condyle (**d**). These steps set internal-external rotation and anterior-posterior translation of the femoral component to the natural articular surface of the posterior femur (**e**)

8.6 Technique for Kinematically Aligning the Tibial Component to the Native Articular Surface

Kinematically aligned TKA sets the tibial component at the native internal-external, varus-valgus, flexion-extension, and proximal-distal positions of the articular surface of the tibia with use of an extramedullary tibial guide (Figs. 8.7, 8.8, and 8.9) [3]. The internal-external rotation of the tibial component is set parallel to the flexion-extension plane of the knee with use of either the major axis of the lateral tibial condyle or a kinematic tibial baseplate method [3, 28, 29]. When the major axis of the lateral tibial condyle method is used, the elliptical-shaped boundary of the articular surface of the lateral tibial condyle is identified, and the major axis is drawn (Fig. 8.7) [3, 28, 29]. A guide is used to drill two holes into the medial articular surface parallel to the major axis drawn on the lateral tibial condyle. After the

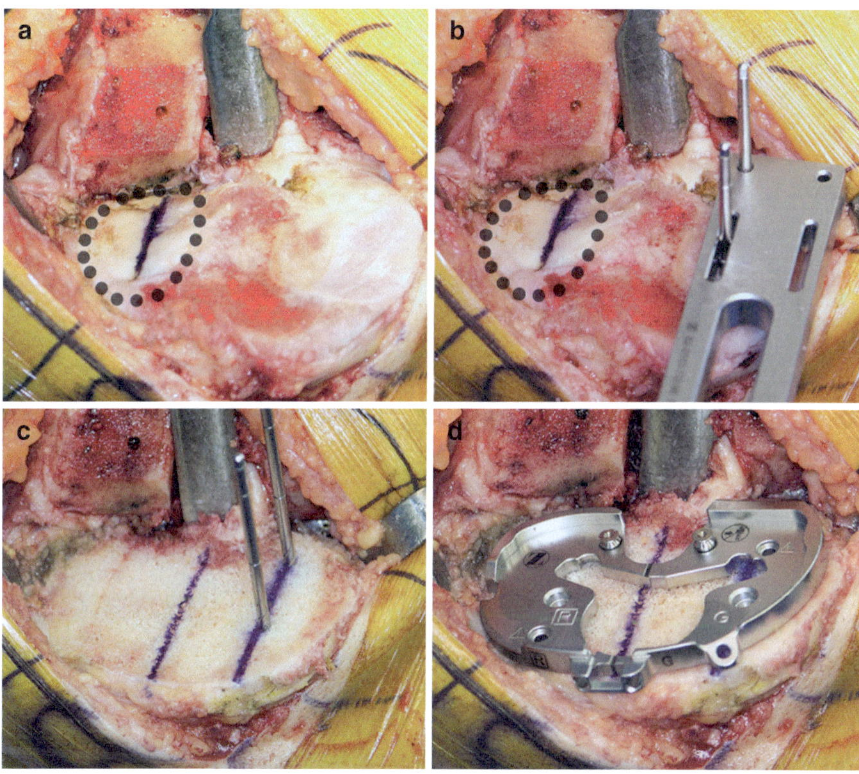

Fig. 8.7 Composite of a right knee shows the major axis of the lateral tibial condyle method for kinematically aligning the internal-external rotation of the trial tibial component to the anterior-posterior axis (*blue line*) of the nearly elliptical-shaped boundary of the articular surface of the lateral tibial condyle (*black dots*) (**a**). A guide is used to drill two pins through the medial tibial articular surface and parallel to the major axis (**b**). The tibial articular surface is resected and removed, the two drill holes are identified (*pins*), and lines parallel to the drill holes are drawn (**c**). The score marks (*green arrows*) indicate that the anterior-posterior axis of the trial tibial baseplate is aligned parallel to these lines (**d**)

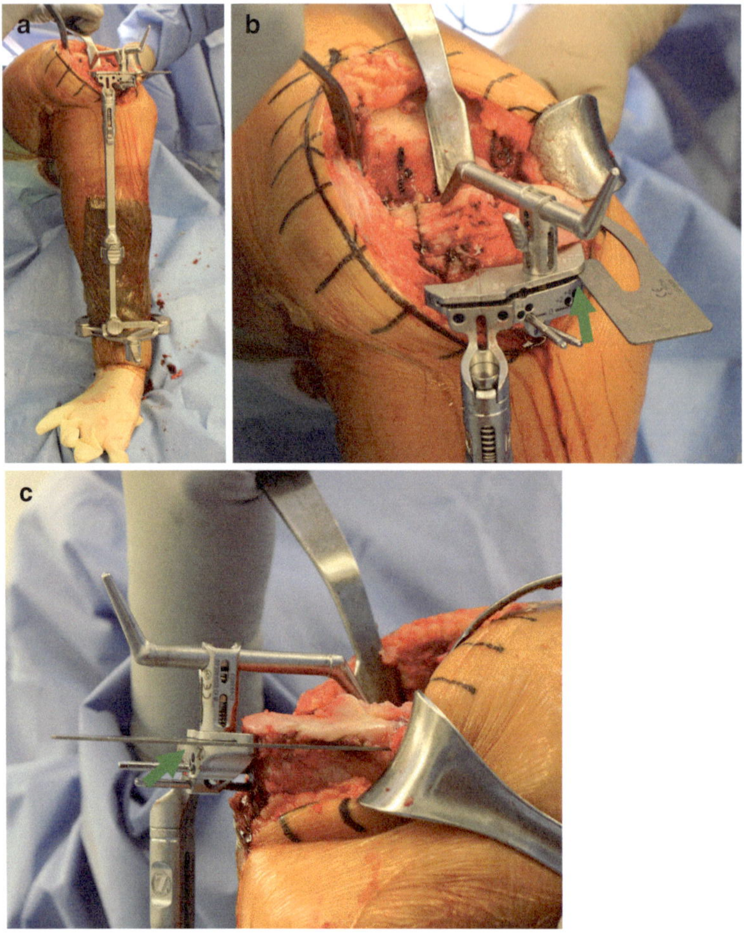

Fig. 8.8 Composite of a right knee shows the steps for kinematically aligning the tibial component. A conventional extramedullary tibial resection guide with a 10 mm offset tibial resection gauge and angel wing (*green arrow*) is applied to the ankle (**a**). The varus-valgus position of the tibial resection is set by adjusting the medial-lateral position of the slider at the ankle end of the guide until the saw slot is parallel to the tibial articular surface after visually compensating for cartilage and bone wear. The proximal-distal translation of the tibial component is set by adjusting the level of the saw slot until there is contact between the 10 mm offset tibial resection gauge and the center of the unworn tibial condyle (**b**). The flexion-extension rotation of the tibial component is set by adjusting the inclination of the angel wing parallel to the slope of the medial joint line (**c**). These steps set the proximal-distal translation and the varus-valgus and flexion-extension rotations of the tibial component parallel to the natural articular surface of the tibia

tibial resection is made, the anterior-posterior axis of the tibial component is aligned parallel to these two holes. This technique uses a rationale similar to Cobb's method, which finds the flexion-extension plane of the knee by fitting circles to the medial and lateral tibial condyles [30]. In contrast to mechanically aligned TKA where the medial border and medial one-third of the tibial tubercle are considered useful

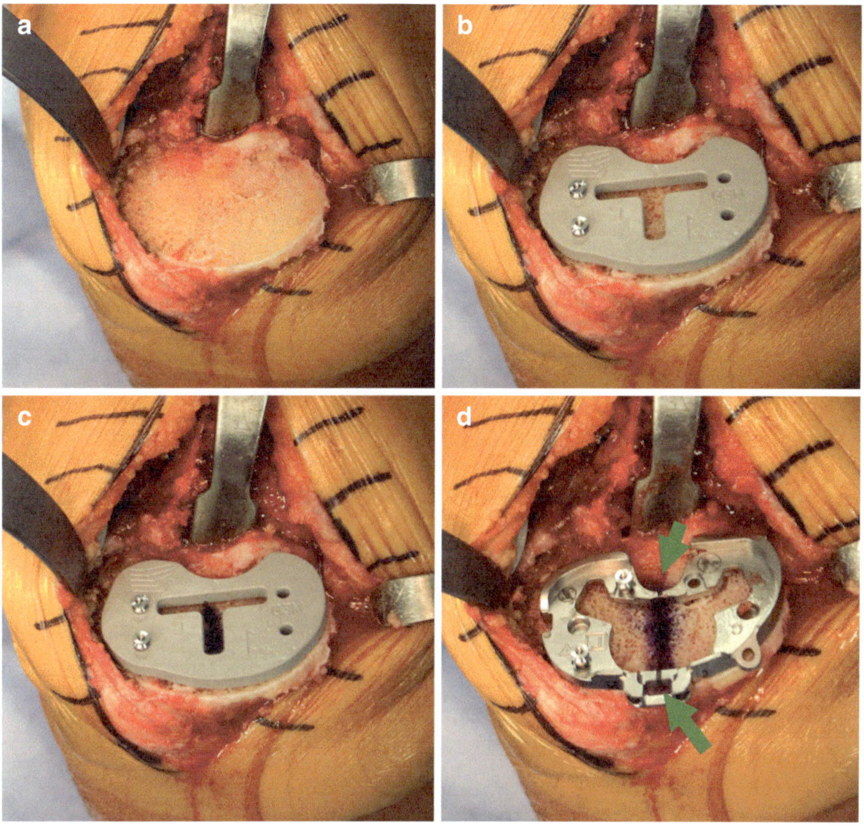

Fig. 8.9 Composite of a right knee shows the steps for aligning the internal-external rotation of the trial tibial component parallel to the flexion-extension plane of the knee with a kinematic tibial baseplate (*gray*). The cortical contour of the anatomic resection of the tibia is shown (**a**). The largest size kinematic tibial baseplate that fits within the contour is selected from the seven kinematic tibial baseplates and is fit within the cortical contour (**b**). The anterior-posterior axis of the kinematic tibial baseplate is marked (*blue line*) (**c**). The score marks (*green arrows*) indicate that the anterior-posterior axis of the trial tibial baseplate is aligned parallel to the *blue line* (**d**)

landmarks, a study of a case series of kinematically aligned TKAs showed that aligning the tibial component to the medial border or medial one-third of the tibial tubercle would have malrotated the tibial component 5° or more from the flexion-extension plane of the knee in 70% and 86% of the knees, respectively [3, 31, 32]. The use of the major axis of the lateral tibial condyle is a reproducible method as shown by a negligible bias (−1° internal) and an acceptable precision (± 5.4°) between the anterior-posterior axis of the tibial component and the flexion-extension plane of the knee and minimal malrotation of the tibial component on the femoral component [28, 29]. Aligning the anterior-posterior axis of the tibial component parallel to the flexion-extension plane of the knee completes Quality Assurance Step 3 [28, 29, 32].

Next, a conventional extramedullary tibial resection guide is applied to the ankle, and an angel wing is placed in the saw slot of the guide (Fig. 8.8). The varus-valgus position of the tibial component is set by medially translating the slider at the ankle of the guide until the saw slot is parallel to the tibial articular surface after a visual compensation for cartilage and bone wear. The flexion extension or slope of the tibial component is set by adjusting the inclination of an angel wing placed in the saw slot until it is parallel to the slope of the medial joint line to reproduce the offset measured first after exposing the knee joint. The proximal-distal translation of the tibial component is set by adjusting the level of the saw slot until the 10 mm tibial resection gauge contacts the center of the unworn tibial condyle [3]. A conservative tibial resection is made while protecting the insertion of the posterior cruciate ligament. When the kinematic tibial baseplate is used to set internal-external rotation of the tibial component, the largest one of the seven available sizes that fits within the cortical contour of the tibial resection is selected and best fit to the anterior and medial cortical edge (Fig. 8.9). The in vitro reproducibility of the kinematic tibial baseplate was evaluated on 166 tibial resections by five arthroplasty surgeons, three orthopedic surgery fellows/residents, and three students and showed a negligible bias (0.7° external) and acceptable precision (± 4.6°) between the anterior-posterior axis of the kinematic tibial baseplate and the flexion-extension plane of the knee. The in vivo reproducibility was evaluated in 63 kinematically aligned TKAs by one arthroplasty surgeon and showed a negligible bias (0.2° external) and an acceptable precision (± 3.6°) between the anterior-posterior axes of the tibial and the femoral components (unpublished study).

8.7 Balancing the Kinematically Aligned Total Knee Arthroplasty

The algorithm for restoring motion and balance to the kinematically aligned TKA is simple, has a logical progression, and has a defined end point, which are predicated on first completing Quality Assurance Steps 1–3 (Fig. 8.10). To determine which options are needed to restore motion and balance the knee, the knee is examined with trial components. When the knee lacks both extension and flexion but has anterior-posterior and varus-valgus stability throughout the motion arc, remove more tibia. When the knee lacks extension, but fully flexes and has anterior-posterior and varus-valgus stability throughout the motion arc, remove posterior osteophytes, and release the posterior capsule. If removal of the posterior osteophytes and releasing the posterior capsule are ineffective, then decrease the posterior slope on the tibia. Additional resection of the bone from the distal femur is not recommended to restore extension unless the distal bone resection is 2 mm or thinner than the posterior bone resection or unless the PCL is inadvertently released. The penalty from additional resection of bone from the distal femur is proximal translation of the femoral component. This moves the proximal-distal position of the primary transverse axis of the femur proximally but leaves the anterior-posterior position of the primary transverse axis of the femur unchanged, which loosens the collateral

Balancing the kinematically aligned TKA has a defined pathway and endpoint

Tight in extension & flexion	Tight in flexion well-balanced in extension	Tight in extension well-balanced in flexion	Well-balanced in extension & loose in flexion	Tight medial & loose lateral in extension	Tight lateral & loose medial in extension
Use thinner liner Recut tibia and remove more bone	Increase posterior slope until natural A-P offset is restored at 90° of flexion	Remove posterior osteophytes Reassess Strip posterior capsule	Add thicker liner and recheck knee extends fully When knee dose not fully extend check PCL tension When PCL is incompetent consider PS implant	Remove medial osteophytes Reassess Recut tibia in 2° more varus Insert 2mm thicker liner	Remove lateral osteophytes Reassess Recut tibia in 2° more valgus Insert 2mm thicker liner

Fig. 8.10 The table shows a stepwise algorithm for balancing the kinematically aligned TKA. The top row lists six malalignments, and the bottom lists the corresponding corrective actions. Notice those corrections that require a recut of bone are performed by fine-tuning the proximal-distal translation and the varus-valgus and flexion-extension (slope) rotations of the tibial resection and not by recutting the femur

ligaments in extension but not in flexion. This limits flexion and kinematically malaligns the knee. When the knee lacks flexion but fully extends and has anterior-posterior and varus-valgus stability throughout the motion arc, increase the posterior slope on the tibia. A kinematically aligned femoral component does not need recession or release of the posterior cruciate ligament to increase flexion.

When the knee is tight medially throughout the motion arc and fully flexes and extends, remove medial femoral and tibial osteophytes. When medial tightness persists, recut the tibia in 1–2° more varus until there is negligible varus-valgus laxity with trial components with the knee in full extension. When the knee is tight laterally throughout the motion arc and fully flexes and extends, remove lateral femoral and tibial osteophytes. When the lateral tightness persists, recut the tibia in 1–2° more valgus until there is negligible varus-valgus laxity with trial components with the knee in full extension. Negligible varus-valgus laxity with the knee in full extension restores the native limb alignment and completes Quality Assurance Step 4 [3, 16, 24].

Finally, adjust the F-E cut of the tibia until the A-P offset of the anterior tibia from the distal medial femur with trial components at 90° of flexion is equal to the osteoarthritic knee at the time of surgical exposure, and there is approximately 14°

of passive internal-external rotation. Restoration of the A-P offset and native passive internal-external rotation completes Quality Assurance Step 5 [3, 16, 24].

In the case where the posterior cruciate ligament is insufficient due to inadvertent release or incompetency, and there is anterior-posterior instability in 90° of flexion, but stability in full extension uses either a liner with an increased anterior slope or a posterior-stabilized component.

8.8 Examples of Severe Varus and Valgus Deformity Treated with Kinematically Aligned Total Knee Arthroplasty

Kinematically aligned TKA can be performed with any severity of varus deformity (Fig. 8.11). The prearthritic native joint line is restored and the native laxities of the soft tissue envelope maintained. The example illustrates a posttraumatic knee with a severe varus deformity, flexion contracture, and chronic posterior cruciate ligament insufficiency. Due to the posterior cruciate ligament insufficiency, we chose a posterior cruciate ligament-substituting implant.

There are special considerations when performing kinematically aligned TKA in the patient with severe fixed valgus deformity (Fig. 8.12). We estimate that 15% of fixed valgus deformities remain in 2–3° of excessive valgus deformity after adjusting the varus-valgus angle and thickness of the tibial component until the varus-valgus laxity is negligible with the knee to 0° of flexion (Fig. 8.12). In this small subset of valgus knees, we perform a careful lengthening of the lateral collateral ligament 2–3 mm by pie crusting with a spinal needle with distraction applied with a laminar spreader to the lateral compartment with knee in 90° of flexion (Fig. 8.13).

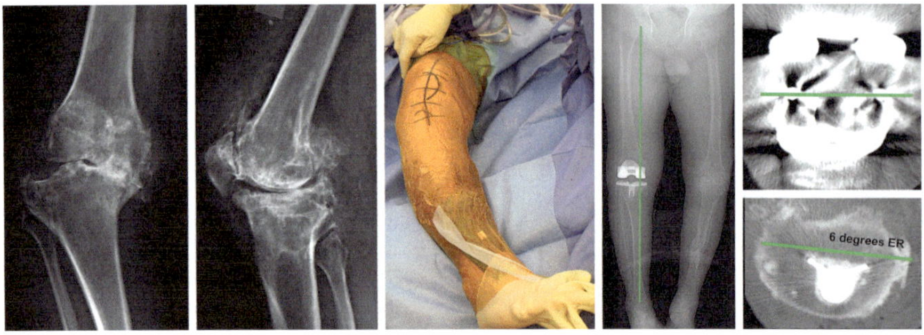

Fig. 8.11 Composite shows the preoperative radiographs of a posttraumatic knee with a severe varus deformity, flexion contracture, and chronic posterior cruciate ligament insufficiency, an intraoperative photograph of the varus deformity, and a postoperative computer tomographic scanogram of the limb and axial views of the femoral and tibial components. The kinematically aligned TKA restored the natural alignment and laxities of the knee without a release of the medial collateral ligament and was performed with posterior cruciate ligament-substituting implants because of the torn posterior cruciate ligament

After completing the lengthening, a recut guide is used to cut the tibia in 2–3° more varus, and a 2 mm thicker liner is inserted. For a tibia of normal length, each degree of varus or valgus correction at the knee joint causes a 6–7 mm medial or lateral translation of the ankle. Therefore, a 3° varus correction at the knee causes an 18–21 mm medial translation at the ankle, which corrects the valgus deformity of the limb and knee. On the rare occasion, these corrective actions do not reduce a chronic lateral patella subluxation or dislocation a lateral release is performed.

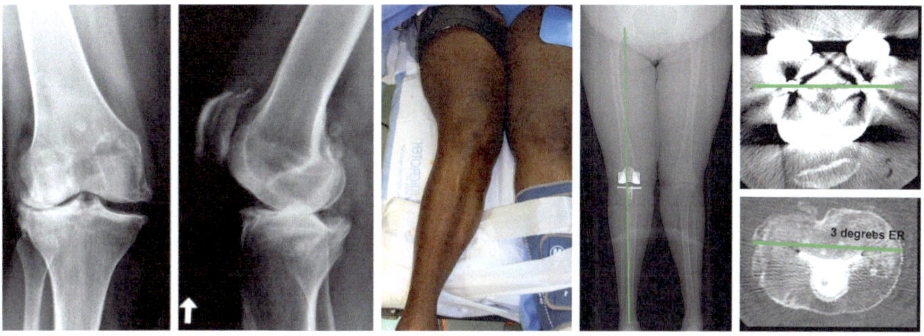

Fig. 8.12 Composite shows the preoperative radiographs of the knee with severe valgus deformity, intraoperative photograph of the severe valgus deformity, and flexion contracture, and postoperative computer tomographic scanogram of the limb and axial views of the femoral and tibial components. The kinematically aligned TKA restored the natural alignment and laxities of the knee without a release of the lateral collateral ligament in this patient with an intact posterior cruciate ligament

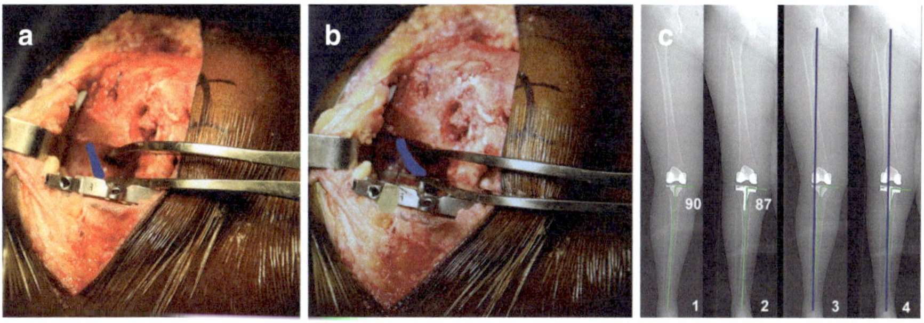

Fig. 8.13 Composite shows the laminar spreader in the lateral side of a right knee before (**a**) and after a 3 mm incremental lengthening of the lateral collateral ligament with use of the pie-crusting technique (*blue*) (**b**) and the use of the pie-crusting technique in another patient to correct the alignment of the knee and limb left too valgus at the time of primary kinematically aligned TKA (**c**). The tibial component in the primary surgery was originally set at 90° to the mechanical axis of the tibia (*1*), which left the leg too valgus (*3*). The revision followed the stepwise algorithm for correcting the valgus deformity by adjusting the varus-valgus alignment of the tibial component and leaving the original femoral component alone (Fig. 8.10). At revision, the varus-valgus alignment of the tibial component tibial component was set at 87° to the mechanical axis of the tibia by lengthening the lateral collateral ligament 3 mm (*2*), and the insertion of a thicker liner moved the ankle 20 mm more medial, which realigned the limb to neutral (*4*)

8.9 Summary

Kinematically aligned TKA is a promising surgical technique that provides significantly better pain relief, function, flexion, a more normal-feeling knee than mechanical alignment with a similar implant survivorship at 2, 3, and 6 years [1, 2, 4, 5, 33]. The three goals of kinematically aligned TKA are to restore (1) the native tibial-femoral articular surfaces, (2) the native knee and limb alignments, and (3) the native laxities of the knee. We presented five Quality Assurance Steps that intraoperatively verify both kinematic alignment of the femoral and tibial components to the native joint lines and correct balancing of the knee even in patients with severe varus and valgus deformities and flexion contractures. The following three links provide video and animated instruction for surgeons interested in learning more about kinematically aligned TKA.

1. YouTube Live surgical demonstration of kinematically aligned TKA performed at ISAKOS 2015 in Lyon, France (www.youtube.com/watch?v=VW9-GdUYBcs) TouchSurgery's free animated surgery application for learning technique and intraoperative decision-making when performing kinematically aligned TKA downloadable to smart phone, iPad, or tablet (www.touchsurgery.com)
2. Dr. Stephen M Howell's website containing PDFs of published papers (http://www.drstevehowell.com/)

References

1. Calliess T, Bauer K, Stukenborg-Colsman C, Windhagen H, Budde S, Ettinger M PSI kinematic versus non-PSI mechanical alignment in total knee arthroplasty: a prospective, randomized study. Knee Surg Sports Traumatol Arthrosc Off J ESSKA. 2016:1–6. doi:10.1007/s00167-016-4136-8.
2. Dossett HG, Estrada NA, Swartz GJ, LeFevre GW, Kwasman BG. A randomised controlled trial of kinematically and mechanically aligned total knee replacements: two-year clinical results. Bone Joint J. 2014;96-B(7):907–13. doi:10.1302/0301-620X.96B7.32812.
3. Howell SM, Papadopoulos S, Kuznik KT, Hull ML. Accurate alignment and high function after kinematically aligned TKA performed with generic instruments. Knee Surg Sports Traumatol Arthrosc Off J ESSKA. 2013;21(10):2271–80. doi:10.1007/s00167-013-2621-x.
4. Howell SM, Papadopoulos S, Kuznik K, Ghaly LR, Hull ML. Does varus alignment adversely affect implant survival and function six years after kinematically aligned total knee arthroplasty? Int Orthop. 2015;39(11):2117–24.
5. Nam D, Nunley RM, Barrack RL. Patient dissatisfaction following total knee replacement: a growing concern? Bone Joint J. 2014;96-B(11 Supple A):96–100. doi:10.1302/0301-620X.96B11.34152.
6. Eckhoff DG, Bach JM, Spitzer VM, Reinig KD, Bagur MM, Baldini TH, Flannery NM. Three-dimensional mechanics, kinematics, and morphology of the knee viewed in virtual reality. J Bone Joint Surg Am. 2005;87(Suppl 2):71–80. doi:10.2106/JBJS.E.00440.
7. Pinskerova V, Iwaki H, Freeman MA. The shapes and relative movements of the femur and tibia at the knee. Orthopade. 2000;29(Suppl 1):S3–5.
8. Iwaki H, Pinskerova V, Freeman MA. Tibiofemoral movement 1: the shapes and relative movements of the femur and tibia in the unloaded cadaver knee. J Bone Joint Surg Br. 2000;82(8):1189–95.

9. Weber WE, Weber EFM. Mechanik der menschlichen Gehwerkzeuge. Göttingen: Verlag der Dietrichschen Buchhandlung; 1836.
10. Hollister AM, Jatana S, Singh AK, Sullivan WW, Lupichuk AG. The axes of rotation of the knee. Clin Orthop Relat Res. 1993;290:259–68.
11. Coughlin KM, Incavo SJ, Churchill DL, Beynnon BD. Tibial axis and patellar position relative to the femoral epicondylar axis during squatting. J Arthroplasty. 2003;18(8):1048–55.
12. Iranpour F, Merican AM, Baena FR, Cobb JP, Amis AA. Patellofemoral joint kinematics: the circular path of the patella around the trochlear axis. J Orthop Res Off Pub Orthop Res Soc. 2010;28(5):589–94. doi:10.1002/jor.21051.
13. Eckhoff D, Hogan C, DiMatteo L, Robinson M, Bach J. Difference between the epicondylar and cylindrical axis of the knee. Clin Orthop Relat Res. 2007;461:238–44. doi:10.1097/BLO.0b013e318112416b.
14. Howell SM, Howell SJ, Hull ML. Assessment of the radii of the medial and lateral femoral condyles in varus and valgus knees with osteoarthritis. J Bone Joint Surg Am. 2010;92(1):98–104. doi:10.2106/JBJS.H.01566.
15. Gu Y, Roth JD, Howell SM, Hull ML. How frequently do four methods for mechanically aligning a total knee arthroplasty cause collateral ligament imbalance and change alignment from normal in white patients? AAOS Exhibit Selection. J Bone Joint Surg Am. 2014;96(12):e101.
16. Roth JD, Howell SM, Hull ML. Native knee laxities at 0 degrees , 45 degrees , and 90 degrees of flexion and their relationship to the goal of the gap-balancing alignment method of total knee arthroplasty. J Bone Joint Surg Am. 2015;97(20):1678–84. doi:10.2106/JBJS.N.01256.
17. Hutt J, Masse V, Lavigne M, Vendittoli PA. Functional joint line obliquity after kinematic total knee arthroplasty. Int Orthop. 2016;40(1):29–34. doi:10.1007/s00264-015-2733-7.
18. Ji HM, Han J, Jin DS, Seo H, Won YY. Kinematically aligned TKA can align knee joint line to horizontal. Knee Surg Sports Traumatol Arthrosc Off J ESSKA. 2016;24(8):2436–41. doi:10.1007/s00167-016-3995-3.
19. Vanlommel L, Vanlommel J, Claes S, Bellemans J. Slight undercorrection following total knee arthroplasty results in superior clinical outcomes in varus knees. Knee Surg Sports Traumatol Arthrosc Off J ESSKA. 2013;21(10):2325–30. doi:10.1007/s00167-013-2481-4.
20. Victor JM, Bassens D, Bellemans J, Gürsu S, Dhollander AA, Verdonk PC. Constitutional varus does not affect joint line orientation in the coronal plane. Clin Orthop Relat Res. 2014;472(1):98–104.
21. Bellemans J, Colyn W, Vandenneucker H, Victor J. The Chitranjan Ranawat award: is neutral mechanical alignment normal for all patients? The concept of constitutional varus. Clin Orthop Relat Res. 2012;470(1):45–53. doi:10.1007/s11999-011-1936-5.
22. Delport H, Labey L, Innocenti B, De Corte R, Vander Sloten J, Bellemans J. Restoration of constitutional alignment in TKA leads to more physiological strains in the collateral ligaments. Knee Surg Sports Traumatol Arthrosc Off J ESSKA. 2015;23(8):2159–69. doi:10.1007/s00167-014-2971-z.
23. Blazek K, Favre J, Asay J, Erhart-Hledik J, Andriacchi T. Age and obesity alter the relationship between femoral articular cartilage thickness and ambulatory loads in individuals without osteoarthritis. J Orthop Res Off Pub Orthop Res Soc. 2014;32(3):394–402. doi:10.1002/jor.22530.
24. Roth JD, Hull ML, Howell SM. Rotational and translational limits of passive motion are both variable between and unrelated within normal tibiofemoral joints. J Orthop Res Off Pub Orthop Res Soc. 2015;33 (11):n/a–n/a. doi:10.1002/jor.22926
25. Freeman MA, Pinskerova V. The movement of the normal tibio-femoral joint. J Biomech. 2005;38(2):197–208. doi:10.1016/j.jbiomech.2004.02.006.
26. Nedopil AJ, Howell SM, Hull ML. What clinical characteristics and radiographic parameters are associated with patellofemoral instability after kinematically aligned total knee arthroplasty?. Int Orthop. 2016. [Epub ahead of print]. PMID: 27619673.
27. Nam D, Lin KM, Howell SM, Hull ML. Femoral bone and cartilage wear is predictable at 0 degrees and 90 degrees in the osteoarthritic knee treated with total knee arthroplasty.

Knee Surg Sports Traumatol Arthrosc Off J ESSKA. 2014;22(12):2975–81. doi:10.1007/s00167-014-3080-8.
28. Nedopil AJ, Howell SM, Hull ML. Does malrotation of the tibial and femoral components compromise function in kinematically aligned total knee arthroplasty? Orthop Clin North Am. 2016;47(1):41–50. doi:10.1016/j.ocl.2015.08.006.
29. Nedopil AJ, Howell SM, Rudert M, Roth J, Hull ML. How frequent is rotational mismatch within 0±10 in kinematically aligned total knee arthroplasty? Orthopedics. 2013;36(12):e1515–20.
30. Cobb JP, Dixon H, Dandachli W, Iranpour F. The anatomical tibial axis: reliable rotational orientation in knee replacement. J Bone Joint Surg Br. 2008;90(8):1032–8. doi:10.1302/0301-620X.90B8.19905.
31. Brar AS, Howell SM, Hull ML. What are the bias, imprecision, and limits of agreement for finding the flexion-extension plane of the knee with five tibial reference lines? Knee. 2016; doi:10.1016/j.knee.2016.01.005.
32. Howell SM, Chen J, Hull ML. Variability of the location of the tibial tubercle affects the rotational alignment of the tibial component in kinematically aligned total knee arthroplasty. Knee Surg Sports Traumatol Arthrosc Off J ESSKA. 2013;21(10):2288–95. doi:10.1007/s00167-012-1987-5.
33. Howell SM, Howell SJ, Kuznik KT, Cohen J, Hull ML. Does a kinematically aligned total knee arthroplasty restore function without failure regardless of alignment category? Clin Orthop Relat Res. 2013;471(3):1000–7. doi:10.1007/s11999-012-2613-z.
34. Dossett HG, Swartz GJ, Estrada NA, LeFevre GW, Kwasman BG. Kinematically versus mechanically aligned total knee arthroplasty. Orthopedics. 2012;35(2):e160–9. doi:10.3928/01477447-20120123-04.
35. Nunley RM, Ellison BS, Zhu J, Ruh EL, Howell SM, Barrack RL. Do patient-specific guides improve coronal alignment in total knee arthroplasty? Clin Orthop Relat Res. 2012;470(3):895–902. doi:10.1007/s11999-011-2222-2.
36. Roth JD, Howell SM, Hull ML. Native knee laxities at 0°, 45°, and 90° of flexion and their relationship to the goal of gap-balancing a TKA. J Bone Joint Surg. 2015;97(20):1678–84. (In Press).

Part III

Operative Procedure 2: Primary TKA

Operative Procedure: Varus Knee

9

David Figueroa and Francisco Figueroa

Contents

9.1 Introduction

In varus OA knees, TKA often involves the release of the medial structures in order to realign the leg and also achieve balance and stability. In rare occasions it requires tensing lateral structures to achieve this goal. Correct soft tissue balance is essential to the success of TKA surgery [1].

A knee can be described as "balanced" when the normal motion of the knee is not hindered by the soft tissue constraint, so that normal knee motion (kinematics) is allowed by the soft tissue envelope. On the other hand, sufficient tension of the ligaments should be present to provide stability. Incorrect soft tissue balancing can result in a number of complications, including instability, abnormal polyethylene wear, aseptic loosening, altered patellofemoral biomechanics, and pain [1].

D. Figueroa, MD (✉) • F. Figueroa, MD
Facultad de Medicina Clínica Alemana, Universidad del Desarrollo, Concepción, Chile
e-mail: dhfigueroa@gmail.com

S. Matsuda et al. (eds.), *Soft Tissue Balancing in Total Knee Arthroplasty*,
DOI 10.1007/978-3-662-54082-4_9

While medial release is the standard intraoperative mode of balancing, its sequence and extent is not clear, but according to different studies it is necessary in 76–88% of OA varus knees [2–4].

We present here our method for balancing of a varus TKA. As no clear guidelines has been published, the order is not mandatory, and it is obviously dependent of the gap affected (flexion or extension).

9.2 Step 1: Cruciate Retaining (CR) or Posterior Stabilized (PS)

The first decision that has to be made when dealing with a varus TKA is to retain or sacrifice the posterior cruciate ligament (PCL). The PCL is both a posterior and a medial structure; thus, it may be contracted in a varus-deformed lower extremity. When the PCL is retained as in CR arthroplasty, it must be assessed and balanced. The PCL could be released from the intercondylar notch in the femur or from its insertion in the tibia.

The PCL supports the flexion gap. Thus, the release of the PCL results in a flexion gap that is larger than the extension gap. Therefore, it is recommended that the distal femoral bone resection be increased to aid in equalizing the gap [5].

When sacrificing the PCL as in PS TKA, less medial soft tissue release typically offers better balance. For that reason we recommend in severe varus knees to use a PS TKA, simplifying the procedure (Fig. 9.1).

9.3 Step 2: Osteophytes

The presence of osteophytes on the medial aspect of the tibial plateau and on the medial femoral condyle can have a significant tightening effect on the structures that make up the medial soft tissue sleeve. For this reason, all osteophytes should be removed before any soft tissue release is performed. Removal of the osteophytes that impede on the medial soft tissue sleeve is often enough to provide a balanced flexion and extension gap in the mild varus knee [5] (Fig. 9.2).

9.4 Step 3: Superficial Medial Collateral Ligament

The critical stabilizers on the medial side of the knee include the superficial medial collateral ligament (sMCL) fibers on the anterior aspect and posterior structures such as the posterior oblique ligament (POL) and the semimembranosus (SM) tendon fibers that merge into the posterior capsule [6].

The sMCL has its origin on the medial epicondyle and its tibial insertion on the medial aspect of the upper tibia. It affects both the flexion (anterior fibers) and the

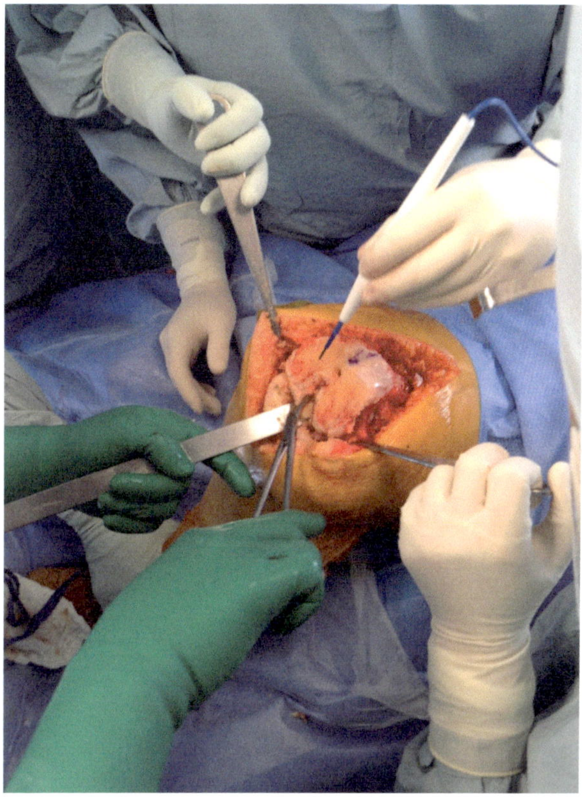

Fig. 9.1 Sacrificing the posterior cruciate ligament in a PS total knee replacement

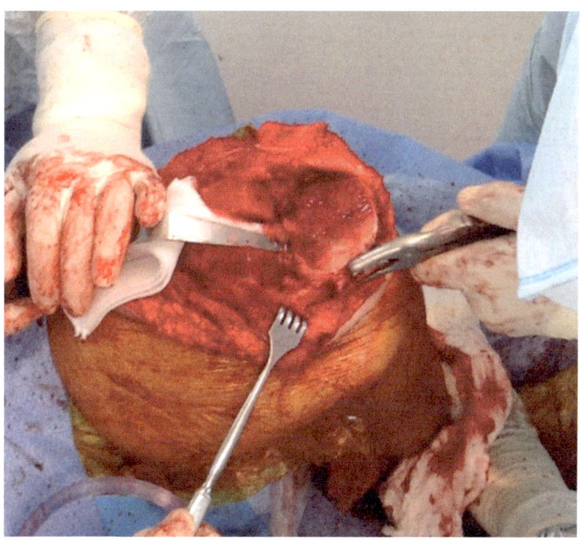

Fig. 9.2 Resection of the medial osteophytes in the tibial plateau in a varus knee

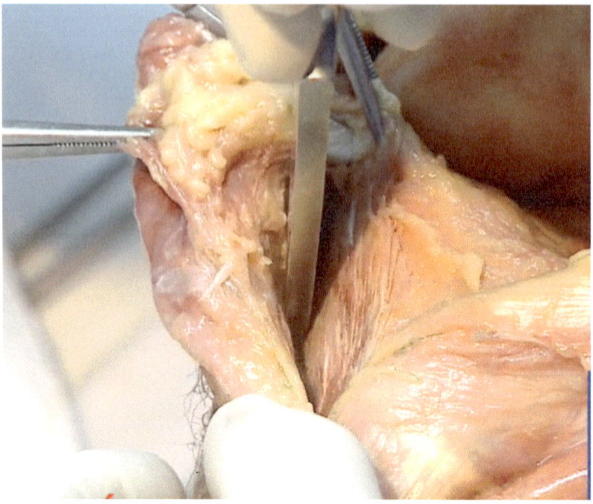

Fig. 9.3 Release of the superficial layer of the medial collateral ligament (sMCL)

extension (posterior fibers) gap. A subperiosteal technique is used to release the sMCL off the tibial insertion from just medial to the pes anserine tendon insertion to the medial aspect of the upper tibia (Fig. 9.3). The surgeon should begin by performing a gentle release and then reassess the flexion and extension gaps so that the appropriate amount of release can be obtained without causing overcorrection or instability resulting from an excessive amount of release.

9.5 Step 4: Posterior Oblique Ligament

The POL fibers run in an oblique fashion from the upper posterior aspect of the sMCL fibers into the posteromedial aspect of the medial flare of the proximal tibia. The POL should be the first structure released when the knee is tight only in extension and not in flexion in a varus TKA.

Another indication for release of the POL occurs when, after release of the posterior fibers of the sMCL, the knee remains tight in extension. The insertion of the POL is released in a subperiosteal fashion from the medial-most point of the tibial cut. This release is directed at a 45° angle in the posterior direction [5].

9.6 Step 5: Semimembranosus (SM)

The SM tendon has a complex attachment to the posteromedial aspect of the tibia, with five described insertion sites. The posterior nature of its blended insertion with the capsule means that the release of the SM tendon affects the extension space more than it does the flexion space.

If the knee remains tight in full extension after the release of the posterior sMCL fibers and the POL, then the release of the SM tendon should be considered.

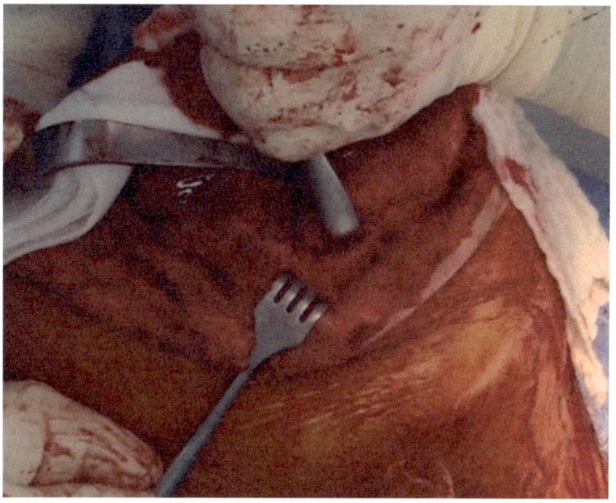

Fig. 9.4 Release of the semimembranosus in the posterior medial corner of the tibial plateau

A subperiosteal technique is performed to release the insertion from the posteromedial aspect of the proximal tibia. Although that classically release of the SM tendon was reserved for knees with significant varus deformity or combined varus and flexion contracture deformity, new publications confronts these guidelines. Koh et al. [7] presented a SM release as the second step of their algorithm ((1) release of the deep MCL, (2) release of the SM, (3) release of the sMCL) describing that after realizing the first two steps, only a 6.7% of the patients still required a release of the sMCL to achieve a correct balance, decreasing the risk of instability associated with this procedure (Fig. 9.4).

9.7 Step 6: Pes Anserinus, Medial Epicondyle Osteotomy, Medial Tibial Plateau Resection, and Lateral Collateral Ligament Advancement

Other possible releases exist for certain cases but are rarely used in regular practice.

Pes anserinus release should be reserved only for very severe varus knees; their release affects extension more than flexion.

Osteotomy of the medial epicondyle has also been reported to aid in balancing and providing exposure of the varus knee with flexion contracture, but Mihalko et al. [8] in a recent cadaveric study demonstrated that knee specimens in the laboratory treated with medial epicondylar osteotomy were significantly more lax in flexion than a standard sMCL release raising concerns about the use of an epicondylar osteotomy because of the risk of instability.

Another option for the knee with a severe varus deformity involves resection of the bone along the medial tibial plateau, with downsizing and relative lateralization of the tibial baseplate. The final effect is a relative medialization of the tibial tubercle, which may enhance patellar tracking, too. Recently Ahn et al. [9] compared this option to a traditional release in 40 patients. They concluded that in severe varus knees, bony resection of proximal medial tibia can be considered as an alternative technique, with less total operation time and a comparable soft tissue balance.

If, after complete release of medial-sided structures, imbalance persists and the medial gap is tight, the surgeon should consider advancing the lateral collateral ligament (LCL) to correct the imbalance. This can be accomplished on the fibular side of the joint by osteotomizing the proximal fibula and advancing it distally to tighten the LCL.

9.8 Recent Evidence

A recent review of the literature available was done by Hunt et al. [1]. They conclude that there is a lack of evidence to support extensive medial release for routine varus knee replacement as the better option of treatment. Regarding surgical methods used or algorithms, they report that methods can vary between surgeons and the level of detail provided in published articles is often very limited producing a lack of consensus for quantification of such releases on the medial side, so interpretation of surgical procedures remains difficult. Furthermore, they describe that the description of the methods and also the subjective approach normally adopted to assess the stability of the joint by "feel" can make it difficult for relatively inexperienced surgeons to achieve balance confidently and accurately.

Regarding the release techniques, Goudarz et al. [10] compared an algorithmic approach proposed by Bellemans et al. [11] that consisted in pie crust releases of the anteromedial or posteromedial structures of the knee depending on the gap affected to a group where classical subperiosteal releases were made. They concluded that the pie crust releases obtained better stability, requiring a lower need of constrained inserts (8% vs. 18%) and with similar outcomes at 1 year follow-up.

Mihalko et al. [12] latter did a biomechanical validation of the pie crust release for medial side structures in TKA. In their study they reported that ligament release pie crust release produced symmetric changes in the extension and flexion gaps compared to a traditional release which produced greater gaps in flexion that could lead to a flexion instability. Therefore, they advocated for the use of pie crust releases over classical subperiosteal releases.

Conclusion

Medial releases are the standard method for balancing a varus TKA. There are no strict guidelines published, and even a consensus of the better method of release does not exist. Recently the pie crust method of release has been described as a more secure method for releasing the medial-sided structures and avoiding complications related to overcorrection.

References

1. Hunt NC, Ghosh KM, Athwal KK, Longstaff LM, Amis AA, Deehan DJ. Lack of evidence to support present medial release methods in total knee arthroplasty. Knee Surg Sports Traumatol Arthrosc. 2014;22(12):3100–12.
2. Aunan E, Kibsgård T, Clarke-Jenssen J, Röhrl SM. A new method to measure ligament balancing in total knee arthroplasty: laxity measurements in 100 knees. Arch Orthop Trauma Surg. 2012;132(8):1173–81.
3. Griffin FM, Insall JN, Scuderi GR. Accuracy of soft tissue balancing in total knee arthroplasty. J Arthroplasty. 2000;15(8):970–3.
4. Whiteside LA, Saeki K, Mihalko WM. Functional medical ligament balancing in total knee arthroplasty. Clin Orthop Relat Res. 2000;380:45–57.
5. Mihalko WM, Saleh KJ, Krackow KA, Whiteside LA. Soft-tissue balancing during total knee arthroplasty in the varus knee. J Am Acad Orthop Surg. 2009;17(12):766–74.
6. Meloni MC, Hoedemaeker RW, Violante B, Mazzola C. Soft tissue balancing in total knee arthroplasty. Joints. 2014;2(1):37–40.
7. Koh HS, In Y. Semimembranosus release as the second step of soft tissue balancing in varus total knee arthroplasty. J Arthroplasty. 2013;28(2):273–8.
8. Mihalko WM, Saeki K, Whiteside LA. Effect of medial epicondylar osteotomy on soft tissue balancing in total knee arthroplasty. Orthopedics. 2013;36(11):e1353–7.
9. Ahn JH, Back YW. Comparative study of two techniques for ligament balancing in total knee arthroplasty for severe varus knee: medial soft tissue release vs. bony resection of proximal medial tibia. Knee Surg Relat Res. 2013;25(1):13–8.
10. Goudarz Mehdikhani K, Morales Moreno B, Reid JJ, de Paz NA, Lee YY, González Della Valle A. An algorithmic, pie-crusting medial soft tissue release reduces the need for constrained inserts patients with severe varus deformity undergoing total knee arthroplasty. J Arthroplasty. 2016;31(7):1465–9.
11. Bellemans J. Multiple needle puncturing: balancing the varus knee. Orthopedics. 2011;34(9):e510–2.
12. Mihalko WM, Woodard EL, Hebert CT, Crockarell JR, Williams JL. Biomechanical validation of medial pie-crusting for soft-tissue balancing in knee arthroplasty. J Arthroplasty. 2015;30(2):296–9.

Valgus Knee: Severe Cases Included

10

Jaroslaw Czekaj, Timothy Lording, and Sébastien Lustig

Contents

10.1 Introduction

Valgus deformity is less common than varus deformity in the arthritic knee, with an incidence of 10–15% in the population undergoing primary total knee arthroplasty (TKA) [1]. In cases of valgus knee, the surgeon uses the same set of instruments; however, the choice of approach, strategy for soft tissue balancing, order

J. Czekaj • S. Lustig, MD, PhD (✉)
Albert Trillat Center, Lyon North University Hospital, Lyon, France
e-mail: sebastien.lustig@gmail.com

T. Lording
Melbourne Orthopaedic Group, Melbourne, VIC, Australia

S. Matsuda et al. (eds.), *Soft Tissue Balancing in Total Knee Arthroplasty*,
DOI 10.1007/978-3-662-54082-4_10

of ligament release, positioning of implants, and the degree of constraint required may vary considerably in comparison to the varus knee. These issues, as well as the management of bone defects caused by wear, must be considered during preoperative preparation and may require adaptation of the surgical plan according to the intraoperative situation. We emphasize the essential place of preoperative planning based on radiological and physical examination, which allows for staging of the deformity and choice of the proper surgical strategy.

The most essential difficulties in the arthritic valgus knee are correct flexion-extension gap balancing, responsible for knee stability, achieving the right patella position, and assuring sufficient contact at the bone-implant interface.

In the following chapter, we discuss the abovementioned concerns and concentrate on the particularities of primary TKA in arthritic valgus knees.

10.2 Valgus Knee Deformity

The normal mean hip-knee-ankle (HKA) angle is 178.8° ± 2.2°, with values greater than 181° considered valgus knee deformity [2]. Correct knee alignment is marked by passage of the gravity line slightly medial to knee joint center. During the single-leg stance phase of gait, the knee joint must resist large forces, exceeding 4–6 times body weight and unequally distributed across the compartments in a ratio of three fourths through the medial and one fourth through the lateral compartment [3]. In the valgus knee, overloading of the lateral femorotibial compartment results in its cartilage and bone wear in the frontal plane and progressively also in the sagittal plane, affecting primarily the posterolateral parts of the tibia and femur.

The early, reducible stages of the deformity advance to a rigid, non-corrigible state due to progressive tightening of the lateral structures, accompanied by the contraction of the lateral biarticular muscle group, which has an additional external rotational action on the tibia. In the advanced stages described above, changes are accompanied by distention and incompetence of the medial structures, notably the medial collateral ligament (MCL) (Fig. 10.1).

External rotation of the tibia in relation to the femur has an important influence on the femoropatellar joint, increasing the Q-angle and lateral displacement forces on the patella, which overloads its lateral side and negatively impacts patellar tracking, leading even to dislocation.

The structural changes described above must be taken into account during bone resection, ligament balancing, and rotational positioning of implants during TKA, in order to avoid unsatisfactory limb alignment, patellar maltracking, or knee instability (Fig. 10.2).

Valgus deformity may be constitutional or acquired.

Constitutional deformity is most frequently bilateral, with an extra-articular origin of the deformity, usually on the femoral side. In cases of significant tibial or femoral contribution to valgus deformity, correctional osteotomy should be considered.

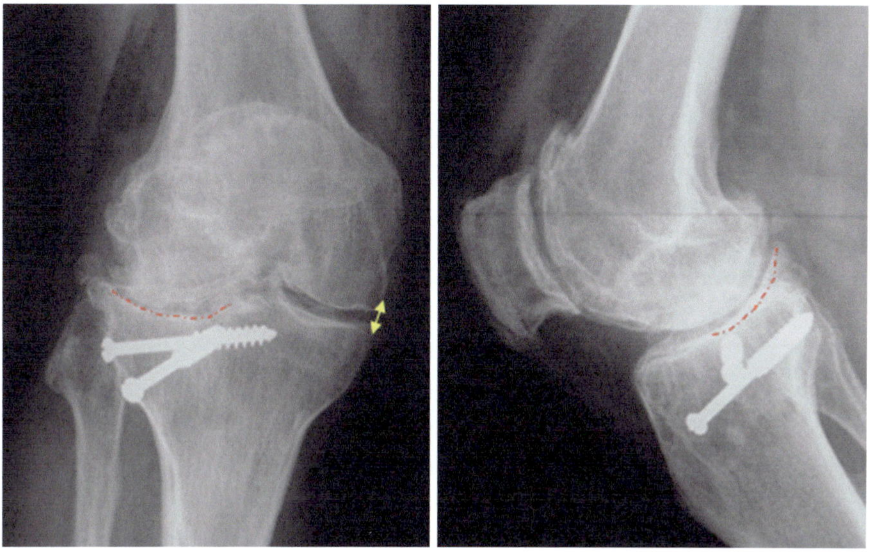

Fig. 10.1 Anteroposterior and lateral X-rays of valgus knee demonstrating the biplanar (frontal and sagittal) bone wear of the lateral tibial plateau (*red dotted lines*) with distraction of the medial side (*yellow arrow*)

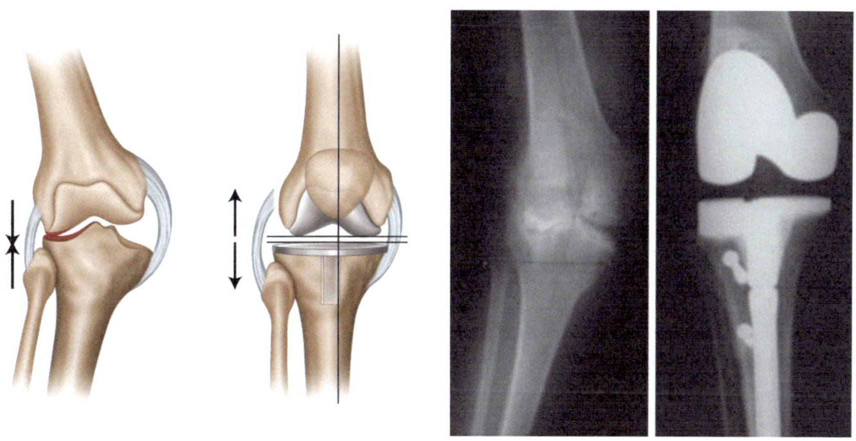

Fig. 10.2 Case of a female patient with severe valgus knee, reconstruction with augment of the lateral tibial plateau, anterior tibial tuberosity osteotomy, and release of the lateral structures to achieve soft tissue balance without the need for a constrained implant

Acquired valgus may be secondary to primary osteoarthritis, rheumatoid arthritis, metabolic disorders such as rickets or renal dystrophy, osteonecrosis, and overcorrection after proximal tibial osteotomy. There are also post-traumatic cases resulting mostly from malunion of tibial plateau fractures.

10.3 Anatomy of the Lateral Compartment of the Knee

The ligaments, capsules, and muscles all contribute to stability of the lateral compartment. The ligamento-capsular elements are represented by the lateral collateral ligament (LCL) and the posterolateral angle complex. The muscles of the lateral aspect of the knee can be divided into anterolateral (iliotibial band (ITB)) and posterolateral groups (the popliteus, biceps femoris, lateral head of the gastrocnemius) (Fig. 10.3).

The *ITB* inserts principally onto Gerdy's tubercle, but it runs also toward the patella as the iliopatellar band and to the lateral intermuscular septum, fibula, and biceps femoris. The ITB is the lateral stabilizer of the first 30° of knee flexion, acting against varus deformation forces, and also has a role in stabilizing internal rotation during knee flexion [4].

The *LCL* runs from the lateral epicondyle of the distal femur to the anterolateral surface of fibular head and acts between 0° and 90° of knee flexion.

The *posterolateral angle complex* is a musculoligamentous unit consisting of the popliteus tendon (POP) and the elements reinforcing the posterolateral capsule (PLC): the oblique popliteal ligament (OPL), arcuate ligament, popliteofibular ligament, and fabellofibular ligament. All stabilize the knee between 0° and 30° of flexion.

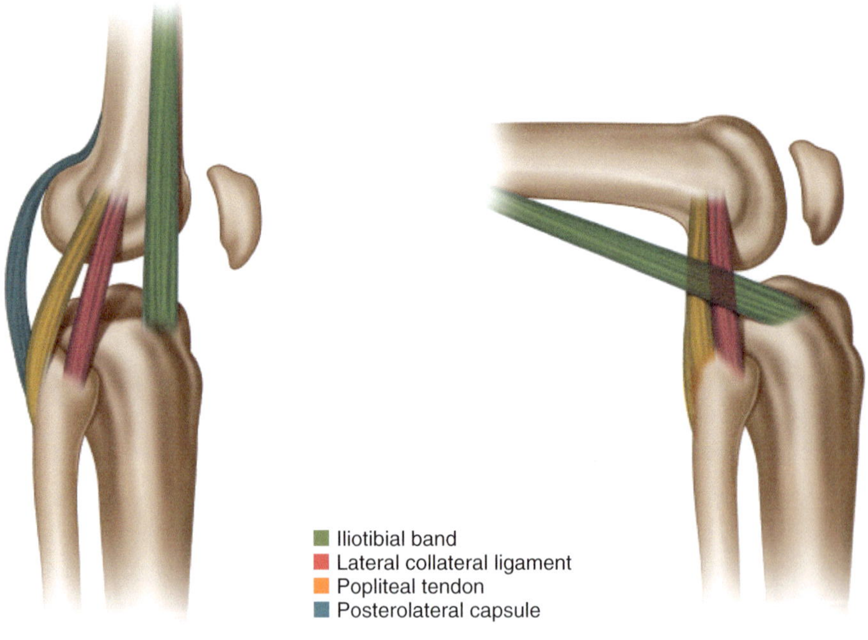

Fig. 10.3 Schematic representation of lateral knee anatomy

The *popliteus muscle tendon* runs obliquely, passing under the LCL to insert anterior to it on the lateral femoral condyle. It is active between 60° and 90° of flexion and its contraction causes internal tibial rotation [5].

The *biceps femoris* is an important landmark for the common peroneal nerve, which is at risk during extensive lateral release [6, 7] or release of biceps femoris from the proximal fibula.

The *posterior articular capsule* works in extension and is located just in front of the lateral gastrocnemius. It may be released in a subperiosteal manner in cases of fixed flexion.

To simplify, the lateral elements can be divided into two groups: those inserting near the transepicondylar axis (LCL and POP), important in both extension and flexion, and those inserting at more distally (ITB, posterolateral capsule, biceps, and lateral gastrocnemius), acting only in extension [8].

Isolated sectioning of one of the aforementioned structures does not destabilize the lateral compartment, and differential opening of the lateral compartment is observed, most notably after LCL section. However, extensive release by sectioning of all these elements will cause the substantial widening of lateral space, further increased if the posterior cruciate ligament (PCL) is sacrificed [8–11]. This effect is more significant in flexion than in extension, making balancing of the resulting asymmetric gaps complicated.

Lateral femoral condyle hypoplasia is the subject of controversy. Brihault et al. [12] demonstrated the predominant importance of femoral valgus over hypoplasia. However, the reduced size of the condyle has implications for "filling in" the lateral space with a more bulky implant and overstuffing. As a consequence it implies closure of the capsular plane problematic during lateral approach (Fig. 10.4).

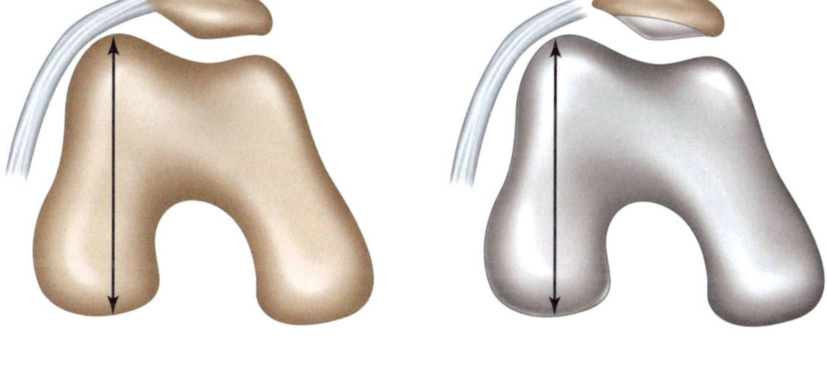

Fig. 10.4 Lateral condyle modification in valgus knee with hypoplasia or wear and the implication for femoral implant placement

10.4 Radiological Assessment of the Arthritic Valgus Knee

Radiological diagnosis of the valgus knee is based on weight-bearing anteroposterior radiographs in extension and lateral radiographs in 30° of flexion, Rosenberg (Schuss) views for femorotibial space assessment, and weight-bearing full-length radiographs for HKA angle evaluation. This last view also permits determination of the femoral and tibial mechanical axes and precise determination of the origin of the valgus deformity. Significant flexion deformity or lower extremity rotational deformities may cause error in HKA angle measurement. It has been shown, however, that rotation of up to 20° has little effect on HKA [13]. Stress valgus-varus radiographs should be performed to evaluate reducibility of the deformation and to judge any associated degree of ligament laxity. Lateral radiographs show the tibial slope. Coexisting patellofemoral OA is evaluated on the patella skyline (Merchant) view at 30° of flexion (Fig. 10.5). The frequent lateral subluxation of the patella, and its diminished thickness in the advanced stages, can be appreciated, influencing the decision for patella resurfacing.

The radiological evaluation helps moreover to appreciate the distribution and amount of osteophytes and loose bodies, the presence of extra-articular deformities or pathologies, and the general bone quality.

10.5 General Considerations in TKA Management in Valgus Knee

When planning TKA in valgus knee, the surgeon must make several decisions concerning:

- The approach, being medial or lateral, and the requirement for tibial tubercle osteotomy
- The amount and order of soft tissue releases and the requirement for condylar osteotomy
- Level of implant constraint
- Extra-articular deformity correction, either simultaneous or two stage

Many factors influence these decisions, including the magnitude and location of deformity, the degree of rigidity, the presence of medial laxity, the amount of bone loss, the preexisting knee flexion deformity, and the condition of the patellofemoral joint.

According to Krackow et al. [10], at least three situations can be apparent (Fig. 10.6):

First – isolated wear of the lateral femorotibial compartment, reducible or not, with competent medial structures

Second – lateral bone wear associated with medial laxity

Third – lateral bone wear combined with femoral or tibial extra-articular deformity (previous osteotomy or post-traumatic malunion)

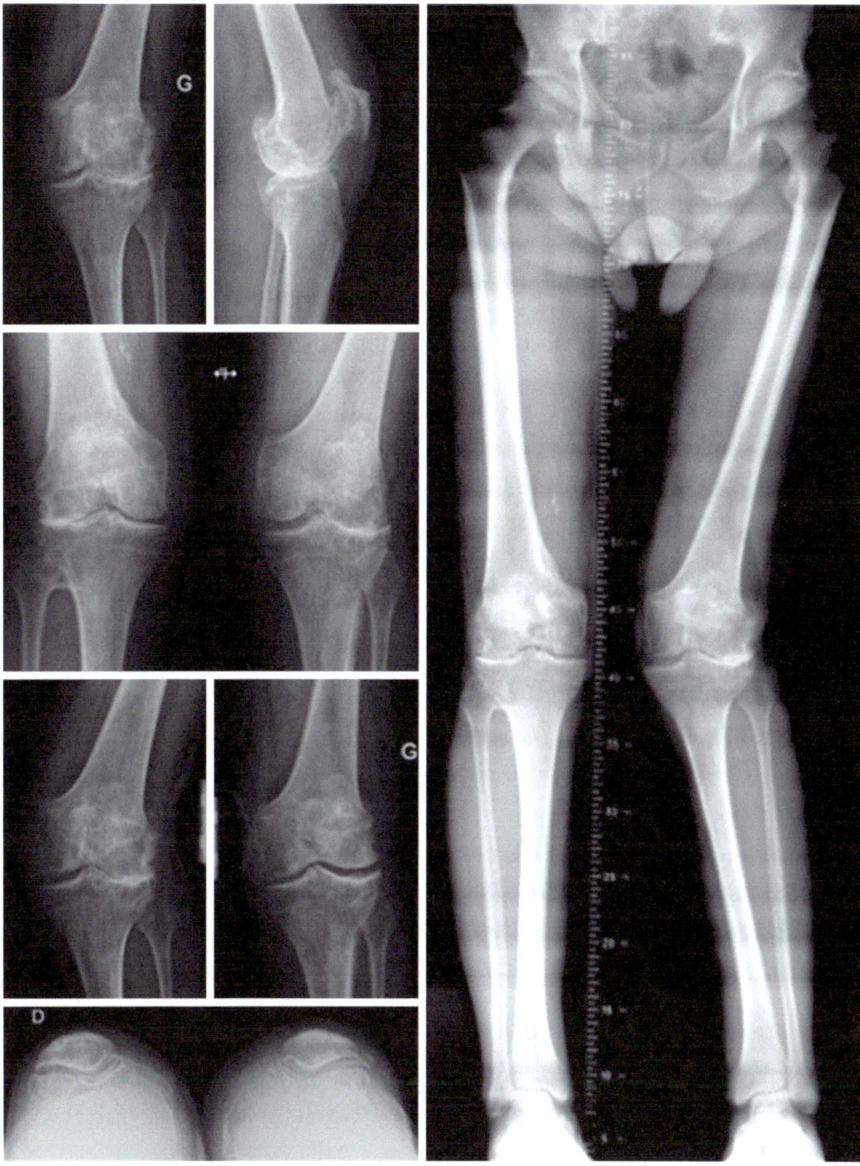

Fig. 10.5 Full set of radiographs required for evaluation and planning TKA in the valgus knee

10.6 Approach Choice

The choice of approach remains controversial. The surgery can be done by either a lateral or medial approach.

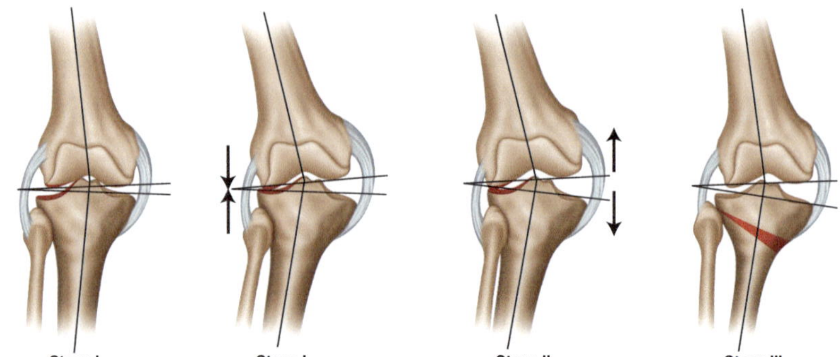

Fig. 10.6 Classification of arthritic valgus knee: *Stage I* – wear of lateral compartment with or without the tightness of lateral structures. *Stage II* – wear of the lateral compartment with laxity of the medial side. *Stage III* – extra-articular deformity (e.g., after valgus-producing osteotomy)

10.6.1 Medial Approach

The medial approach is advantageous in that it is the most commonly used and well-known approach in arthroplasty surgery of the knee. It is easy to perform in valgus knee without tight lateral structures and where there is no flexion deformity. Its usefulness in the valgus knee is improved by the technique of intra-articular or "inside-out" lateral structure release.

It is well described by Ranawat et al. [1]. The medial parapatellar arthrotomy is performed followed by minimal subperiosteal liberation of the medial structures just to allow knee exposure and resection of cruciate ligaments and the menisci.

The osteophytes are removed and the tibial cut is made perpendicular to its anatomical axis. The thickness of resected bone of the unaffected medial part should not exceed 6–8 mm.

The femoral distal cut is performed with the use of an intramedullary guide. The femoral valgus angle is decreased from usual 6–3°, which results in a varus cut of the distal femur. This cut is also minimized and should measure no more than 10 mm on the medial condyle, resulting in a thin or almost no lateral condyle cut.

Ligament balancing is performed firstly in extension by decreasing the tightness of the lateral structures as required in a stepwise manner. The order and degree of release vary according to different authors [1, 9–11, 14–16]. The sequence proposed by Ranawat et al. [1] is the one mostly employed.

The tibiofemoral space is opened in extension with the Meary's spreader. This allows palpation and identification of the tight structures: the posterolateral angle, ITB, and LCL.

Release begins in general with the posterolateral capsule, which is cut at the level of the tibial osteotomy between the posterior border of the ITB and the POP, followed by pie crusting of the capsule above the initial cut (Fig. 10.7). It is at that

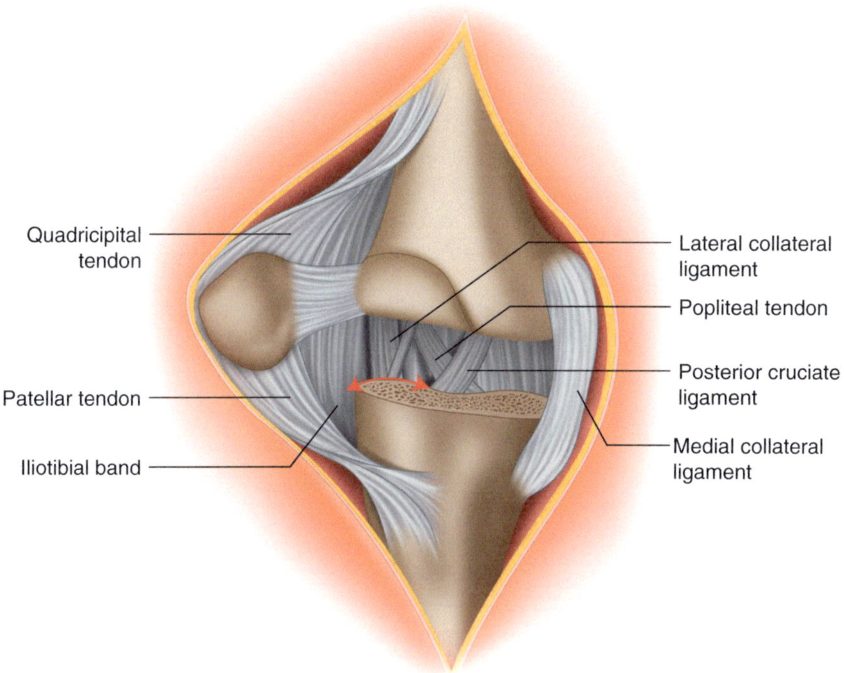

Fig. 10.7 Schematic representation of the right knee with selected structures seen via a medial parapatellar approach, with indication of section level (*red arrow*) of the lateral elements after femoral and tibial cuts. *MCL* medial collateral ligament, *PCL* posterior cruciate ligament, *POP* popliteal tendon, *LCL* lateral collateral ligament, *ITB* iliotibial band, *QT* quadricipital tendon, *PT* patellar tendon

moment the LCL can be elongated according to Elkus et al. [16]. The POP is preserved unless it is too tight. The ITB is elongated with the pie-crusting technique or is liberated from Gerdy's tubercle as required.

At least one lateral structure should be preserved in order to maintain lateral stability. If after ligament balancing in extension there is more than 5 mm of mediolateral laxity, a more constrained prosthesis should be used.

The flexion gap is balanced by adapting the thickness of the posterior femoral condyle cut and rotation of the femoral implant. The knee is flexed to 90° and distracted, and the femoral cutting guide is placed in such a way that its posterior edge is parallel to the tibial cut. The observed asymmetry of the posterior condyle cut creates a systemic gap. To achieve appropriate femoral rotation, in addition to using Whiteside's line as reference, the transepicondylar axis and adequate tensioning in flexion of both compartments should be used [16]. The use of the posterior bicondylar line as reference runs the risk of placement of the femoral implant in internal rotation.

Down- or upsizing of the femoral implant can help in obtaining equality of both spaces. When mediolateral stability in different degrees of flexion is achieved, and after verifying the absence of notching of the anterior femoral cortex, the cutting guide can be fixed and final cuts performed.

The advantage of the medial approach is the choice of which structures are released and in which sequence. The disadvantages are related to weakening of the medial structures and limited access to posterolateral side due to the lateral subluxation of the extensor apparatus, which increases external rotation of the tibia. However, the sliding lateral condyle osteotomy (SLCO) is possible through this approach [17]. Access to the medial structures is easy if medial condyle osteotomy or tensioning of MCL is required.

10.6.2 Lateral Approach

The lateral approach is confusing and more difficult because of anatomical landmark inversion and different management of the soft tissues and the patella. It is, however, logical, giving direct access to the tight lateral structures and conserving the medial structures. It does not allow for tensioning procedures of the MCL [18], which are nonetheless exceptional. On the other hand, it facilitates lateral procedures such as the SLCO [12].

This approach, popularized by Keblish et al. [19] and Buechel et al. [7], follows the lateral border of patellar tendon in its distal part. Keblish proposed a lateral parapatellar arthrotomy with plasty of the lateral femoropatellar retinaculum and the use of the retropatellar fat pad during closure. Mertl et al. [20] pointed out the utility of tubercle osteotomy.

The skin incision is midline, centered on the patella, or slightly eccentric, following its lateral border. The transquadricipital arthrotomy starts proximally between the vastus lateralis and rectus femoris muscles and runs distally to the superolateral corner of the patella. Sectioning of the lateral retinaculum is done in a "Z-plasty" fashion, by separating the retinacular and capsular layers. The retinaculum is sectioned about 3 cm laterally from the patella's edge, whereas the capsule is cut just next to it [19]. The retropatellar fat pad is detached from the patellar tendon and attached to the lateral capsular flap. This allows expansion of the lateral capsular layer and facilitates closure [7, 19]. The capsule is incised distally up to Gerdy's tubercle. The ITB is detached, maintaining continuity with the anterior sural aponeurosis, and soft tissue subperiosteal detachment is continued to the proximal tibiofibular articulation. Special attention must be paid to the common peroneal nerve. In this manner the ITB is loosened, and lateral structure (LCL, POP, and posterolateral capsule) release may be performed depending on the degree of tightness of the involved structures (Fig. 10.8). Initial simultaneous release of both the LCL and POP should be avoided as it results in significant laxity. It may, however, be indispensable in cases with significant flexion deformity.

In general, the patella is inverted, rarely dislocated. In the situation of patella baja or the danger of distal peel off of extensor apparatus, a tibial tubercle osteotomy or detensioning of the quadricipital tendon by the "rectus snip" technique should be

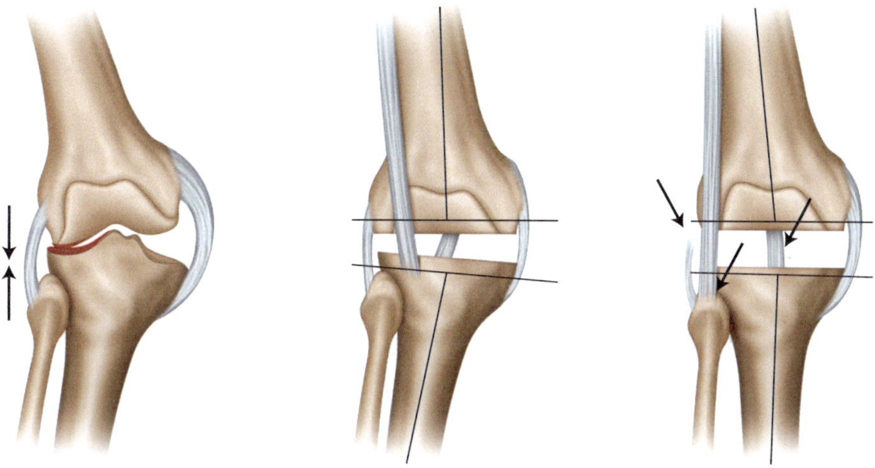

Fig. 10.8 Stage I – wear of the lateral compartment with tightness of lateral structures, release through the lateral approach starting with ITB release, following by the more posterior elements (LCL and/or POP), eventual section of PCL

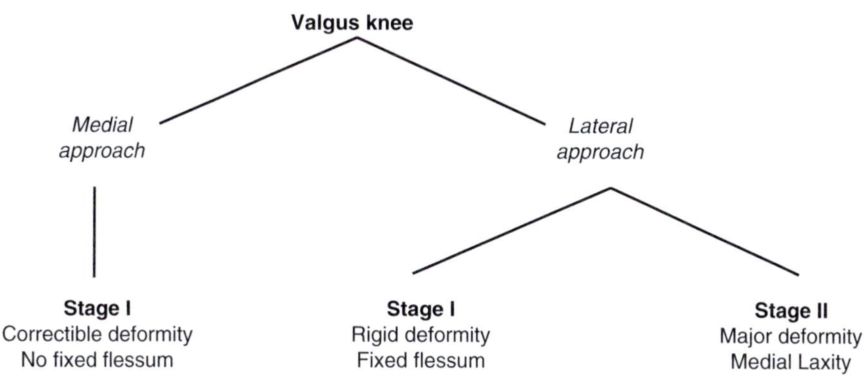

Fig. 10.9 Approach selection algorithm

considered. A tibial tubercle osteotomy is preferred to patella tendon detachment, which has an uncertain prognosis.

In the lateral approach, implant position must take into account the changed orientation of anatomical landmarks. For instance, the tibial implant center should be localized well behind the POP in order to avoid excessive external rotation. Similar caution should be paid when femoral external rotation is assessed.

In conclusion, the medial approach is reserved for minor deformities without medial soft tissue incompetence, while the lateral approach should be employed where there is significant flexion deformity, in cases of major (>10°) valgus or with coexistent medial laxity (Fig. 10.9).

10.7 Bone Cut Management in Valgus Knee

Classically, the extension gap is primary created by proximal tibial and distal femoral osteotomy. Afterward the flexion gap is established, based on a measured resection (independent cuts) or gap balancing (dependent cuts) technique.

To correct the valgus deformity in the frontal plane by keeping the cuts perpendicular to the mechanical axis of the corresponding segment, one is obliged to resect more bone from the medial side. The excessive medial bone resection vis-à-vis the lateral side results in a wider medial femorotibial gap and creation or augmentation of the medial slackness called the "resection laxity." To avoid this, it is important to be conservative with medial bone resection. On the tibial plateau, the resection height should not exceed 6–8 mm. On the distal femur, where the cut is performed with the use of an intramedullary guide, the anatomo-mechanical divergence angle is decreased from the usual 6–7° to 3–4°. This results in a lesser varus cut and decreases the thickness of femoral condyle resection, which should measure no more than 10 mm (Fig. 10.10). Conserving the medial bone leads to very little or even no bone resection on the lateral side. In cases of a marked wear, bone defects may occur, necessitating reconstruction with augments or bone graft.

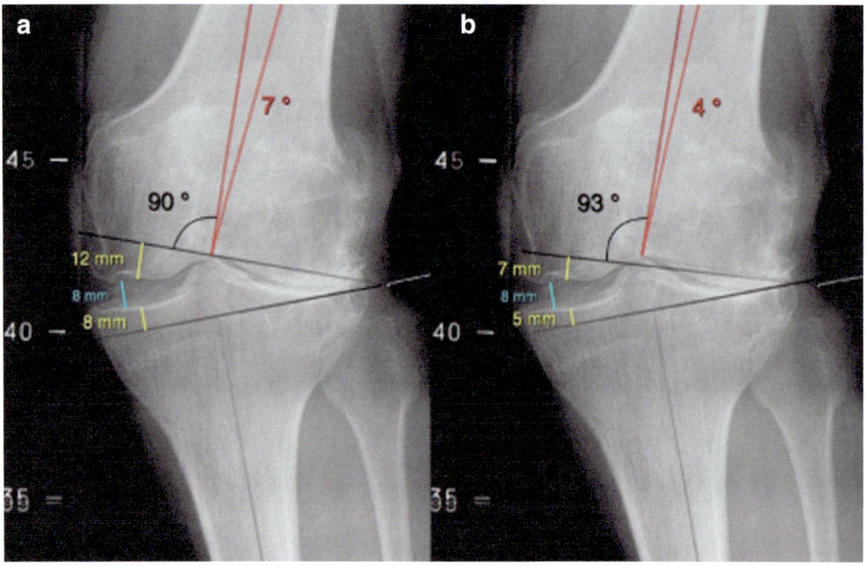

Fig. 10.10 (**a**) Resection thickness of femoral and tibial cut in coronal plane with femoral anatomo-mechanical divergence angle measured at 7° resulting in a wide medial extension gap; (**b**) minimizing the bone cuts and adjusting the femoral anatomo-mechanical divergence angle (decreasing by 3°) resulting in a reduced medial space

In the measured resection technique, the anterior and posterior femoral cuts are performed with the cutting guide on the posterior femoral condyles and after adjustment of external rotation according to anatomical landmarks – Whiteside's line, transepicondylar axis, and condylar posterior line. Separately, these landmarks are not reliable because of lateral bone wear, lateral condyle hypoplasia, and trochlear disturbance. Afterward, a spacer is used to judge the thickness and equality of the resultant medial and lateral spaces in flexion and extension, and ligament release is performed as required.

In the dependent cut or gap balancing technique, the proximal tibial resection is performed first. Subsequently, a tensioner is used to verify the symmetry of the flexion gap in a "flexion first" technique or the extension gap in an "extension first" technique. Soft tissue balancing is performed to equalize each of the tibiofemoral compartments in two reference positions. When all the spaces are symmetrical, the corresponding femoral cutting guide is fixed and the bone resections are performed. The use of the tensioner device helps to establish adequate rotation of femoral component, even though its precision is rather random [21]. Contrary to the varus knee, lateral condyle hypoplasia is often linked to torsional anomalies of the lower extremity, which does not permit the use of fixed values of femoral implant rotation. Rotation balancing is dependent on ligament tensioning in 90° of flexion and is adapted to each case [22].

10.8 Patella Management

The preoperative patella analysis was described above. Femoral trochlea dysplasia and lateral patella displacement are accompanied by tightness of the lateral patellar retinaculum [23]. This may necessitate extensor apparatus realignment when matching of the femoral implant rotation is not enough to obtain correct patellofemoral tracking.

When using the medial approach, the release of the lateral retinaculum is often required to improve patellar tracking [16, 24, 25] and is performed in addition to the division of the medial retinaculum performed during the approach. This introduces the potential for patella devascularization, unless a medial subvastus approach was performed. This risk is not present when using the lateral approach.

Any change to the anterior patellofemoral compartment, for example, by overstuffing or altering the joint line, will affect the tension and isometry of the patellar retinacula. Introduction of thicker polyethylene will lower the patella, whereas distalization of femoral implant will raise the patellar, resulting in increased tension on the retinacula, which can produce pain [21].

As mentioned, patellar tracking is influenced by femoral implant rotation but also by the position of the tibial tray in correspondence to the natural tibial plateau.

Patella resurfacing increases the risk of its fracture if the remaining bone is thin. Patelloplasty may be required, by resection of the lateral facet.

10.9 Ligament Balancing and Matching of Bone Cuts

The aim of ligament balancing is to obtain equal size gaps in extension and in 90° of flexion, with restoration of a normal lower extremity axis and correct positioning of patella. The use of these two reference positions gives information about the relationships between the femoral cuts (distal and posterior) and the proximal tibial cut. It is worth pointing out that before the ligament balancing stage of operation, the removal of all osteophytes, particularly from medially, laterally, and posteriorly, is paramount unless patient-specific instrumentation (PSI) guides are used.

In the normal situation, balance of the knee is maintained by the collateral structures and central pivot. The PCL, if preserved, limits the efficiency of lateral release and may require tensioning of MCL if it is lax [9, 10]. Conserving the PCL is possible if there is no major valgus deformation, no flexion deformity greater than 10°, and no significant lateral compartment bone wear without medial laxity [26, 27]. However, retention of PCL is associated with greater revision rates due to residual medial laxity [28, 29]. Hence, sectioning of the PCL before the other soft tissues makes balancing easier.

Ligaments which are left too taut can become a source of pain and may rupture or progressively stretch. The release of tight structures is better than tensioning of lax elements while they are prone to secondary distension [28]. The order of structures released depends on the objective one wants to reach and often requires compromise between regaining normal limb alignment and achieving knee stability.

In most of the cases, using a lateral arthrotomy, osteophyte removal, and the release done during the approach is sufficient to gain a balanced lateral compartment. In the medial approach, balance is achieved by progressive release of the lateral structures in extension and flexion in an inside-out manner. Massive release is avoided, except in specific cases. Every element must be firstly identified and partially released. In this manner, the degree of release may be controlled before proceeding further.

The structures that may be released include the ITB, LCL, POP, the lateral capsule, and more rarely the distal part of biceps femoris tendon or the proximal origin of the lateral gastrocnemius. ITB release may be performed in an extra- or intra-articular fashion [1, 30]; it may be localized at its insertion on Gerdy's tubercle or performed in more proximal part by way of a pie crusting or Z-plasty [16, 24]. The release is more adequate from the lateral side, while connections to the surrounding structures may be freed more selectively.

In the lateral approach, an ITB release is an integral part of the approach itself in contrast to the medial approach, where its liberation by pie crusting, as proposed by Ranawat et al. [1, 16], is a separate part of the procedure.

A lateral arthrotomy with ITB release is sufficient in the majority of cases to balance the knee and to gain adequate access to the joint.

When the lateral gap is not large enough, the release of the lateral and posterolateral structures should be performed. Some surgeons start with sectioning of the POP while preserving the LCL condylar insertion [31]; others like Lootvoet et al. [32]

release the LCL while conserving the POP. After Kanamya et al. [33], we recall that the LCL is active throughout the range of flexion and that POP section has more influence in flexion than extension. The POP can be freed first when correcting the flexion deformity in a rigid, valgus knee.

Correction from the intra-articular side is limited in its effect. Even a complete release of LCL does not always allow adequate balancing if the MCL is lax. A correction of, for example, 20° requires a lengthening of 3 cm [7, 18], running the risk of stretching the neurovascular structures on the lateral side. The other consequences of significant ligament release are lowering the patellar height and lengthening the limb.

The alternative to lateral ligament release is the sliding lateral condyle osteotomy (SLCO) as proposed by Brilhault et al. [34]. The tight lateral side makes the osteotomized condyle slide downward and posteriorly, usually around 1 cm, with the correction effect more pronounced in flexion (Fig. 10.11). This technique should be reserved for major deformities with associated flexion deformity. The need for SLCO is quite easy to predict during the assessment of required ligament releases, before release of the LCL and POP.

To conclude, during ligament balancing, the release is more reliable than tensioning. The step-by-step approach permits controlled release and avoids too much lengthening, resulting the uncertain results or the need for a more constrained implant. The soft tissue release is influenced by the chosen approach. In lateral approach, release is made constantly from anterior to posterior [19, 20], while in the medial approach, it is done more variably [1, 10, 11, 15, 16, 35].

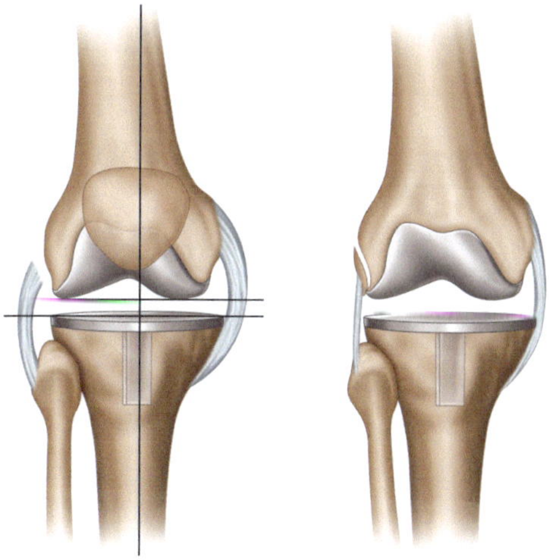

Fig. 10.11 Soft tissue balance by subperiosteal detachment of lateral structures from lateral femoral condyle or by sliding lateral condyle osteotomy (SLCO)

The alternative to soft tissue procedures is the SLCO, which respects the insertion of LCL-POP complex.

Most guiding systems take into account two reference gaps created after the bone cuts and ligament balancing. These gaps should be rectangular and maintain their equality throughout the range of motion.

Soft tissue balance is easy to obtain in cases without contracted lateral structures, no matter the approach used and with the possibility of PCL conservation.

In valgus knees with bony wear associated with tightness of the lateral structures or the flexion deformity of at least 20°, ligament balancing is required first in extension and then in flexion, by inside-out release of the LCL followed by POP and additionally the ITB and/or PLC. However, in the lateral approach, the release begins with the ITB and continues with the LCL and/or POP and finally the PLC if flexion deformity persists. The PCL is sacrificed at the beginning. In the absence of medial laxity, no action on medial side is required, but it may be judged that a more constrained implant (mediolateral condylar constrained) is suitable. The alternative SLCO allows almost simultaneous balancing in extension and in flexion.

In cases of valgus knee with medial laxity, the schema of lateral liberation is the same. We systematically employ the lateral approach and PCL resection before balancing. The implantation of a less constrained implant is preferred in younger, fitter patients with a longer life expectancy, whereas in subjects with bad health conditions, a hinge prosthesis allows more rapid recovery (Fig. 10.12).

The tensioning techniques for the MCL described by Williot and Healy [8, 36], by tightening the MCL on its tibial or femoral insertion, are avoided where possible.

In cases of valgus knee with associated extra-articular deformity, corrective osteotomy may be inevitable, especially if the deformation is localized in the diaphyseal or metaphyseal segment and is secondary to trauma or previous valgus-producing osteotomy.

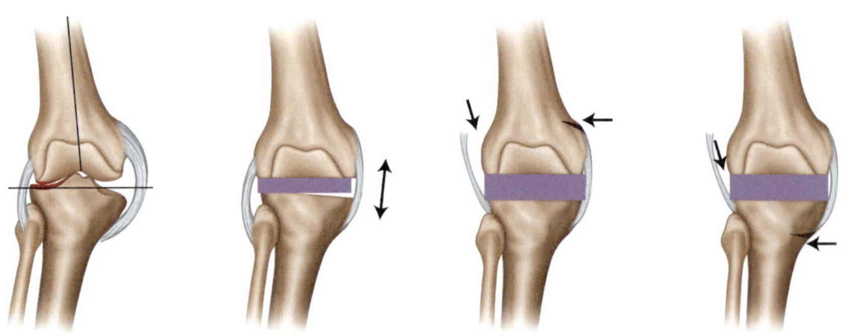

Fig. 10.12 Stage II valgus knee with medial laxity, persistent valgus after the distal femoral and proximal tibial cuts, gaps balancing by lateral release or by tightening the medial side (MCL tensioning at the femoral or tibial insertion)

10.10 Type of Implants Used in Complex Valgus TKA

Complex cases are related to a major degree of valgus, associated medial laxity, or preexisting bone deformities. The results of TKA in valgus knees [37] show that frontal laxity of 5° or more and major preoperative valgus deformity of more than 10° are the principal factors predicting the use of a more constrained implant in primary cases.

10.10.1 TKA in Major Valgus Knee

In cases of significant deformation, correction should be made at its origin. If it is intra-articular, it may be corrected with adequate bone cuts and ligament release, while if it is extra-articular, a corrective osteotomy of the tibia or femur is performed [23]. The corrective osteotomy may be performed simultaneously with TKA, or as two-stage surgery, depending on patient factors (age and health condition).

Two-stage procedures are not well tolerated by elderly subjects, due to the time required for osteotomy consolidation and the duration of reduced weight bearing.

For a one-stage approach, the surgical technique is adjusted on a case-by-case basis. In our institution we prefer to perform the osteotomy first and to fix it prior to implantation of the prosthesis.

When facing major valgus deformation in younger, active patients, preservation of the soft tissue envelope and correct balance are paramount, to allow the implantation of a less constrained implant.

In patients over 75 years old, in mediocre health condition, and in patients with reduced autonomy, single surgery is advised, permitting complete weight bearing as soon as possible and immediate rehabilitation. Extensive lateral release may require the placement of a prosthesis with augmented mediolateral constraint or even a hinge-type implant if the posterolateral capsule was sacrificed (Fig. 10.13).

10.10.2 TKA After High Tibial Osteotomy

High tibial valgus-producing osteotomy creates some knee joint modifications which need to be taken into account: postsurgery scar, collateral ligament violation, alteration of the proximal epiphyseal architecture by external subtraction or medial addition, and the presence of osteosynthesis implants. Excessive valgus often exists because of overcorrection at the time of surgery, or sometimes the osteotomy aggravates itself with time.

TKA after excessive valgus-producing osteotomy or after its secondary deterioration is particular, and the risks are different depending on the type of osteotomy. In all situations, bone cuts must be conservative, to not engender lateral or medial laxity.

After the medial opening type of osteotomy, the risk of the rupture of MCL during TKA is not negligible, so the possible need for a more constrained implant must

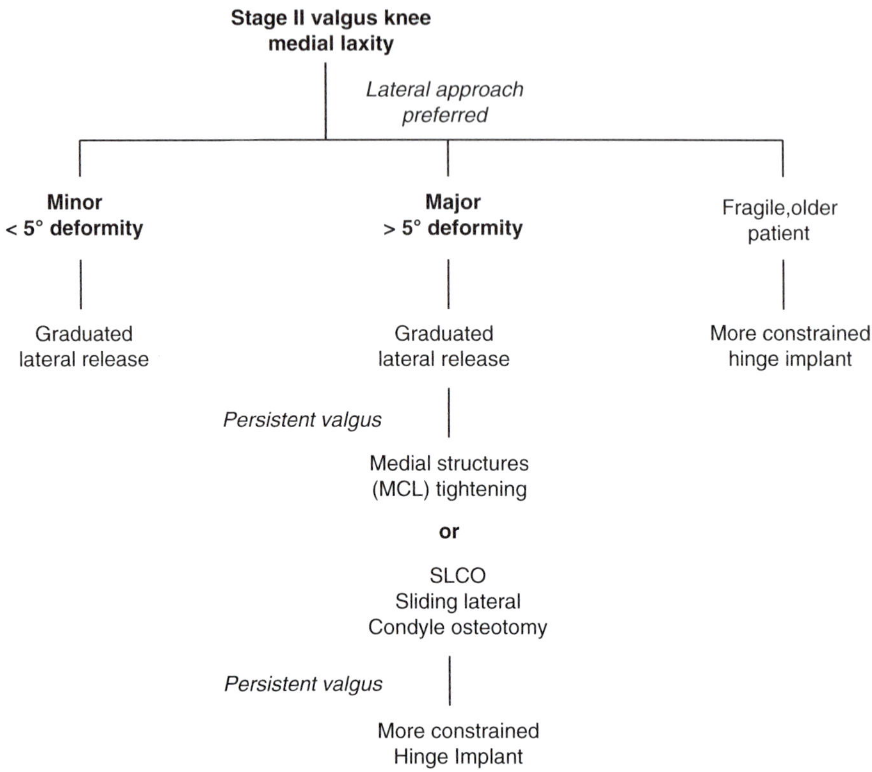

Fig. 10.13 Algorithm for the management of the Stage II valgus knee with medial laxity

be anticipated. In the younger patient, a tibial varus-producing osteotomy may be discussed, whereas in an older patient, a more constrained prosthesis is preferred.

After a lateral closing type of osteotomy, deformation of tibial metaphysis in relation to the diaphysis may create impingement of the prosthetic stem with the lateral cortex; thus, the use of a stem with offset is advisable. As previously described, the condition of the ligaments defines the type of implant, with residual laxity requiring an increased level of constraint in the prosthesis.

Conclusions

Lateral and medial approaches may both be used. The lateral approach is our choice in complex cases and major deformities.

In valgus deformity due only to bone wear and without tight lateral structures, the medial and lateral approaches are equivalent. The matched release of PLC, LCL, or POP associated with partial liberation of ITB is sufficient. The use of bone graft or augments to fulfill the bone deficit on the lateral side may be necessary.

In the valgus deformities with tightness of lateral structures, the lateral approach is preferable, with direct release of ITB, followed by the LCL, the POP as required, and the PLC. If after the mobilization of the ITB a rigid valgus of more than 5° persists, SLCO may be performed, provided mediolateral constrained implants are available.

In cases of valgus knee with medial laxity, the lateral approach is advisable. The mediolateral constrained prosthesis is mainly used after successful ligament balancing; otherwise, a hinge implant is the solution. The technique of medial ligament tensioning may be useful even though their reliability is uncertain.

If the valgus deformation has an extra-articular component of more than 5°, then a corrective osteotomy is required.

References

1. Ranawat AS, Ranawat CS, Elkus M, Rasquinha VJ, Rossi R, Babhulkar S. Total knee arthroplasty for severe valgus deformity. J Bone Joint Surg Am. 2005;87 Suppl 1(Pt 2):271–84.
2. Hsu RW, Himeno S, Coventry MB, Chao EY. Normal axial alignment of the lower extremity and load-bearing distribution at the knee. Clin Orthop Relat Res. 1990;255:215–27.
3. Castaing J, Burdin P. Le genou. In: Anatomie fonctionnelle de l'appareil locomoteur. Paris: Vigot; 1960.
4. Desmé D, Galand-Desmé S, Besse JL, Henner J, Moyen B, Lerat JL. Axial lower limb alignment and knee geometry in patients with osteoarthritis of the knee. Rev Chir Orthop Reparatrice Appar Mot. 2006;92(7):673–9.
5. Mihalko M. Anatomic and biomechanical aspects of pie crusting posterolateral structures for valgus deformity correction in total knee arthroplasty: a cadaveric study. J Arthroplasty. 2000;15(3):347–53.
6. Clarke HD, Schwartz JB, Math KR, Scuderi GR. Anatomic risk of peroneal nerve injury with the " pie crust " technique for valgus release in total knee arthroplasty. J Arthroplasty. 2004;19(1):40–4.
7. Buechel FF. A sequential three-step lateral release for correcting fixed valgus knee deformities during total kneearthroplasty. Clin Orthop Relat Res. 1990;260:170–5.
8. Williot A, Rosset P, Favard L, Brilhault J, Burdin P. Total knee arthroplasty in valgus knee. Orthop Traumatol Surg Res. 2010;96S:S37–42.
9. Whiteside LA. Correction of ligament and bone defects in total arthroplasty of the severely valgus knee. Clin Orthop Relat Res. 1993;288:234–45.
10. Krackow KA, Jones MM, Teeny SM, Hungerford DS. Primary total knee arthroplasty in patients with fixed valgus deformity. Clin Orthop Relat Res. 1991;273:9–18.
11. Whiteside LA. Selective ligament release in total knee arthroplasty of the knee in valgus. Clin Orthop Relat Res. 1999;367:130–40.
12. Brilhault J, Ledu C, Rousselle JJ, Burdin P. Femoral shaft bowing in valgus knees: an anatomic study. Rev Chir Orthop Reparatrice Appar Mot. 2006;92(2):133–9.
13. Swanson KE, Stocks GW, Warren PD, Hazel MR, Janssen HF. Does axial limb rotation affect the alignment measurements in deformed limbs? Clin Orthop Relat Res. 2000;371:246–52.
14. Boettner F, Renner L, Arana D, Claus N, Faschingbauer M. Total knee arthroplasty for valgus osteoarthritis: the results of a standardized soft – tissue release technique. Knee Surg Sports Traumatol Arthrosc. 2016;24(8):2525–31.
15. Clarke HD, Fuchs R, Scuderi GR, Scott WN, Insall JN. Clinical results in valgus total knee arthroplasty with the "pie crust" technique of lateral soft tissue releases. J Arthroplasty. 2005;20(8):1010–4.
16. Elkus M, Ranawat CS, Rasquinha VJ, Babhulkar S, Rossi R, Ranawat AS. Total knee arthroplasty for severe valgus deformity. Five to fourteen-year follow-up. J Bone Joint Surg Am. 2004;86-A(12):2671–6.

17. Hadjicostas PT. Computer-assisted osteotomy of the lateral femoral condyle with non-constrained total knee replacement in severe valgus knees. J Bone Joint Surg Br. 2008;90(11):1441–5.
18. Krackow KA, Mihalko WM. Flexion-extension joint gap changes after lateral structure release for valgus deformity correction in total knee arthroplasty: a cadaveric study. J Arthroplasty. 1999;14(8):994–1004.
19. Keblish PA. The lateral approach to the valgus knee. Surgical technique and analysis of 53 cases with over two-year follow-up evaluation. Clin Orthop Relat Res. 1991;271:52–62.
20. Mertl P, Jarde O, Blejwas D, Vives P. Lateral approach of the knee with tibial tubercle osteotomy for prosthetic surgery. Rev Chir Orthop Reparatrice Appar Mot. 1992;78(4):264–7.
21. Gougeon F. Traitement de la gonarthrose associée au genu valgum (options thérapeutiques). In: Conférences d'enseignement 2009, in Cahiers d'Enseignement de la SOFCOT 98. 2009. p. 94–110.
22. Chou W, Siu K, Ko J, Chen J, Wang C, Wang F, Wong T. Preoperative templating and computer-assisted total knee arthroplasty for arthritic valgus knee. J Arthroplasty. 2013;28(10):1781–7.
23. Lonner JH, Siliski JM, Lotke PA. Simultaneous femoral osteotomy and total knee arthroplasty for treatment of osteoarthritis associated withsevere extra-articular deformity. J Bone Joint Surg Am. 2000;82(3):342–8.
24. Politi J, Scott R. Balancing severe valgus deformity in total knee arthroplasty using a lateral cruciform retinacular release. J Arthroplasty. 2004;19(5):553–7.
25. Miyasaka KC, Ranawat CS, Mullaji A. 10- to 20-year followup of total knee arthroplasty for valgus deformities. Clin Orthop Relat Res. 1997;345:29–37.
26. Mcauley JP, Ms MBC, Hamilton WG, Ms ET, Engh GA. Posterior cruciate-retaining total knee arthroplasty for valgus osteoarthritis. Clin Orthop Relat Res. 2008;466:2644–9.
27. Misra AN, Hussain MRA, Fiddian NJ, Newton G. The role of the posterior cruciate ligament in total knee replacement. J Bone Joint Surg Br. 2003;85-B:10–3.
28. Koskinen E, Remes V, Paavolainen P, Harilainen A, Sandelin J, Tallroth K. The knee Results of total knee replacement with a cruciate-retaining model for severe valgus deformity — A study of 48 patients followed for an average of 9 years ☆. Knee. 2011;18(3):145–50.
29. Kubiak P, Archibeck MJ, White Jr RE. Cruciate-retaining total knee arthroplasty in patients with at least fifteen degrees of coronal plane deformity. J Arthroplasty. 2008;23(3):366–70.
30. Whiteside LA, Roy ME. Anatomy, function, and surgical access of the iliotibial band in total knee arthroplasty. J Bone Joint Surg Am. 2009;91(Suppl 6):101–6.
31. Easley ME, Insall JN, Scuderi GR, Bullek DD. Primary constrained condylar knee arthroplasty for the arthritic valgus knee. Clin Orthop Relat Res. 2000;380:58–64.
32. Lootvoet L, Blouard E, Himmer O, Ghosez JP. Complete knee prosthesis in severe genu valgum. Retrospective review of 90 knees surgically treated through the anterio-external approach. Acta Orthop Belg. 1997;63(4):278–86.
33. Kanamiya T, Whiteside LA, Nakamura T, Mihalko WM, Steiger J, Naito M. Ranawat Award paper. Effect of selective lateral ligament release on stability in knee arthroplasty. Clin Orthop Relat Res. 2002;404:24–31.
34. Brilhault J, Lautman S, Favard L, Burdin P. Lateral femoral sliding osteotomy lateral release in total knee arthroplasty. J Bone Joint Surg Br. 2002;84(8):1131–7.
35. Aglietti P, Lup D, Cuomo P, Baldini A, De Luca L. Total knee arthroplasty using a pie-crusting technique for valgus deformity. Clin Orthop Relat Res. 2007;464:73–7.
36. Healy WL, Iorio R, Lemos DW. Medial reconstruction during total knee arthroplasty for severe valgus deformity. Clin Orthop Relat Res. 1998;356:161–9.
37. Girard J, Amzallag M, Pasquier G, Mulliez A, Brosset T, Gougeon F, Duhamel A, Migaud H. Total knee arthroplasty in valgus knees : Predictive preoperative parameters influencing a constrained design selection. Orthop Traumatol Surg Res. 2009;95:260–6.

Complicated Cases: Recurvatum and Severe Contracture

11

Ricardo Varatojo, Ricardo Telles de Freitas, and Mário Vale

Contents

11.1 Introduction

Patients proposed for total knee arthroplasty (TKA) present severe pain, limited function, loss of motion, and increasing deformity.

The two main goals in TKA are complete pain relief and improving mobility which results in restoring patient function and ensuring patient satisfaction. Mobility after TKA is related to four parameters: the patient, the implant, the surgical management, and the postoperative rehabilitation protocol.

Most patients present fixed varus and valgus deformities in the coronal plane. The sagittal plane deformities are mostly flexion contractures, and a few are recurvatum.

R. Varatojo, MD (✉) • R.T. de Freitas, MD • M. Vale, MD
Knee, Ankle and Sports Trauma Unit, Orthopedic Department, Hospital Cuf Descobertas, Lisbon, Portugal
e-mail: jricardovaratojo@gmail.com

S. Matsuda et al. (eds.), *Soft Tissue Balancing in Total Knee Arthroplasty*,
DOI 10.1007/978-3-662-54082-4_11

11.2 Severe Contracture

A flexion contracture is by definition an inability to bring the knee to full extension passively. In the examination for full extension, the patient must be recumbent with both legs exposed and the heel on the table. If the knee is fully extended, the examiner cannot be able to pass his hand or fingers behind the popliteal space, but in the presence of flexion contracture deformity, the examiner can do it.

The etiology of flexion contractures is related to the recurrent effusions present in the end-stage degenerative or inflammatory joint disease. These effusions cause increased pressure within the knee, resulting in pain and discomfort. Patients will seek for a position of comfort with the knee in slight flexion that increases the intra-articular volume and consequently feeling less pain by having inferior pressure inside the knee and relaxing the posterior capsule.

This is a self-perpetuating process that leads to a greater degree of contracture as the disease progresses. Patients limit full extension in their daily activities as the disease progresses as they spend more time seated, sometimes sleep with a pillow under the knee and even walking do not extend the knee. All these actions increase the flexion contracture deformity.

Severe flexion contraction deformities are found in rheumatoid arthritis, juvenile rheumatoid arthritis, ankylosing spondylitis, hemophilia, posttraumatic sequela, and end-stage arthritis. Hemophilia is a factor of poor prognosis [14].

One of the goals for the total knee surgeon is to obtain full extension because during normal gait, the knee is at full extension at the time of heel strike and then gradually flexes during stance phase and swing phase [11]. A patient that cannot fully extend the knee must contract his quadriceps to prevent the knee from buckling during early stance, and this increases the work of walking.

Rehabilitation in the early stage of flexion contracture deformity has a role with quadriceps strengthening and stretching techniques, and they can also be used in the preoperative period preparing and teaching the patients for the postoperative recovery.

Patients must have a prearthroplasty conditioning program and be informed of all the phases of the surgical intervention.

Patients presenting spasticity of the hamstrings, frequently occurring in cerebral palsy, must have neurologic evaluation and can be candidates for botulism toxin injection. This treatment can be also an option on the preoperative approach in patients with severe flexion contracture.

A complete radiological exam is mandatory, including lateral and AP view of the knee, a full limb, and sky-view radiographs. Bony deformity, osteophytes, patella height, and the alignment of the lower limb should be analyzed.

Flexion contracture greater than 30° can be defined as a severe one, imposing a complex surgical procedure with the use of implants with increased constraint, and patients must be informed of the risks.

The treatment involves a combination of bone resection and soft tissue balance, trying as much as possible to preserve the tibial and the femoral joint lines with limited bone sacrifice [2, 3, 10, 13, 17].

11.2.1 Surgical Technique

A spinal or a general anesthetic procedure can be used; we prefer the first one that allows us to keep an epidural catheter to control the immediate postoperative pain. We begin the rehabilitation protocol at 24–48 h in the immediate postoperative period depending on patient compliance.

After induction of the anesthesia, the surgeon should evaluate the degree of the deformity present and the ability to correct the deformity. Can the varus or valgus malalignment be corrected to neutral, and what is the status of the medial and lateral collateral ligaments?

Holding the extremity by the heel and raising the leg, is there a flexion contracture, is it reducible, and what is the degree of the deformity on both the coronal and sagittal planes?

The goals of the surgical procedure are to achieve balanced flexion/extension gap with reconstruction of the mechanical axis. A standard surgical approach is done aiming the best exposure and the least soft tissue damage.

A fixed varus deformity associated with moderate to severe flexion contracture implies immediately an extensive release from the proximal medial tibia including the deep collateral ligament, meniscal capsular ligament, semimembranosus, and sometime some of the superficial medial collateral ligament [13]. The next step is the removal of the osteophytes from the distal femur and proximal tibia.

Distal femoral preparation needs the identification of the AP and the transepicondylar axis of the femur. Using standard sizing guide, with a posterior or anterior referencing system, we try to choose the largest femoral size when the femur is between sizes. The result will be a smaller flexion gap which allows overcorrection of the tibial surface to correct the flexion contracture.

The distal femur correction is one of the keys to the successful correction of a severe flexion contracture, beginning by removing the amount of the bone that is being replaced by metal, thereby maintaining the joint line. These severe deformities to obtain full extension need distal femur resection up to 6 mm if all other techniques to obtain full extension fail [2, 3, 13]. Raising the joint line adversely affects knee kinematics and can result in extensor lag and, in the extreme damage, the collateral ligament's femoral insertions.

After finishing the femoral resections, the most important steps are the removal of posterior osteophyte and reestablishment of the posterior recess of the knee by the release of the posterior capsule from the femur done by subperiosteal stripping with a curved osteotome [11, 13, 25] (Figs. 11.1 and 11.2).

We can either use a custom femorotibial spreader or a femoral suspension device introduced in the intramedullary canal to elevate the femur at 90° of knee flexion, allowing a good view of the posterior segment of the joint, taking care to avoid damage to the popliteal vessels and nerves. A curved osteotome and bone nibbler can be used sequentially, medially, and laterally, changing the position of the laminar spreader for osteophyte removal and elevation of the capsule from the posterior femur.

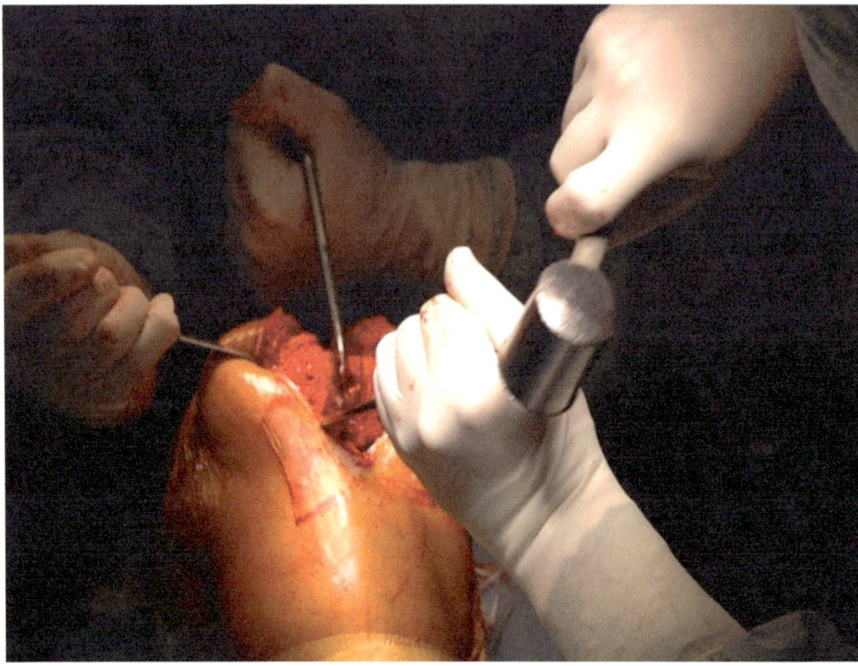

Fig. 11.1 Osteophytes removal with a curved osteotome

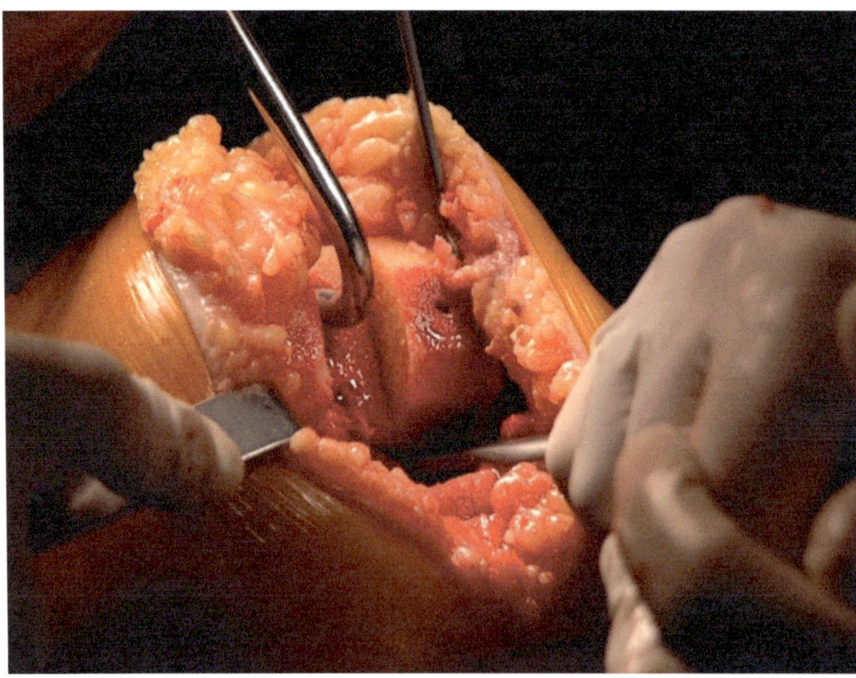

Fig. 11.2 Release of the posterior capsule

For severe flexion contractures, greater than 40°, this approach can be used to elevate the tendinous origins of the gastrocnemius muscles medially and laterally [12, 13].

Techniques of transverse sectioning of the posterior capsule, initially described by Insall, should not routinely be used. Zaidi [26] described that with knee flexion, the neurovascular bundle is displaced anteriorly and can lie tethered against the posterior capsule, representing a major risk of damage.

We prefer to do tibial resection after distal femoral cut is complete. The goal of tibial resection is also to reestablish the tibial joint line, planned to be perpendicular to the tibial shaft axis in the coronal plane. The amount of resection required depends on the degree of the deformity and ligamentous tension.

The amount of posterior slope depends also on the deformity and the type of implant used. When using a posterior cruciate-retaining TKA, the slope should be set at 5–10°, whereas in cruciate-substituting designs, the slope should be set to neutral because the PCL cut increases the flexion gap by 2 mm more than the extension gap (9).

The flexion contracture deformity presents a flexion gap that is generally greater than the extension gap, and therefore, a resection without posterior slope will facilitate the flexion/extension gap balancing [13].

After bone resections and osteophyte removal are completed, the next step will be balance of the flexion/extension gaps and of the medial and lateral collateral ligaments with either spacer blocks or trial components [3, 13, 21, 25]. A step-by-step adjustment of the soft tissue releases and further removal of osteophytes should be perfomed (Fig. 11.3).

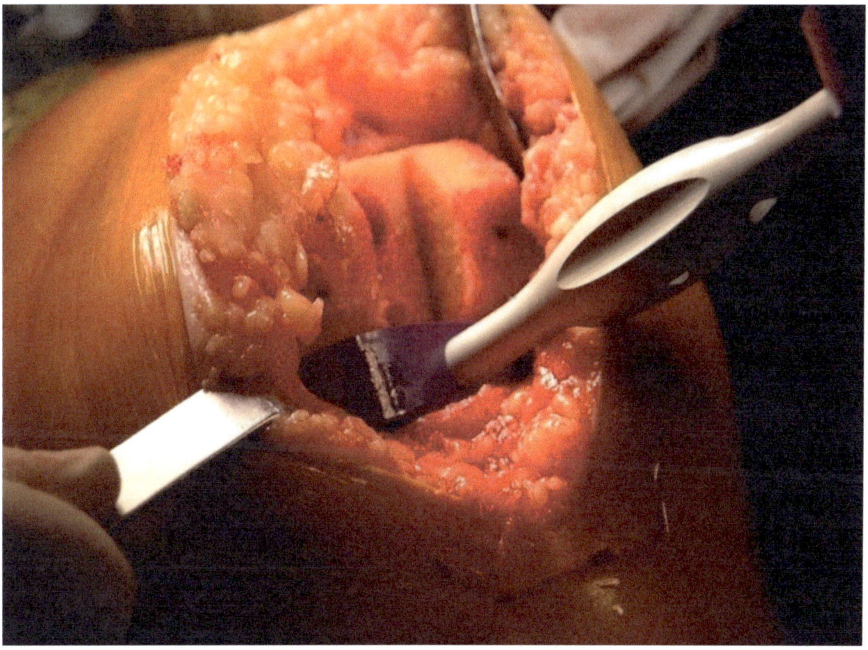

Fig. 11.3 Evaluation of the flexion gap with a spacer block

If flexion contracture deformity remains after all releases are done, then further distal femoral resection must be done to balance the flexion/extension gap and obtain full extension [2, 13, 17]. Additional 2 mm of bone resection in posterior cruciate-retaining design, but in the presence of severe flexion contracture deformity the joint line elevation can be rarely extended by 4 or 6 mm [14]. This purpose can be better accomplished with posterior cruciate-sacrificing design [14], because in these severe cases the PCL is contracted and difficult to balance (Fig. 11.4).

With severe flexion contracture, where greater amounts of distal femoral resection are required to obtain full extension, all structures anterior to the posterior

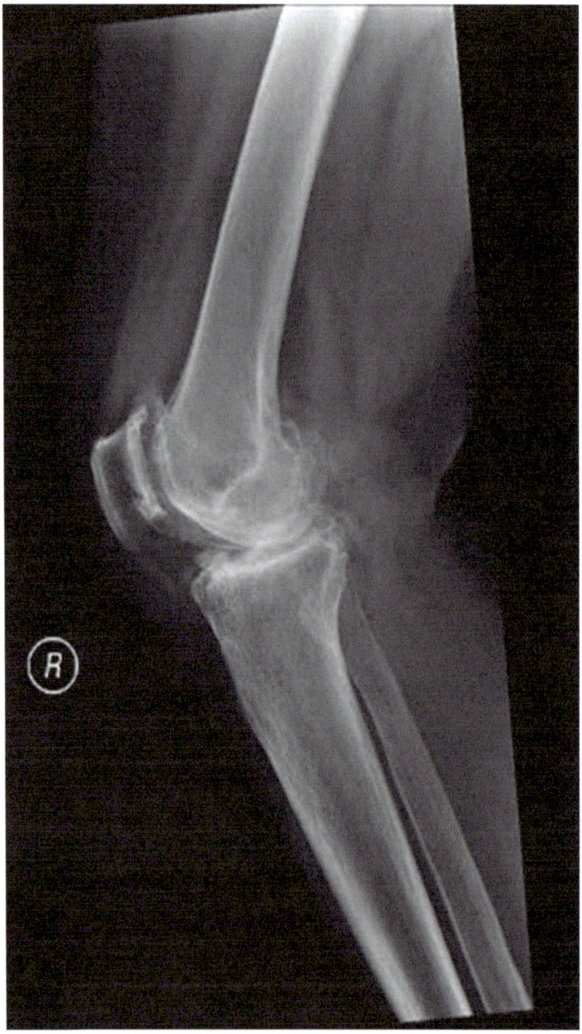

Fig. 11.4 Severe flexion contracture deformity

capsule are lax in full extension. A posterior stabilized constrained device may be required for varus/valgus stabilization during all the arc of motion.

A common error is to begin by resecting too much distal femur resulting in an elevation of the joint line and midflexion instability. Our attention must first be directed to soft tissue balancing, posterior capsule release, and osteophyte removal [2, 3, 11, 13].

Our philosophy is to use an implant system offering a continuum of constraint or at least to have on the operating theater options for specific indications presented by the patients after major ligament releases or bone resection. It is advisable to have a hinged implant ready when undertaking such surgery.

A surgical algorithm was proposed by Bellemans and associates consisting of four steps: (1) mediolateral ligament balancing with resection of all osteophytes and overcorrection of 2mm of the distal femur, (2) progressive posterior capsule release and gastrocnemius release, (3) additional resection of up to a maximum of 4 mm of the distal femur, and (4) hamstrings tenotomy. With flexion contractures greater than 35°, additional resection of the distal femur and hamstrings tenotomy were performed in only 28.6 % and 22.9 % of cases, respectively.

The surgical concept seems to be that over-resection of the distal femur by more than 2 mm should be avoided until all osteophytes have been removed and the knee is correctly balanced medially and laterally. Complete correction of the deformity, with no help from the surgeon, must be obtained intraoperatively at the end of the procedure [3, 11, 13].

Preoperative flexion contracture severity does not correlate with the residual contracture. That is to say, a mild flexion contracture is not easier to correct than a severe one [14]. Long ago Firestone et al. [4] showed that the degree of perioperative residual flexion contracture impacts final extension recovery.

In patients with flexion contractures greater than 45/60° [11], reaching full extension is not possible without marked shortening of the femur. In these rare patients nowadays in developed countries, a preoperative traction can often decrease the contracture below 30/45° [12]. The options are to perform a femoral shortening and accept an extensor lag or allow a residual 10–15° of flexion contracture [13] often reasonably well tolerated by the patients. This minimized the risk of stretch injuries of neurovascular structures.

With bilateral severe flexion contracture, as in deformities over 10°, the TKA must be done simultaneously [11]. If not, the operated knee becomes longer than the contralateral side, and to compensate for the leg discrepancy, the patient will walk with the operated knee flexed. Over a period of several months, even with the proper rehabilitation program, this leads to a flexion contracture.

When patient's medical problems do not allow for a simultaneous TKA, then the optional treatment is to place a heel lift on the shoe of the nonoperated leg until the time for its surgery.

The presence of severe flexion contracture deformity may require at the end of the procedure a proximal realignment of the extensor mechanism to strengthen it, giving the quadriceps muscle some mechanical advantage and minimizing the risk of extensor lag. This can be done by lateral and distal advancement of the vastus medialis obliquus [13].

11.2.2 Postoperative Regimen

Patients with major flexion contracture deformity must reach full extension at the final of the surgical procedure. There are different rehabilitation protocols and regimens, ranging from 3 to 6 weeks of knee immobilization in extension associated or not to modified CPM programs that can be used, but the main focus must be to obtain full extension. These immobilization devices can be removed only for rehabilitation with range-of-motion exercises, strengthening of the quadriceps, and stretching protocols.

Finally, the importance of prolonged postoperative rehabilitation is to be stressed, progress still being possible between 6 months and 1 year postoperatively [14, 21].

11.2.3 Results

Bellemans and associates using a posterior referencing technique combined with a four-step treatment algorithm reported excellent results in 130 knees in moderate (15–30°) and severe (more than 30°) deformities. All patients having less than 10° of residual contracture at 2-year follow-up and two patients who underwent biceps tenotomy for severe contracture sustained peroneal nerve injury.

Whiteside and Mihalko [17] presented a retrospective study of 103 knees with major flexion contracture deformity ranging from 20 to 60°. The average preoperative flexion contracture was 27.1° and 2.7° at postoperative period with an average follow-up of 70.4 months. The data suggest that a contracted collateral ligament is the most likely primary structure whose effective release allows correction of the flexion contracture in most cases. Only 2 % of the patients needed an additional 4 mm distal femur resection.

Berend et al. [3] in 52 knees with a mean preoperative flexion contracture of 28° manage to correct the deformity down to less than 10 % in over 94 % of cases in his series, compared to 59 % of cases in a study from Massin [14].

11.3 Recurvatum

Degenerative knees presenting for a total knee arthroplasty with hyperextension >5° or genu recurvatum are uncommon, occurring in 0.5–1 % [10, 15]. This deformity may be secondary to a congenital hypoplasia of distal femur, posttraumatic or postinfection osteoarthritis, rheumatic diseases, an inversion of the tibia slope after a high tibial osteotomy, or extensor mechanism weakness or paralysis [6, 18].

Genu recurvatum may be associated with fixed valgus deformity because of a contracture of the iliotibial band and cruciate and collateral ligament laxity [10, 22]. Patients with poliomyelitis commonly suffer from quadriceps weakness, and they rely on locking the knee in hyperextension to walk [5]. Because of posterior capsule and ligament stretching and also because of compensatory changes like hip extension and ankle plantar flexion with foot equinus deformity, these patients with neuromuscular diseases likely recur the recurvatum after surgery and have been considered relatively contraindicated for TKA [5, 7, 15].

Therefore, when considering a knee replacement in a patient with hyperextension deformity, special attention should be given to evaluate the strength of quadriceps, hamstrings, and gastrocnemius complex [16]. Gait analysis and whether medial or lateral instability exists are also crucial since residual instability after TKA increases the risk of recurrence of recurvatum [15].

Radiographic analysis must include a long-standing lower limb lateral view, besides the standard evaluation, to determine femur and/or tibia contributions in the deformity.

11.3.1 Surgical Technique

In recurvatum deformity, the knee can be considered to have an excessively large extension gap compared to flexion gap.

Several authors have suggested techniques to correct genu recurvatum when performing a total knee replacement. Insall [6] suggested that correction may be obtained by underresection of bone ends and using a thicker femoral or tibial component. Krackow [10] and Krackow and Weiss [9] suggested that posterior capsule plication and proximal and posterior transfer of the collateral ligaments may be required for surgical correction of the recurvatum. Whiteside and Mihalko [25] described their protocol for recurvatum knee, downsizing femoral component, when in between sizes, which allows for underresection of the tibia, improving stability in extension.

Like in flexion contracture, the goals of surgery are to balance the flexion/extension gap and restore the mechanical axis of the limb. Appropriate bone resections and soft tissue releases will accomplish that. The distal femoral cut is crucial in recurvatum knees, and depending on the degree of laxity and hyperextension deformity, 2–5 mm less than implant thickness should be resected. When sizing femoral component, the smaller one should be chosen when in between sizes. After the posterior condylar resection, proximal osteophytes must be removed to accommodate deep flexion, but posterior capsule should not be released. On the tibial side, bone cut should be minimized, and slope can be slightly increased to facilitate balance of flexion/extension gap. As previously noted, one must remember that sacrificing the posterior cruciate ligament will increase the flexion gap by 2 mm more than the extension gap [13].

In severe cases with recurvatum >20°, distal femoral augmentation or rotating-hinge devices with a built-in stop to hyperextension may be required.

In patients with neuromuscular disorders and extensor mechanism weakness, hinge prosthesis should be used, because of the high rate of failure with the conventional implants [5, 19]. However, surgeons must keep in mind that the ability to lock the knee in hyperextension is often essential for those patients who can walk. Therefore, special hinged implants that allow few degrees of hyperextension should be preferred in those cases.

Using constrained devices has been a concern, regarding increased stress transfer to the fixation interface and subsequent loosening, but more recent rotating-hinge prosthesis allows more physiological kinematics by a better distribution of the shearing forces, and encouraging results are available [1, 20, 23, 24].

11.3.2 Results

In patients with well-functioning extensor mechanism, genu recurvatum tends not to recur after TKA [7, 16]. Whiteside et al. [25] reported ten knees with preoperative recurvatum (6–25°, mean 11°), treated successfully, with no recurrence after 2 years.

Meding et al. [15] reported the results of 57 cruciate-retaining TKAs performed in patients with a mean preoperative recurvatum of 11°. Their results at a mean follow-up of 4.5 years were excellent, and only two cases had a recurrent deformity, related to a residual medial instability after surgery. Mullaji et al. [18] showed their results in 45 TKAs in recurvatum knees of 11°, and they had no recurrence, after 2 years (Figs. 11.5 and 11.6).

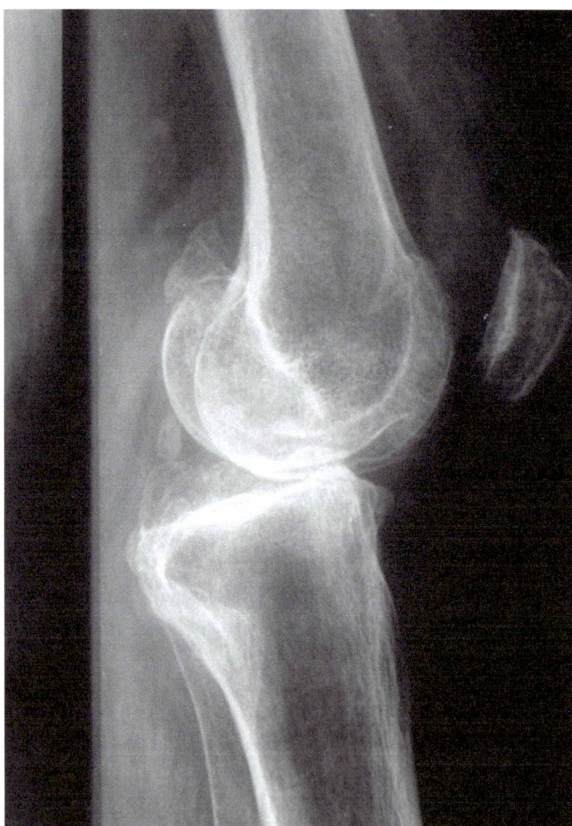

Fig. 11.5 Recurvatum (Courtesy Gamelas J)

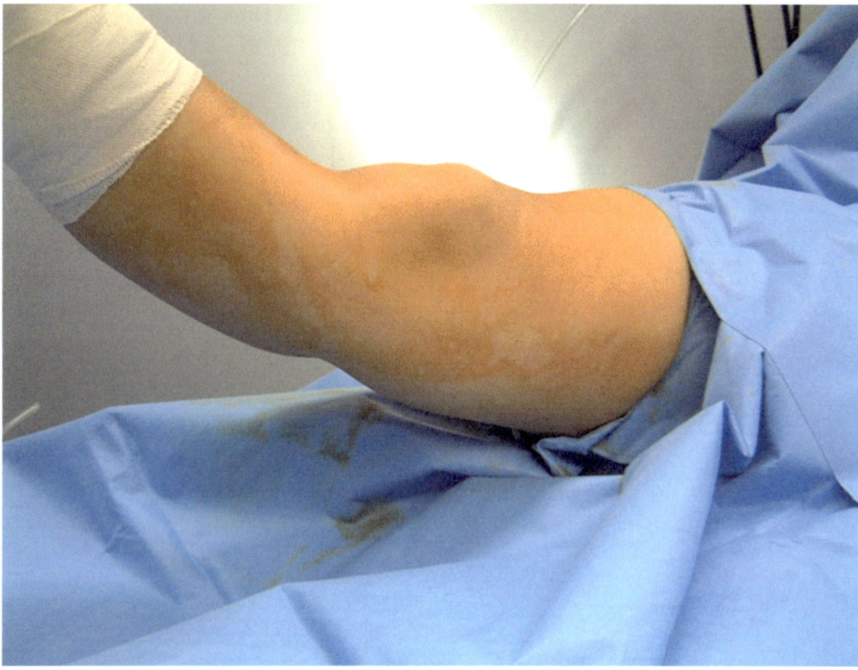

Fig. 11.6 Recurvatum (Courtesy Gamelas J)

Jordan et al. [8] published the largest series on TKA in patients with poliomyelitis. They treated 17 TKAs with only one hinge prosthesis and had no loosening or recurrence at follow-up. However, just two cases had a muscle power less than 3/5. Giori and Lewallen [5] reported that functional deterioration and recurrence of hyperextension instability occur when quadriceps strength is less than antigravity. Tigani et al. [23] had excellent results using rotating-hinge implants in ten TKAs at a mean follow-up of 4 years.

Conclusion

In conclusion, genu recurvatum is no more a contraindication for TKA, but etiology should be elucidated. In the absence of neuromuscular disease, hyperextension deformities tend not to recur after surgery, if adequate gap balancing technique is performed. When quadriceps strength is compromised, rotating-hinge prosthesis is advised, and surgeons must not forget that a slight hyperextension is needed for those who can be able to walk.

References

1. Barrack RL. Evolution of the rotating hinge for complex total knee arthroplasty. Clin Orthop. 2001;392:292–9.
2. Bellemans J, Vandenneucker H, Victor J, Vanlauwe J. Flexion contracture in total knee arthroplasty. Clin Orthop Relat Res. 2006;452:78–82.

3. Berend J, Lombardi Jr AV, Adams JB. Total knee arthroplasty in patients greater than 20 degrees flexion contracture. Clin Orthop Relat Res. 2006;452:83–7.
4. Firestone TP, Krackow KA, Davis JD, Teeny SM, Hungerford DS. The management of fixed flexion contractures during total knee arthroplasty. Clin Orthop Relat Res. 1992;284:221–7.
5. Giori NJ, Lewallen DG. Total knee arthroplasty in limbs affected by poliomyelitis. J Bone Joint Surg. 2002;84A:1157–61.
6. Insall JN. Surgical techniques and instrumentation in total knee arthroplasty. In: Insall JN, Windsor RE, Scott WN, Kelly MA, Aglietti P, editors. Surgery of the knee. New York: Churchill Livingstone; 1993. p. 739–804.
7. Insall JN, Haas SB. Complications of total knee arthroplasty. In: Insall JN, Windsor RE, Scott WN, Kelly MA, Aglietti P, editors. Surgery of the knee. New York: Churchill Livingstone; 1993. p. 891–934.
8. Jordan L, Kligman M, Sculco TP. Total knee arthroplasty in patients with poliomyelitis. J Arthroplasty. 2007;22:543–8.
9. Krackow KA, Weiss AP. Recurvatum deformity complicating performance of total knee arthroplasty: a brief note. J Bone Joint Surg. 1990;72A:268–71.
10. Krackow KA. The technique of total knee arthroplasty. CV Mosby: St Louis; 1990.
11. Laskin RS, Beksac B. Assess and achieve maximal extension. In: Bellemans J, Ries MD, Victior J, editors. Total knee arthroplasty, vol. 30. Heidelberg: Springer; 2005. p. 194–7.
12. Lu H, Mow CS, Lin J. Total knee arthroplasty in the presence of severe flexion contracture: a report of 37 cases. J Arthroplasty. 1999;14:775–80.
13. Lombardi AV, Berend KR. Recurvatum/flexion contracture in total knee arthroplasty. In:Advanced reconstruction knee, vol. 22. Rosemont: AAOS; 2011. p. 189–97.
14. Massin P, Petit A, Odri G, Ducellier F, Sabatier C, Lautridou C, Cappelli M, Hulet C, Canciani JP, Letenneur J, Burdin P. Total knee arthroplasty in patients with greater than 20 degrees flexion contracture. Orthop Traumatol Surg Res. 2009;95(4 Suppl 1):S7–12.
15. Meding JB, Keating EM, Ritter MA, Faris PM, Berend ME. Total knee replacement in patients with genu recurvatum. Clin Orthop. 2001;393:244–9.
16. Meding JB, Keating EM, Ritter MA, Faris PM, Berend ME. Genu recurvatum in total knee replacement. Clin Orthop. 2003;416:64–7.
17. Mihalko WM, Whiteside LA. Bone resection and ligament treatment for flexion contracture in knee arthroplasty. Clin Orthop Relat Res. 2003;406:141–7.
18. Mullaji A, Lingaraju AP, Shetty GM. Computer-assisted total knee replacement in patients with arthritis and a recurvatum deformity. J Bone Joint Surg Br. 2012;94-B:642–7.
19. Patterson BM, Insall JN. Surgical management if gonarthrosis in patients with poliomyelitis. J Arthroplasty. 1992;(Suppl)7:419–26.
20. Petrou G, Petrou H, Tilkeridis C, Stavrakis T, Kapetsis T, Kremmidas N, Gavras M. Medium-term results with a primary cemented rotating-hinge total knee replacement. A 7- to15-year follow-up. J Bone Joint Surg Br. 2004;86(6):813–7.
21. Scuderi GR, Kochhar T. Management of flexion contracture in total knee arthroplasty. J Arthroplasty. 2003;22(4suppl 1):20–4.
22. Tew M, Forster IW. Effect of knee replacement on flexion deformity. J Bone Joint Surg. 1987;69B3:395–9.
23. Tigani D, Fosco M, Amendola L, Boriani L. Total knee arthroplasty in patients with poliomyelitis. Knee. 2009;16:501–6.
24. Westrich GH, Mollano AV, Sculco TP, Buly RL, Laskin RS, Windsor R. Rotating hinge total knee arthroplasty in severely affected knees. Clin Orthop. 2000;379:195–208.
25. Whiteside LA, Mihalko WM. Surgical procedure for flexion contracture and recurvatum in total knee arthroplasty. Clin Orthop Relat Res. 2002;404:189–95.
26. Zaidi SH, Cobb AJ, Bentley G. Danger to the popliteal artery in high tibial osteotomy. J Bone Joint Surg Br. 1995;77:384–6.

Operative Procedure for Primary TKR: How to Increase ROM

12

Samih Tarabichi, Ahmed El-Naggar, and Mohamed Adi

Contents

12.1 Introduction

Deep knee flexion is a real concern for Middle Eastern and Asian patients undergoing total knee replacement (TKR). Since many daily activities, such as praying, dining, or using the oriental toilet, and many social encounters such as attending the Shaikh's majlis are carried out on the ground [1, 2] (Fig. 12.1). It has been shown that during prayers, people routinely flex the knee between 150 and 165°, 20–30 times each day [3]. Often, patients in these societies tend to refuse TKR because of

S. Tarabichi (✉)
Burjeel Hospital for Advanced Surgery, Dubai, United Arab Emirates
e-mail: samtarabichi@yahoo.com

A. El-Naggar
Dubai Hospital, Dubai, United Arab Emirates

M. Adi
Strasbourg University Hospital, Strasbourg, France

S. Matsuda et al. (eds.), *Soft Tissue Balancing in Total Knee Arthroplasty*,
DOI 10.1007/978-3-662-54082-4_12

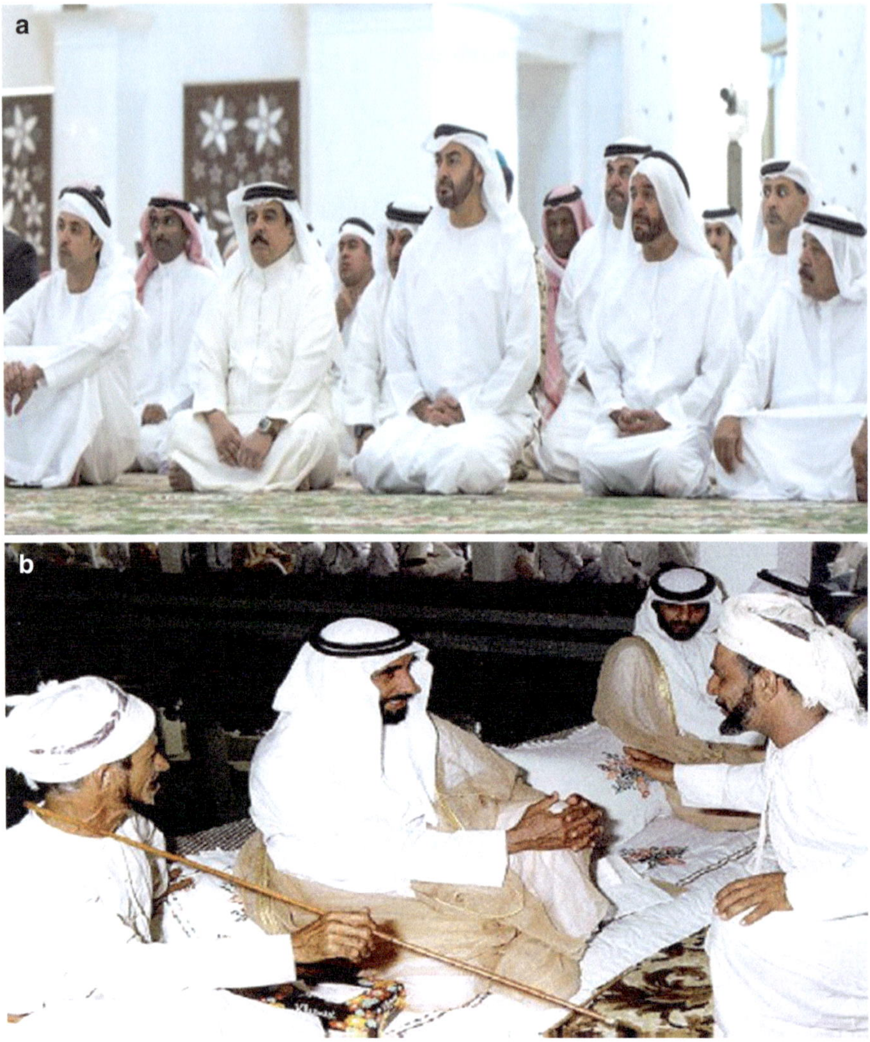

Fig. 12.1 Deep knee flexion activities including kneeling, squatting, and sitting cross-legged are considered crucial to people in this region (**a**) His Highness Sheikh Mohamed bin Zayed Al Nahyan and His Majesty King of Bahrain with the royal family during prayer (Wam). (**b**) The founder of United Arab Emirates Sheikh Zayed Bin Sultan Al Nahyan sitting on the floor in his "Majlis," which is part of social activity in our region for receptions and also to address grievances

concerns that the postoperative range of motion (ROM) will be less than adequate for their daily living [4]. Therefore, high ROM post-TKR should be pursued when possible on patients whose daily activities require a higher ROM to enable them to maintain their lifestyles. In fact, high-flexion activities post-TKA are safe and do not increase the complication rate as compared to the other series [5].

12.2 Factors Affecting Knee Flexion

In order to achieve full flexion post-TKR, many factors, in addition to the surgical technique, should be addressed. Some of these factors can be controlled by the surgeon such as the implant design, surgical techniques, postoperative pain management, and rehabilitation. Other factors such as preoperative ROM, patient's body mass index, and patient's physical ability unfortunately cannot be controlled by the surgeon [6].

The implant design has the least direct effect on obtaining full flexion, and the implant is only useful in being more accommodating to full flexion. However, in order to accomplish full flexion in any patient, it's important to remember that pain management and good rehabilitation program and multidisciplinary approach to the patient should be established in the hospital on a solid basis. Aggressive rehabilitation and adequate pain control are important in preventing postoperative contracture of the soft tissue and achieving better flexion [7].

We truly believe that surgical procedure is quite important to improve the ROM after TKR, and in this chapter, we will focus on quadriceps release technique. We still consider preoperative ROM has a great effect on the outcome of the TKR as many of the international studies so far claim that the ROM postoperatively averages the same as preoperatively [8]. However, in our series which are more than 6000 cases, we were able to obtain a better average ROM postoperatively compared to preoperatively. We consider that this is mainly due to the fact that we have performed routinely a modified quadriceps release (Tarabichi's maneuver) in all our patients to increase the ROM intraoperatively [9]. In the literature, no one has discussed before the importance of the quadriceps release in achieving better flexion in TKR. The purpose of this chapter again is to discuss the anterior knee release and how to obtain a better flexion intraoperatively. Nevertheless, always be reminded that the other factors should be met in order to obtain a better ROM.

12.3 Quadriceps Muscle Release (The Forgotten Release)

Quadriceps release has been used by sports medicine in order to increase the ROM. It is normally done through arthroscopy to increase the mobility for patients who suffer from posttraumatic and postsurgical knee stiffness. The stiffness is typically developed after a period of inactivity in the lower limbs [10]. It has been demonstrated that the restriction in ROM of stiff knee is frequently caused by adhesions that tether the distal quadriceps tendon and/or muscle to the bone surface, thereby preventing the quadriceps muscle and tendon from its normal excursion during flexion [11].

We have done analysis of knee movement; on average in order for the knee to bend from 0 to 90°, the quadriceps tendon normally stretches 6 cm which varies depending on femur size; the larger the femur, the more quadriceps stretching is needed to achieve the flexion (Fig. 12.2). The stretching of the quadriceps per 1° of knee flexion is more on the extreme ends of ROM. The quadriceps have to stretch

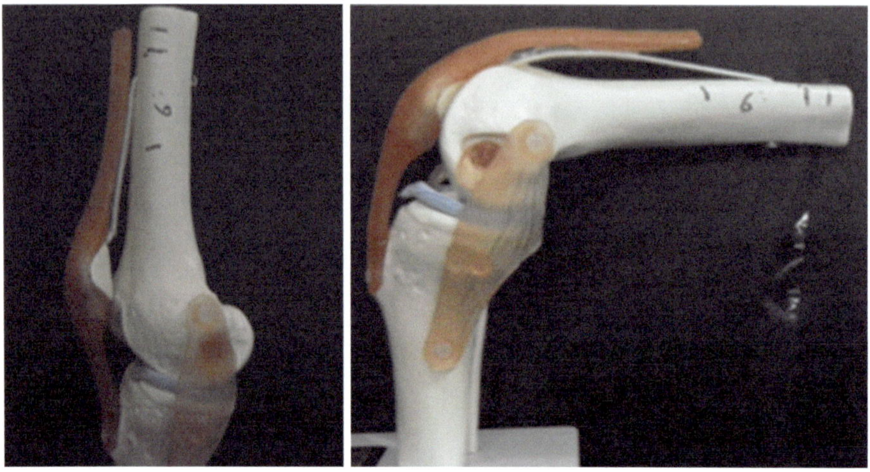

Fig. 12.2 Quadriceps tendon stretches 6 cm on average when the knee bends from 0 to 90°

1.5 cm in order for the knee to bend from 135–155°; the average stretching is 0.7 mm per 1° compared to 0.4 mm per 1° in the ROM of 80–110°.

In our experience, as in the case of posttraumatic stiff knee, the anterior adhesions between the quadriceps muscle and the anterior surface of the femur are the main responsible factors for the restriction of ROM in the stiff arthritic knee. Therefore, we adapted our surgical techniques to address these adhesions and to improve the ROM in all our patients who undergo TKR (Fig. 12.3).

In another study, we performed 42 modified quadriceps muscle releases on patients with advanced osteoarthritis scheduled for TKR. The ROM was documented intraoperatively both before and immediately after the release. Passive flexion improved significantly in all patients (mean, 32.4° of improvement, *P*: 0.001) following a modified quadriceps release only, before doing any ligamentous release and excision of posterior osteophytes [9]. These results strongly suggest that adhesions of the quadriceps muscle to the underlying femur are the major factors which prevent the distal excursion of the quadriceps tendon, thereby preventing deep flexion in patients with osteoarthritis.

12.4 Surgical Technique

Our technique is a standard subvastus approach, initiated with an anterior midline skin incision. Once the extensor mechanism is mobilized, the underlying suprapatellar pouch can be identified and is subsequently excised along with any adhering bands or fibrotic tissue (Fig. 12.4a, b). Doing so provides direct access to the deep interface of the quadriceps muscle and the anterior surface of the femur, allowing the release to be carried out (Fig. 12.4c, d).

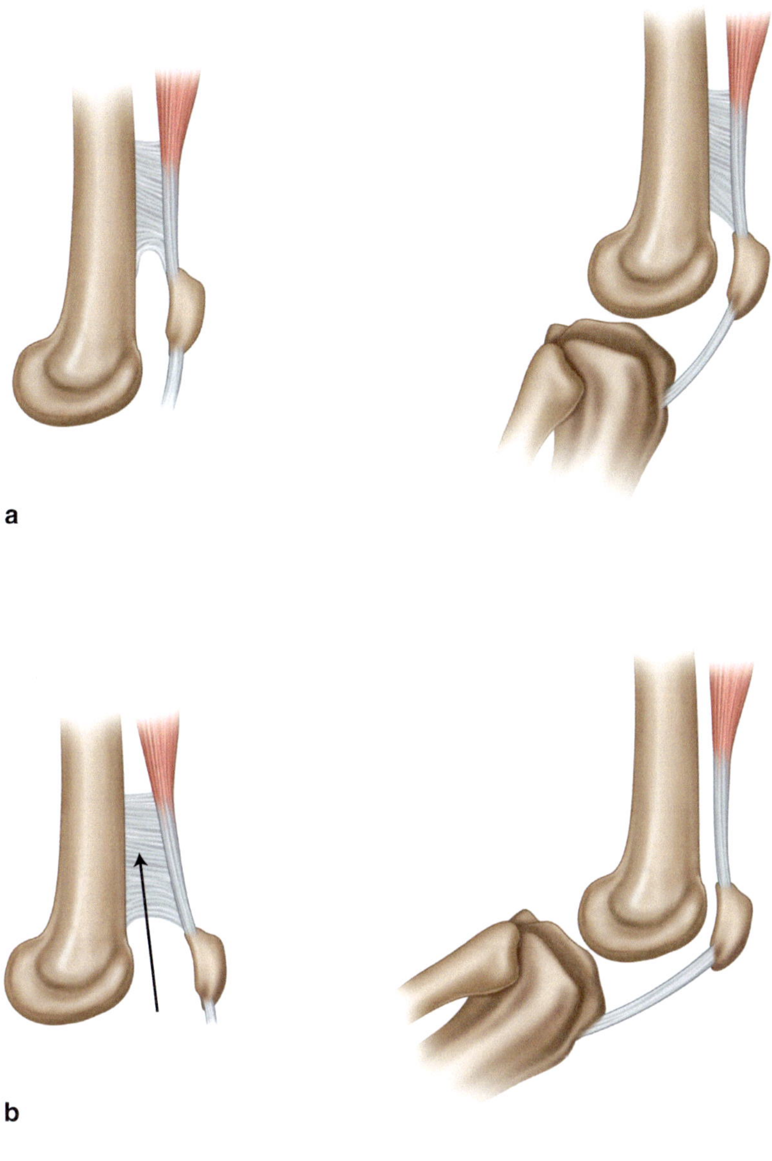

a

b

Fig. 12.3 Simplified illustrations demonstrating the basic principle of our approach. (**a**) How fibrotic adhesions between the quadriceps and the distal femur (*left*) can limit flexion substantially (*right*) by limiting quadriceps excursion. The suprapatellar pouch is represented by the inverted "U" distal to the aforementioned adhesions. (**b**) How a modified quadriceps release, demonstrated by the cartoon arrow above (*left*), would allow the extensor mechanism further excursion, leading to a greater ROM (*right*)

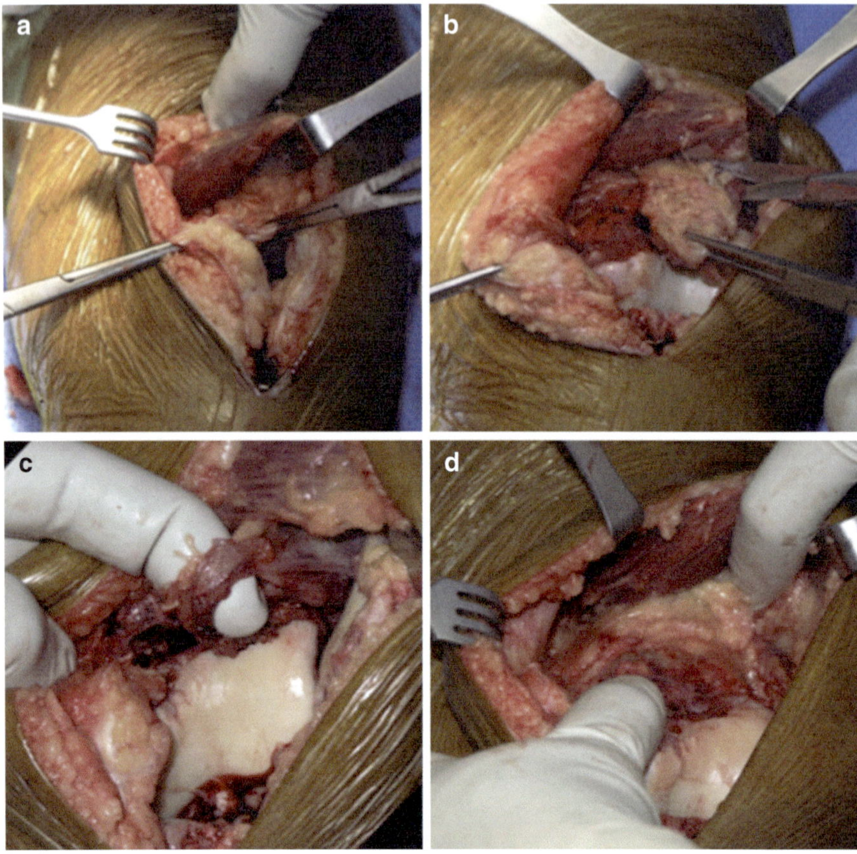

Fig. 12.4 Photographs of the knee anterior aspect while undergoing quadriceps release prior to bone cut. (**a**, **b**) The extensor mechanism being retracted laterally while the surgeon identifies and completely resects the suprapatellar pouch. (**c**) A fibrotic band found tethering the underbelly of the quadriceps muscle to the distal femur during the blunt release, which was subsequently excised. (**d**) The net outcome of the release, which is the removing of the majority of adhesions between the quadriceps muscle and the distal anterior aspect of the femur

The release is carried out in a stepwise fashion where the knee is flexed after each release. If the ROM is estimated to be below 130°, the release is progressed further proximally until a ROM of over 130° is obtained (Fig. 12.5). No bony resection, ligament releases, or lateral/medial retinacular releases were performed at that point in time, as was described by Nicoll in his conventional quadricepsplasty [12].

In our institution, we actually do not proceed with surgery and bone cut until we get a good ROM of the knee through anterior quadriceps release, and this has some advantages.

The first is the fact that obtaining better flexion will make the surgery much easier. There will be less tension on the soft tissue which will prevent skin necrosis

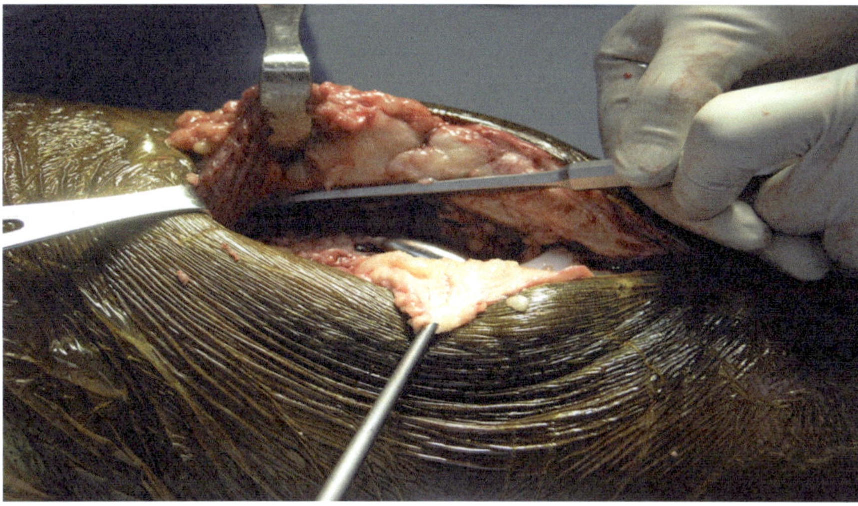

Fig. 12.5 Photo of the knee anterior aspect; the release is progressed proximally until a ROM of over 130° is obtained

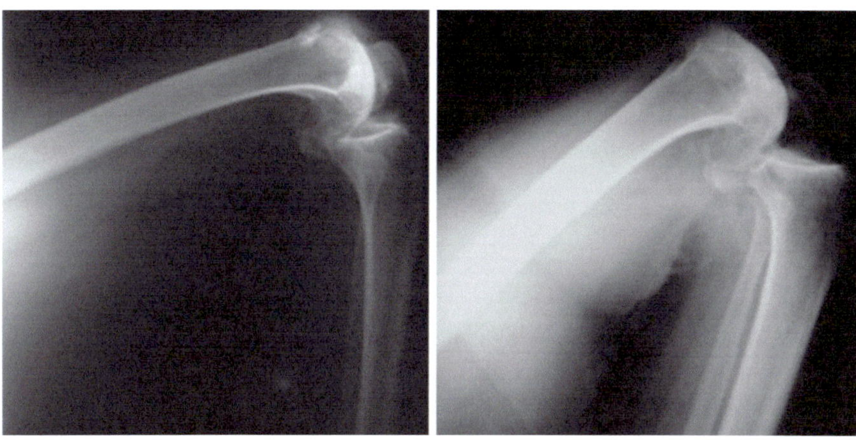

Fig. 12.6 A 74-year-old woman who underwent quadriceps release prior to start TKR. Despite the large posterior osteophytes that can be seen in the prerelease lateral x-ray (*left*), we were able to truly improve flexion from 105° to 140° as shown in the post-release lateral x-ray (*right*)

and damages to the edges of the bone because of the hard retraction and it also decreases the tension on the patellar tendon; hence it prevents the incidental avulsion of patellar tendon in case of arthritic stiff knee.

Second, it will make the surgery more precise, and while the knee is fully bent, the surgeon will be able to visualize the knee well. The third advantage of obtaining full flexion intraoperatively is that we are giving the patient a better chance in obtaining better ROM postoperatively (Figs. 12.6 and 12.7).

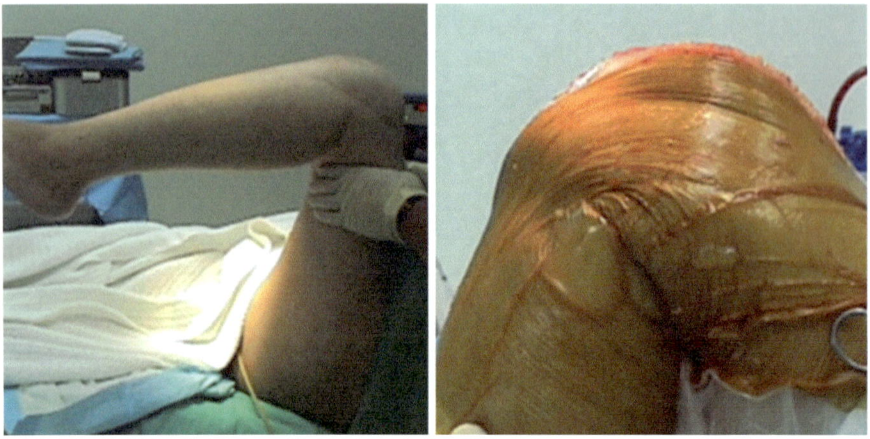

Fig. 12.7 A 58-year-old woman who had quadriceps release prior to bony resection. Photos of the lateral aspect of the left knee in passive flexion before (*left*) and after (*right*) release

12.5 Results of Quadriceps Release

Our results of follow-up over 1028 patients show 3% of our cases (198 patients) have poor ROM (flexion less than 90°) preoperatively. This group dropped to 0.10% after 3 months postoperatively (Table 12.1). We found 88% of our patients (878 patients) achieved excellent ROM (flexion more than 125°) after 3 months postsurgery. Similarly, 30% of them were able to achieve full flexion 3 months after surgery (Figs 12.8 and 12.9).

12.6 Discussion

Some surgeons claim that if we do the tibial tubercle osteotomy and move it proximally about 1 cm which is the maximum, we can improve the ROM in patients especially with patella baja. We have tried that on the model; moving the tibial tubercle osteotomy 1 cm proximally will improve the ROM only about 10°. Subsequently, doing tibial tubercle osteotomy on osteoarthritic stiff knee will allow the surgeon to perform the TKR easily, but when he returns the tibial tubercle back even with 1 cm proximally, the knee will be stiff again. Therefore, we are doing quadriceps muscle release techniques in all our TKR patients to improve the ROM.

Although the quadriceps release technique is an easy and safe procedure, some surgeons have concerns about the postoperative heterotopic ossification (HO) following quadriceps release. The formation of HO after TKR is known to be associated with loss of ROM, stiffness, as well catching and snapping in the patella-femoral joint [13]. In our series of over 6000 cases, we had six patients which developed HO postsurgery. The ROM in our HO patients was not affected, which is the same

Table 12.1 Show significant increase in the number of patient who had a good to excellent ROM 3 months postsurgery (more than 85%)

ROM	Degree	Pre–op (%)	3 months post–op (%)
Poor	<90	3	0.10
Acceptable	90–105	21	2.50
Good	110–125	40	12.50
Excellent	>125	36	88

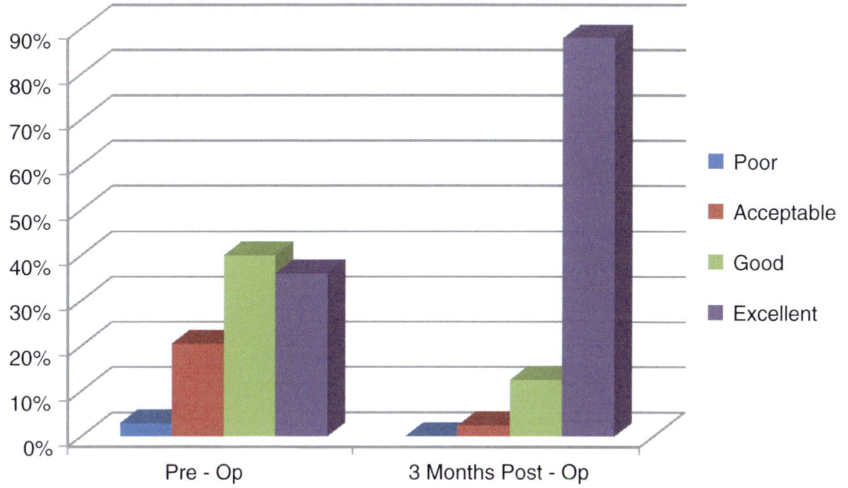

There is a significant decrease in number of patients who had poor range of motion (less than 0.10%)

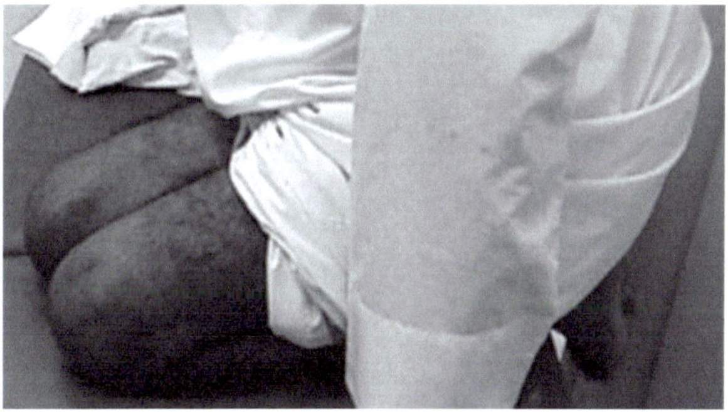

Fig. 12.8 Patient with bilateral TKR kneeling with full flexion, as per definition, 3 months postoperatively

finding in the Toyoda study (Fig. 12.10). Toyoda group found that the ROM in the knees with HO has some limitation at early post-op evaluation. However, there was no significant difference in ROM compared to the knees without HO after 1 year of surgery [14].

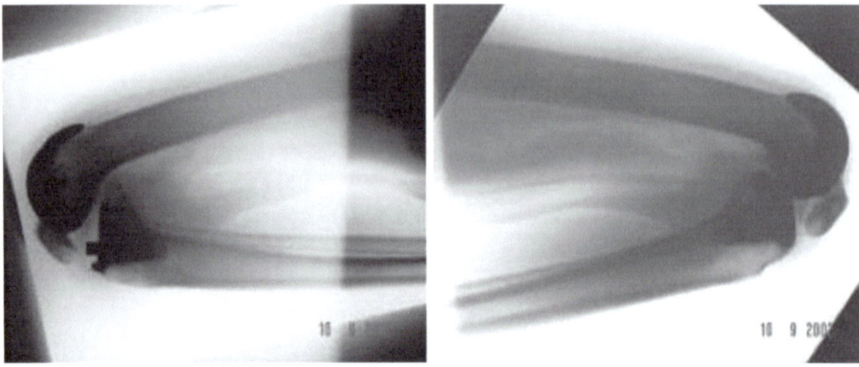

Fig. 12.9 Lateral x-ray of the same patient, 3 months postoperatively

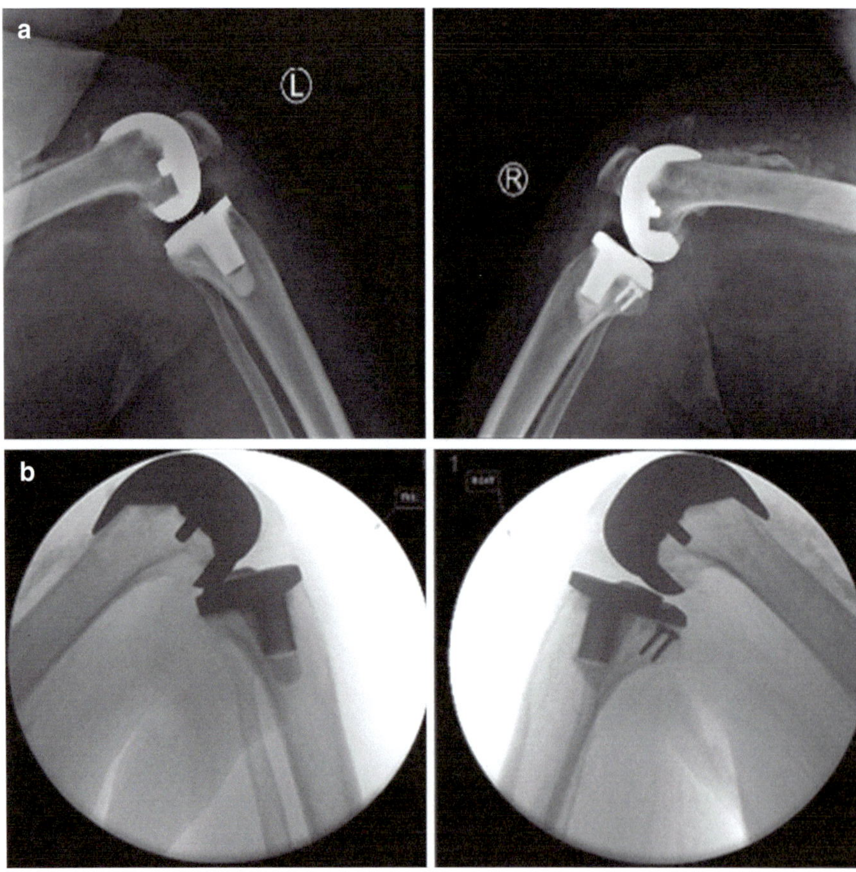

Fig. 12.10 (**a**) A 59-year old female patient 3-month post-bilateral TKR with extensive HO as seen in the lateral x-rays. (**b**) C-arm shows same patient has a good ROM on both knees despite the presence of HO

Conclusion

High ROM post-TKR is important for many patients, and it should be done whenever it is possible to enable our patients to continue their lifestyles as normal as possible. Quadriceps muscle release is an essential surgical technique in TKR which improves ROM in arthritic stiff knee.

The success in obtaining an immediate and significant improvement in ROM by only releasing the quadriceps muscle from its tethering adhesions and keeping other pathological changes such as large osteophytes, severe knee deformities, and irregular articular surfaces intact clearly demonstrates that the inadequate excursion of the quadriceps muscle and tendon is the principal limiting factor to improve knee flexion [9].

We strongly recommend performing quadriceps muscle release in all TKR especially in stiff knee. Our experience has shown a meticulous and careful quadriceps release will enable the surgeon to do his entire primary TKR plus revision on stiff knees without requiring to do the tibial tubercle osteotomy. At our institute, we have not needed to perform the tibial tubercle osteotomy for the last 9 years.

References

1. Tarabichi S, Tarabichi Y, Tarabish A, Hawari M. Importance of full flexion after total knee replacement in Muslims' daily a lifestyle. J Indian Med Assoc. 2006;38:17–22.
2. Tarabichi S, Acker SM, Cockburn RA, Krevolin J, Li RM, Wyss UP. Knee kinematics of high-flexion activities of daily living performed by male Muslims in the Middle East. J Arthroplasty. 2011;26(2):319–27.
3. Hefzy MS, Kelly BP, Cooke TD. Kinematics of the knee joint in deep flexion: a radiographic assessment. Med Eng Phys. 1998;20:4.
4. Villar RN, Solomon VK, Rangam J. Knee surgery and the Indian knee. The importance of the preservation of flexion. Trop Doct. 1989;19:1.
5. Tarabichi S, Tarabichi Y, Tarabish A, Hawari M. Achieving deep flexion after primary total knee arthroplasty. J Arthroplasty. 2010;25(2):220–4.
6. Kansara D, Markel D. The effect of posterior tibial slope on range of motion after total knee arthroplasty. J Arthroplasty. 2006;21(6):809–14.
7. Mauerhan DR, Mokris JG, Ly A, et al. Relationship between length of stay and manipulation rate after total knee arthroplasty. J Arthroplasty. 1998;13:896.
8. Collins JE, Rome BN, Daigle ME, Lerner V, Katz JN, Losina E. A comparison of patient-reported and measured range of motion in a cohort of total knee arthroplasty patients. J Arthroplasty. 2014;29(7):1378–82.
9. Tarabichi S, Tarabichi Y. Can an anterior quadriceps release improve range of motion in the stiff arthritic knee. J Arthroplasty. 2010;25(4):571–5.
10. Epps CE. Complications in orthopaedic surgery. Philadelphia: JB Lippin- cott Co; 1978. p. 498.
11. Smillie IS. Injuries of the knee joint. 4th ed. Williams & Wilkins: Baltimore; 1973. p. 365.
12. Nicoll EA. Quadricepsplasty. J Bone Joint Surg. 1963;45- B:183.
13. Iorio R, Healy WL. Heterotopic ossification after hip and knee arthroplasty: risk factors, prevention, and treatment. J Am Acad Orthop Surg. 2002;10:409.
14. Toyoda T, Matsumoto H, Tsuji T, Kinouchi J, Fujikawa K. Heterotopic ossification after total knee arthroplasty. J Arthroplasty. 2003;18(6):760–4.

Part IV

Assessment in Primary TKA

Assessment in Primary TKA: Intraoperative Assessment Tensor

13

Tomoyuki Matsumoto, Hirotsugu Muratsu, and Ryosuke Kuroda

Contents

13.1 Introduction

Total knee arthroplasty (TKA) is a well-established procedure, which generally provides pain relief, improved physical function, and a high level of satisfaction to patients with end-staged osteoarthritis. Whereas surgeons could achieve accurate osteotomy and implant positioning using a navigation system,

There are no conflicts of interest or financial disclosures related to the article.

T. Matsumoto, MD, PhD (✉) • R. Kuroda, MD, PhD
Department of Orthopaedic Surgery, Kobe University Graduate School of Medicine, Kobe, Japan
e-mail: mastun@m4.dion.ne.jp

H. Muratsu, MD, PhD
Department of Orthopaedic Surgery, Steel Memorial Hirohata Hospital, Himeji, Japan

S. Matsuda et al. (eds.), *Soft Tissue Balancing in Total Knee Arthroplasty*,
DOI 10.1007/978-3-662-54082-4_13

patient-specific instrumentation, or the development of a surgical jig, the management of soft tissue balance during TKA remains difficult, leaving much to the surgeon's subjective feel. Knee instability after primary TKA is considered an important factor for early TKA failure, as shown in registry data [65]. Fehring et al. studied 279 revision surgeries within 5 years of their index arthroplasty and reported 74 revision cases (27%) caused by instability [15]. In a retrospective study of revision surgery, Sharkey et al. reported instability in 21.2% of their early revision knee arthroplasty failures [74]. They concluded that the instability might be due to inadequate correction of soft tissue imbalances in both the sagittal and coronal planes. As a result, soft tissue balancing has been recognized as an essential surgical intervention for improving the outcomes of TKA.

13.2 Traditional Soft Tissue Balance Assessment

Although several methods and devices for assessing soft tissue balance, such as manual distraction [18], traditional tensor [18], space block [24], and lamina spreaders [16], have been described in previous publications, assessment has not been quantitative and has mainly depended on the subjective feeling of the surgeons. The second generation of tensor devices that were quantitatively applied and objective, with the measurement made under fixed torque or load, were commercially available [5, 8, 69, 84, 88] or individually developed or modified [21, 85, 86, 89]. Asano et al. [4] used a commercially available tensor combined with their original torque driver, in which the load at every 1-mm interval of gap distance could be measured. However, their method could only be used for measurement with an everted, and thereby unphysiological, patellar orientation, without the prosthesis, and only in extension or 90° of flexion.

D'Lima et al. developed a knee arthroplasty tibial tray, with force transducers and a telemetry system, to measure tibiofemoral compressive forces directly in vivo [11, 57]. From 1996, the study group spent time refining manufacturing techniques, improving durability, and testing safety, after which they reported the first electronic knee prosthesis implant in 2004. Recently, they summarized the design, development, and in vivo use of two generations of electronic knee prostheses with activities associated with daily living, rehabilitation, exercise, and athletics from their many studies [10]. Although this device provides a lot of useful information on kinematics after TKA, it is too specialized and expensive for routine clinical use. The implantable tibial tray with force transducers and telemetry system is useful for research but needs a bulky implant with an extension stemlike structure and cannot be used with other TKA systems limiting the population in which it can be used.

13.3 Soft Tissue Balance Assessment with an Offset-Type Tensor

13.3.1 Design and Parameters

In order to permit soft tissue balancing under physiological conditions in a surgeon-friendly manner, a new tensor was developed to obtain soft tissue balancing throughout the range of motion with reduced patellofemoral (PF) and aligned tibiofemoral (TF) joints [59]. The offset-type tensor consists of the following three parts: an upper seesaw plate, a lower platform plate with a spike, and an extra-articular main body (Fig. 13.1). Both plates are placed at the center of the knee, and we apply one of the two tensioning devices that are catered to appropriately fit either a cruciate-retaining (CR) or a posterior-stabilized (PS) TKA. The PS TKA tensor consists of a seesaw plate with a proximal post along the center that fits the intercondylar space as well as a cam for the femoral trial prosthesis. This post and cam mechanism controls the tibiofemoral position in both the coronal and sagittal planes. The CR TKA tensor consists of a seesaw plate with a proximal convex-shaped centralizer that fits the intercondylar space and controls the coronal joint alignment. These mechanisms permit us to reproduce the joint constraint and alignment after implanting the prostheses. This device is ultimately designed to permit surgeons to measure the

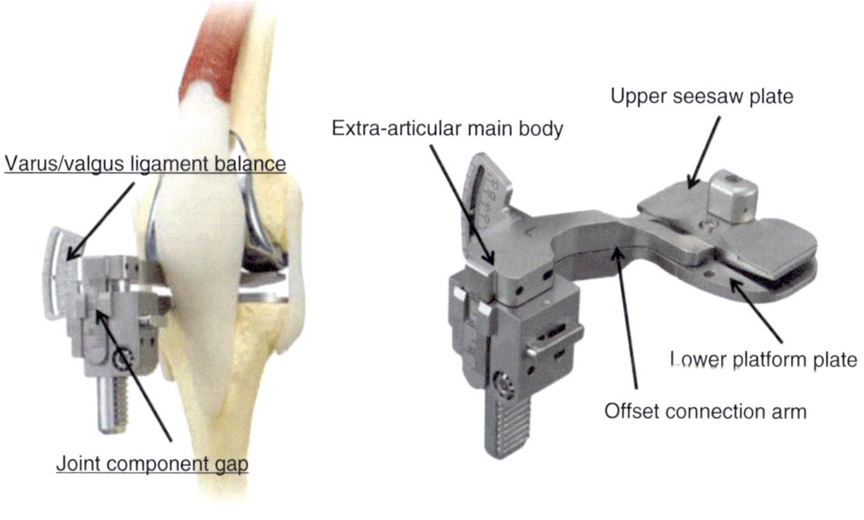

Fig. 13.1 Offset-type tensor. The tensor consists of three parts: upper seesaw plate, lower platform plate, and extra-articular main body. Two plates are connected to the extra-articular main body by the offset connection arm

varus/valgus ligament balance and joint center/joint component gap while applying a constant joint distraction force. Joint distraction forces ranging from 30 lb. (13.6 kg) to 80 lb. (36.3 kg) can be exerted between the seesaw and platform plates through a specially made torque driver, which can change the applied torque value. After sterilization, this torque driver is placed on a rack that contains a pinion mechanism along the extra-articular main body, and the appropriate torque is applied to generate the designated distraction force. Once appropriately distracted, attention is focused on the following two scales that correspond to the tensor: the angle (°, positive in value in varus ligament balance) between the seesaw and platform plates and the distance (mm) between the center midpoints of upper surface of the seesaw plate and the proximal tibial cut (mm, joint center/joint component gap). By measuring these angular deviations and distances under a constant joint distraction force, the ligament balance and joint center/joint component gaps can be measured, respectively.

13.3.2 Soft Tissue Balance with a Reduced PF Joint

We reported our experience using this device for intraoperative measurement with the PS TKA and further discussed the importance of the patellar orientation during the measurement [43, 49, 50]. First, we reported joint component gap kinematics in PS TKA with and without patellar eversion. The component gap showed an accelerated decrease during full knee extension. With the PF joint everted, the component gap increased throughout knee flexion. In contrast, the component gap with a reduced PF joint increased with knee flexion but decreased after 60° of flexion [49]. Second, we reported that intraoperative joint component gap kinematic assessment with a reduced PF joint has the possibility to predict the postoperative flexion angle and thus allows evaluation of the surgical technique throughout a range of knee motion. Both an increased value during the extension to flexion gap and a decreased value during the flexion to deep flexion gap with PF joint reduced, not everted, showed inverse correlations with the postoperative knee flexion angle, not with the preoperative flexion angle [43]. Third, we demonstrated that the correlations between the soft tissue balance, assessed by the tensor, and the navigation system were higher with a reduced PF joint than those with an everted PF joint. This suggests that surgeons should assess soft tissue balance during PS TKA with the PF joint reduced when using a navigation system [50]. In a series of intraoperative soft tissue balance assessments, we emphasized the importance of maintaining a reduced and anatomically oriented PF joint in order to obtain accurate and more physiologically relevant soft tissue balancing.

In addition to our reports, some recent studies have emphasized the importance of the physiological postoperative knee condition in assessing soft tissue balance with PF joint reduction [17, 26, 91]. Using our tensor with a 5-mm-long minute uniaxial foil strain gauge, Gejo et al. reported a similar kinematic pattern of the intraoperative joint component gap; when the patella was reduced, the joint gap was decreased at 90 and 135° of flexion (by 1.9 mm and 5.5 mm, respectively) compared with the gap with the patella everted. Patellar tendon strain at 90° of flexion, increasing with knee flexion, correlated with the joint gap difference with the patella in the everted and reduced positions. Based on their study, they concluded that the knee extensor mechanism might have an influence on the joint gap and be important in achieving the optimal joint gap balance during TKA [17]. With the use of an original tensor device that can measure the load of the spread joint gap, Yoshino et al. reported a significant difference between the loads in the patella-everted position and the reset position in flexion, but not in extension, in PS TKA. However, in CR TKA, they reported no significant difference between the loads in the patella-everted position and in patella-reset position at either extension or flexion. Therefore, they concluded that the load in the flexion gap will increase in PS TKA or, in other words, the flexion gap distance will decrease by resetting [91]. With the use of an offset-type tensor that has been developed based on our tensor, Kamei et al. reported a joint gap size and inclination measured intraoperatively on a knee in 90° flexion, with and without patellar eversion [26]. After the tibial and distal femoral cuts were made, they showed that the joint gap with the patella in situ (17.0 ± 3.4 mm) was significantly greater than that with patellar eversion (15.4 ± 3.0 mm), as was gap inclination at 90° flexion with the patella in situ (4.9° ± 3.1°) compared with that observed with patellar eversion (4.0° ± 2.9°). Based on these results, they speculated that the steeper flexion gap inclination obtained without patellar eversion induced more externally rotated femoral positioning in the absence of patellar eversion. They emphasized that these results ought to be taken into account by surgeons considering a switch from conventional to minimal incision surgery (MIS) TKA.

13.3.3 Soft Tissue Balance with Femoral Component Placement

The main concepts of measurement using the new tensor are different from the conventional tensioning device with the femoral trial component in place as well as a reduced PF joint. As the next step, accordingly, we focused on the difference in soft tissue balancing between the placement of femoral trial component and the conventional osteotomized condition. In the intraoperative assessment of soft tissue balance, the joint gap showed a significant decrease in extension, but not flexion, after femoral trial prosthesis placement. Varus ligament balances were significantly reduced in extension and increased in flexion after femoral trial placement [58]. These changes in extension might be caused by the tensed posterior structures of the knee, associated with the posterior condyle of the externally rotated, aligned femoral trial. At knee flexion, a medial tension in the extensor mechanisms might be increased after femoral trial placement with PF joint repaired and increased ligament balance in varus. We measured the "joint component gap," which is remarkably different from the more conventional gap measurement. The joint component gap is measured with the femoral component in place, whereas the conventional gap measurement is made between the cutting surfaces of the femur and tibia. By keeping the femoral component in place, the knee is afforded a greater degree of extension because of its curving arc. In this arrangement, the posterior condyles of the component tighten the posterior capsule, resulting in a smaller joint gap at full extension. In addition, because of the 7-degree posterior slope of the tibia and a slight femoral anterior bowing, we can consider the "conventional extension gap" to be at about 10° of the knee flexion angle. Mitsuyama et al. similarly reported on 80 varus-type osteoarthritic knees with the offset-type tensor that selecting a larger size femoral component as well as femoral component placement reduced the extension gap [55]. They reported that the placement of the femoral component reduced the medial and lateral extension gaps by 1.0 mm and 0.9 mm, respectively. The medial and lateral gaps further decreased by 2.1 mm and 2.8 mm, respectively, when a specially made femoral component with a posterior condyle enlarged by 4 mm was tested. Mihalko et al. found in a cadaver study that the release of more posterior structures had a greater effect on the extension gap than on the flexion gap, explaining the importance of the relationship between posterior structures and the extension gap [54]. Sugama et al. reported in their operative study that a bone cut from the posterior femoral condyles could change the tension of the posterior soft tissue structures and so alter the width and shape of the extension gap [75]. These previous reports support our hypothetical mechanism.

13.4 Different Patterns of Soft Tissue Balance in Specified Conditions

13.4.1 Soft Tissue Balance in CR and PS TKA

Our abovementioned series of studies were only implemented with PS TKA. The long-term results of CR and PS TKAs have shown an ability to relieve pain and improve function. Nevertheless, the superiority of the CR or PS TKA remains a source of great controversy in the field of TKA. Proponents of the CR TKA advocate maintaining the posterior cruciate ligament (PCL) in order to increase stability, promote femoral rollback, and thereby enhance the patient's ability to climb stairs [1, 2, 6, 13, 37], while proponents of the PS TKA highlight studies in which patients with a resected PCL display a greater postoperative range of motion [23, 25, 37]. It is important to note in this debate, however, that investigators have been unable to show a difference in clinical outcome between these types of knees [6, 13, 83]. We have previously shown that, among patients undergoing bilateral TKAs performed by the same surgeon and including a CR and PS TKA in alternate knees of the same patient, there was no difference in the postoperative knee score, yet the postoperative range of motion was significantly superior after resecting the PCL [40]. Accordingly, we extended our previous study and report on our experience with this device for the intraoperative soft tissue balance measurements of CR and PS TKAs, performed with both a reduced and everted patella.

While the joint component gap measurements made with a reduced patella of PS TKA increased from extension to flexion, these values remained constant for CR TKA throughout the full range of motion. Additionally, the joint component gaps at deep knee flexion were significantly smaller for both types of prosthetic knees when the PF joint was reduced [42]. From our data, the CR TKA had stable joint kinematics from extension into deep flexion, while the joint kinematics for the PS TKA were more dynamic. Our data thereby support prior studies, indicating that the CR TKA affords patients greater stability. Our data further indicate that compared with a CR TKA, a PS TKA with a reduced patella results in significantly larger gaps when the arc of motion ranges from mid- to deep flexion.

In the assessment of varus/valgus balance, while the measurements of varus ligament balance with a reduced patella in PS TKA slightly increased from extension to flexion, these values slightly decreased for CR TKA from extension to flexion [46]. The data showed that CR TKA produced constant soft tissue tension from extension into deep flexion, whereas PS TKA produced soft tissue tension that tended to be more in varus during flexion. The PCL in the knees with osteoarthritis is considered relatively rigid and shortened, despite being macroscopically intact. Our findings indicate that compared with CR TKA, PS TKA with the patella reduced results in a significantly larger varus angle when the arc of motion is between midrange and deep flexion. After performing the independent cut procedure, we applied 3° or 5° of external rotation in the series of studies when setting the femoral component, which may have caused a decreasing varus balance in flexion in patients who underwent CR TKA. Some studies indicated that the flexion gap in healthy knees is not rectangular and that the lateral joint gap is significantly lax [39, 56, 72, 79]. The use of both a traditional soft tissue release and the measured resection technique for the knees with osteoarthritis in varus produces a pattern of soft tissue tension that may at least partly explain why PS TKA produces a better postoperative range of motion.

Taken together, the kinematic patterns of soft tissue balance differ between the patellae everted and reduced as well as between PS and CR TKA. In light of these findings, we should carefully select patients according to the condition of their PCL, set an appropriate angle of external rotation, or do both if we wish to obtain good outcomes in CR TKA.

13.4.2 Soft Tissue Balance in Minimal Incision Surgery TKA

MIS TKA is widely promoted as a possible improvement over the conventional TKA. Its major advantages are the requirement of a smaller skin incision and the avoidance of patellar eversion and quadriceps muscle splitting, leading to reduced blood loss, less perioperative pain, shorter length of hospital stay, and earlier return of knee function [9, 20, 27, 32, 35, 36, 71, 82]. Although traditional TKA allows for excellent visualization, component orientation, and fixation and has been associated with remarkable long-term implant survival, MIS TKA is attractive because of the small incision, minimal or absent pain, and discomfort associated with surgery. However, while there is some evidence that these short-term benefits occur with MIS TKA, there is concern because of more complications associated with the MIS technique, including vascular injury [81], patellar tendon injury, condylar fracture, wound dehiscence and necrosis, and component malalignment. In particular, the quadriceps-sparing (QS) approach has been developed as the least-invasive approach to the extensor mechanism by limiting medial parapatellar arthrotomy to the superior pole of the patella [82]. Although new surgical instrument designs enable surgeons to use this approach, this technique remains challenging to perform without causing damage to the vastus medialis obliquus due to the limited working space [63, 68].

Accordingly, we compared intraoperative soft tissue balance measurements of MIS QS and conventional TKA, performed with the patella and femoral component in place. Whereas the joint component gap in MIS QS-TKA was significantly larger through the entire arc of flexion compared with that of conventional TKA, the pattern of joint looseness (joint component gap-polyethylene insert thickness) showed no difference between the two procedures. The varus ligament balance in MIS QS-TKA was significantly larger than that in conventional TKA at 0°, 90°, and 135° of knee flexion [48]. The study suggested that MIS TKA may lead to ligament imbalance due to the difficulties induced by a limited working space. Furthermore, different approaches seemed to result in a different pattern of intraoperative soft tissue balance. The intraoperative patterns of soft tissue balance differ between the laterally retracted and reduced patella as well as between QS and mini TKA [62]. The results indicate that surgeons performing conventional soft tissue balance evaluation with the patella laterally retracted in MIS TKAs are at a greater risk for underestimating joint gap and varus ligament imbalance depending on the joint exposures compared with those performing the evaluation in the postoperative condition after TKA with the patella reduced. Similarly, Niki reported on parapatellar, midvastus, subvastus, and lateral subvastus approaches and found that the joint gap in mid-flexion to flexion showed a large value with the medial parapatellar approach and a laterally shifted patella, while the subvastus approach caused a reduction of the flexion gap [61].

13.4.3 Soft Tissue Balance in Gap Technique

In the abovementioned study, soft tissue balance measurements were made only in PS or CR TKAs using the measured resection technique. However, the best method to obtain rotational alignment of the femoral component in flexion remains controversial. Some investigators favor a measured resection technique in which bony landmarks (femoral epicondyles, posterior femoral condyles, or the anteroposterior axis) are the primary determinants of femoral component rotation [7, 19, 38, 66, 70, 87]. Others recommend a gap-balancing methodology in which the femoral component is positioned parallel to the resected proximal tibia with each collateral ligament equally tensioned [12, 14, 28]. Given this debate, several surgeons recently reported more consistent equalization of extension and flexion gaps with the use of a computer-assisted gap-balancing technique and compared it with the conventional measured resection technique [64, 73]. In contrast, in a comparison between the navigation-assisted measured resection and navigation-assisted gap-balancing techniques, some surgeons reported a better restoration of the joint line position in the navigation-assisted measured resection technique, despite no differences in short-term clinical outcomes [33, 78].

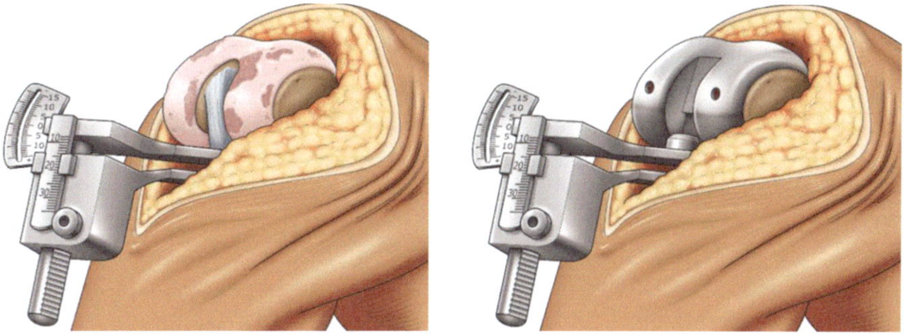

Fig. 13.2 Assessment option. The tensor can be used in the two conditions after tibial bone cut and after femoral bone cut and femoral component placement

Using the offset-type tensor, which can be used in the gap technique [77], we assessed soft tissue balance during CR TKA using the tibia-first gap technique with a navigation system. With the tibia-first gap technique, the kinematics of the component gap showed a similar pattern to the measured resection technique during CR TKA; following a significant increase during the initial 30° of knee flexion, the joint component gap showed a gradual decrease toward 120° of flexion [42, 46]. With the offset-type tensor, soft tissue balance could be assessed after tibial cut and femoral cut were made and the femoral component placed (Fig. 13.2). The basic value of the joint gap before femoral osteotomy reflected the final value, following the femoral cut and with femoral component placement [45]. Accordingly, the tibia-first gap technique may have the advantage of letting surgeons predict the final soft tissue balance even before making the femoral osteotomies. The tibia-first technique, as with the measured resection technique, showed a different intraoperative soft tissue balance pattern associated with different approaches, and soft tissues could easily be balanced in CR TKA [41]. When compared among the four combinations, PS or CR TKA and measured resection or gap technique, CR TKA with the gap technique was found to obtain equalized rectangular gaps in extension and flexion more easily than the other techniques. However, the different patterns in intraoperative soft tissue balance assessment showed no differences in objective clinical scores at 2-year follow-up [44]. A patient-derived subjective scoring system may be useful for identifying the importance of intraoperative soft tissue balance assessment.

13.5 Clinical Relevance of Intraoperative Soft Tissue Balance Assessment

Considering the clinical significance of intraoperative assessment, we should confirm that intraoperative values assessed with the tensor reflect the postoperative soft tissue balance. Hence, we investigated the correlation between the intraoperative values assessed with the tensor and the 5-year postoperative values assessed with stress radiography in extension and flexion [47]. In CR TKA, postoperatively both the joint component gap and ligament balance in extension and flexion showed positive correlations with the intraoperative values of 10° and 90° of flexion. However, in PS TKA, whereas postoperatively both the joint component gap and ligament balance in extension showed positive correlation with the intraoperative values at 10° of flexion, postoperatively neither joint component gap nor ligament balance in flexion correlated with that in 90° of flexion. These results indicate that the intraoperative measurements of soft tissue balance by the tensor reflect the postoperative values assessed by the stress radiographs, even at the 5-year follow-up. However, despite existing correlations in extension, there were no correlations in flexion in either the joint component gap or the ligament balance between intra- and postoperative values in PS TKA. This discrepancy in PS TKA may be caused by flexion instability due to a flexion gap larger than the extension gap [42].

Acquisition of a high flexion angle after TKA is one of the factors leading to patient satisfaction. Therefore, we focused on the relationship between the postoperative flexion angle and the intraoperative soft tissue balance. In the series of studies in PS TKA, the joint gap change value (90–0°) with the PF joint reduced, not everted, showed an inverse correlation with the postoperative knee flexion angle and posterior condylar offset [43]. However, in another series of studies on CR TKA, the postoperative flexion angle was positively correlated with the joint gap change value (90–0°). In either case, multivariate regression analysis among various values, including various joint gap change values, ligament balance, and preoperative knee flexion angle, demonstrated that the preoperative knee flexion angle and the joint gap change value (90–0°) had a significant independent effect on the postoperative knee flexion angle [76]. One of the reasons for this discrepancy may be the different patterns of soft tissue balance between PS and CR TKA [42, 46]. In that report, CR TKA in comparison with PS TKA showed significantly smaller gaps when the arc of movement ranged from mid- to deep flexion [42]. PCL in the osteoarthritic knee is considered relatively rigid and shortened, despite being macroscopically intact. When we consider the flexion gap tightness, Ritter et al. reported that 30% of CR TKA required ligament balancing to obtain a smooth flexion arc [67]. If the PCL was too tight, excessive femoral rollback resulted in anterior lift-off of the tibial trial in flexion, leading to limitation of flexion [29]. Balancing the flexion gap can facilitate postoperative flexion to an increased angle and result in a satisfactory range of motion [3, 34]. In our studies on CR TKA, we found that a 16% increase in flexion gap tightness (smaller flexion gap than extension gap) resulted in a smaller flexion angle. Similarly, using a commercially available knee balancer with the measurement under 80 N distraction force, Higuchi et al. reported that flexion medial/lateral gap tightness led to restriction of the flexion angle [22]. Therefore, in these cases, surgeons are advised to release soft tissues such as the PCL to decrease flexion gap tightness by [29, 67, 90].

Finally, postoperative kinematics such as tibial internal rotation and tibial anterior translation are important to achieve better clinical outcomes, including a high knee flexion angle. With regard to achieving high flexion after TKA, some studies have emphasized that an increase in postoperative tibial internal rotation is observed during knee flexion [31, 88]. Therefore, we investigated the correlation between intraoperative soft tissue balance (assessed by the tensor) and postoperative knee kinematics (assessed by a navigation system) following all prostheses implanted [53]. The results confirmed a positive correlation between varus ligament balance and tibial internal rotation, which may indicate that looseness of the lateral compartment in relation to the medial side at 60° and 90° of flexion permits rotational mobility and results in increased tibial internal rotation. In fact, the positive correlation between the lateral compartment gap and tibial internal rotation from mid- to deep knee flexion was a more sensitive factor than the joint component gap, and the fact that there was no relationship between the medial compartment gap and tibial internal rotation supported this result. Moreover, in another study assessing the correlation between intra- and postoperative knee flexion angle and knee kinematics, postoperative as well as preoperative knee flexion angle was significantly correlated with the postoperative tibial internal rotation [52]. In addition, we reported a positive correlation between intraoperative lateral laxity in flexion and postoperative flexion angle in CR TKA, indicating that medial stability with appropriate lateral laxity was important for achievement of a high flexion angle [60]. Similarly, Kobayashi reported, using postoperative stress radiography, that lateral laxity in flexion (flexion-valgus, 3.4°; flexion-varus, 6.2°) showed a positive correlation with the postoperative knee flexion angle [30]. Other studies also support these findings, indicating that the flexion gap in healthy knees is not rectangular and that the lateral joint gap is significantly lax [39, 56, 72, 80]. In summary, to reproduce medial pivot motion after TKA, medial stability with moderate lateral laxity during flexion might lead to appropriate tibial internal rotation and result in a high flexion angle.

13.6 Perspective

The most important aspect of soft tissue balancing is not just an assessment but also the close interaction between the surgical technique and the assessment, in which surgeons should reflect the surgical technique to attain final soft tissue balance. With the measured resection technique for CR TKA, we recently reported the importance of minimal medial release (osteophyte removal and release of the deep layer of the medial collateral ligament) for varus-type osteoarthritis to maintain an appropriate tibial internal rotation and to gain a high flexion angle [51]. Recently, an offset-type tensor was developed to use with the gap technique as well as the measured resection technique during TKA. With this new system, FuZion™ (Zimmer, Inc.) (Fig. 13.3), surgeons can assess and correct soft tissue balance after making the distal femoral and proximal tibial cut, then adjust femoral rotation based on the tensor measurement, and confirm the final balance throughout the range of motion with femoral component placement. The information, made available by the use of the tensor during surgery, is useful in a real-time manner and is essential for providing insight regarding the true postoperative kinematics. It allows the surgeon to adjust the soft tissue balance more accurately and thereby to expect a better postoperative outcome.

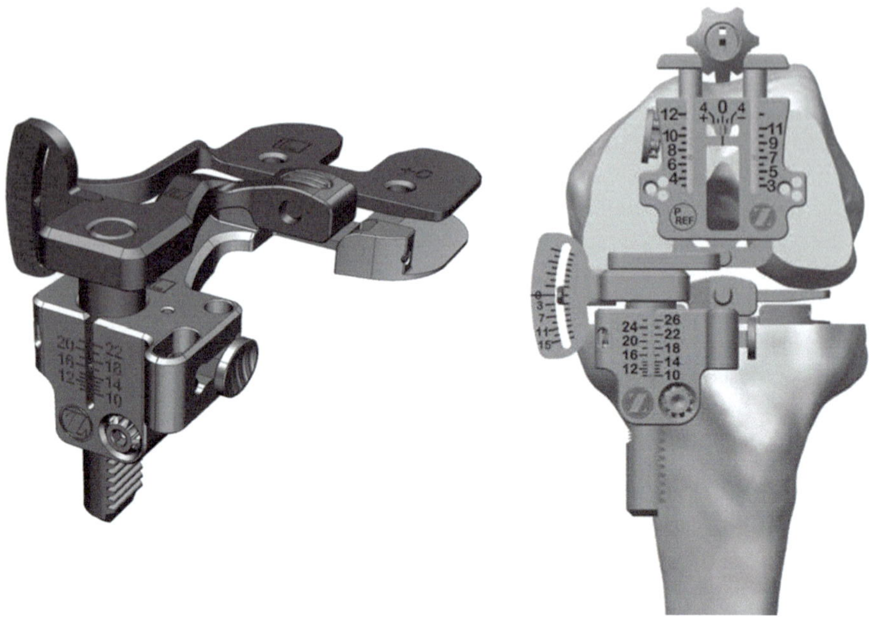

Fig. 13.3 FuZion™ Instrument (Zimmer, Inc.). The FuZion Instruments are based on two platforms, the FuZion Spacer Block and FuZion Tensor, and were specifically designed to provide crossover utility, harmonizing measured resection and gap-balancing philosophies

To achieve successful clinical outcomes, accurate osteotomy/implantation and soft tissue balancing are essential in TKA. Appropriate bone cut and prosthetic implantation have improved due to advances in surgical instrumentations, such as the computer-assisted navigation system, preoperative image-matching technique, or patient-specific instrumentation. Similarly, appropriate soft tissue balancing has become more important than it was previously. With the recent advances in this field described here, improved patient satisfaction after TKA is expected in the near future.

References

1. Andriacchi TP, Andersson GB, Fermier RW, Stern D, Galante JO. A study of lower-limb mechanics during stair-climbing. J Bone Joint Surg Am. 1980;62(5):749–57.
2. Andriacchi TP, Galante JO, Fermier RW. The influence of total knee-replacement design on walking and stair-climbing. J Bone Joint Surg Am. 1982;64(9):1328–35.
3. Arima J, Whiteside LA, Martin JW, Miura H, White SE, McCarthy DS. Effect of partial release of the posterior cruciate ligament in total knee arthroplasty. Clin Orthop Relat Res. 1998;353:194–202.
4. Asano H, Hoshino A, Wilton TJ. Soft-tissue tension total knee arthroplasty. J Arthroplasty. 2004;19(5):558–61.
5. Attfield SF, Warren-Forward M, Wilton T, Sambatakakis A. Measurement of soft tissue imbalance in total knee arthroplasty using electronic instrumentation. Med Eng Phys. 1994;16(6):501–5.

6. Becker MW, Insall JN, Faris PM. Bilateral total knee arthroplasty. One cruciate retaining and one cruciate substituting. Clin Orthop Relat Res. 1991;271:122–4.
7. Berger RA, Rubash HE, Seel MJ, Thompson WH, Crossett LS. Determining the rotational alignment of the femoral component in total knee arthroplasty using the epicondylar axis. Clin Orthop Relat Res. 1993;286:40–7.
8. Booth Jr RE. Tensioners: essential for accurate performance of TKA. Orthopedics. 2003;26(9):962–4.
9. Chen AF, Alan RK, Redziniak DE, Tria Jr AJ. Quadriceps sparing total knee replacement. The initial experience with results at two to four years. J Bone Joint Surg Br. 2006;88(11):1448–53. doi:10.1302/0301-620X.88B11.18052.
10. D'Lima DD, Patil S, Steklov N, Colwell Jr CW. The 2011 ABJS Nicolas Andry Award: 'Lab'-in-a-knee: in vivo knee forces, kinematics, and contact analysis. Clin Orthop Relat Res. 2011;469(10):2953–70. doi:10.1007/s11999-011-1916-9.
11. D'Lima DD, Patil S, Steklov N, Slamin JE, Colwell Jr CW. Tibial forces measured in vivo after total knee arthroplasty. J Arthroplasty. 2006;21(2):255–62. doi:10.1016/j.arth.2005.07.011.
12. Dennis DA. Measured resection: an outdated technique in total knee arthroplasty. Orthopedics. 2008;31(9):940, 943-944.
13. Dorr LD, Ochsner JL, Gronley J, Perry J. Functional comparison of posterior cruciate-retained versus cruciate-sacrificed total knee arthroplasty. Clin Orthop Relat Res. 1988;236:36–43.
14. Fehring TK. Rotational malalignment of the femoral component in total knee arthroplasty. Clin Orthop Relat Res. 2000;380:72–9.
15. Fehring TK, Odum S, Griffin WL, Mason JB, Nadaud M. Early failures in total knee arthroplasty. Clin Orthop Relat Res. 2001;392:315–8.
16. Freeman MA, Todd RC, Bamert P, Day WH. ICLH arthroplasty of the knee: 1968--1977. J Bone Joint Surg Br. 1978;60-B(3):339–44.
17. Gejo R, Morita Y, Matsushita I, Sugimori K, Kimura T. Joint gap changes with patellar tendon strain and patellar position during TKA. Clin Orthop Relat Res. 2008;466(4):946–51. doi:10.1007/s11999-008-0154-2.
18. Griffin FM, Insall JN, Scuderi GR. Accuracy of soft tissue balancing in total knee arthroplasty. J Arthroplasty. 2000;15(8):970–3. doi:10.1054/arth.2000.6503.
19. Griffin FM, Math K, Scuderi GR, Insall JN, Poilvache PL. Anatomy of the epicondyles of the distal femur: MRI analysis of normal knees. J Arthroplasty. 2000;15(3):354–9.
20. Haas SB, Cook S, Beksac B. Minimally invasive total knee replacement through a mini midvastus approach: a comparative study. Clin Orthop Relat Res. 2004;428:68–73.
21. Hetaimish BM, Khan MM, Simunovic N, Al-Harbi HH, Bhandari M, Zalzal PK. Meta-analysis of navigation vs conventional total knee arthroplasty. J Arthroplasty. 2012;27(6):1177–82. doi:10.1016/j.arth.2011.12.028.
22. Higuchi H, Hatayama K, Shimizu M, Kobayashi A, Kobayashi T, Takagishi K. Relationship between joint gap difference and range of motion in total knee arthroplasty: a prospective randomised study between different platforms. Int Orthop. 2009;33(4):997–1000. doi:10.1007/s00264-009-0772-7.
23. Hirsch HS, Lotke PA, Morrison LD. The posterior cruciate ligament in total knee surgery. Save, sacrifice, or substitute? Clin Orthop Relat Res. 1994;309:64–8.
24. Insall JN, Binazzi R, Soudry M, Mestriner LA. Total knee arthroplasty. Clin Orthop Relat Res. 1985;192:13–22.
25. Insall JN, Hood RW, Flawn LB, Sullivan DJ. The total condylar knee prosthesis in gonarthrosis. A five to nine-year follow-up of the first one hundred consecutive replacements. J Bone Joint Surg Am. 1983;65(5):619–28.
26. Kamei G, Murakami Y, Kazusa H, Hachisuka S, Inoue H, Nobutou H, Nishida K, Mochizuki Y, Ochi M. Is patella eversion during total knee arthroplasty crucial for gap adjustment and soft-tissue balancing? Orthop Traumatol Surg Res. 2011;97(3):287–91. doi:10.1016/j.otsr.2011.01.004.
27. Kashyap SN, van Ommeren JW. Clinical experience with less invasive surgery techniques in total knee arthroplasty: a comparative study. Knee Surg Sports Traumatol Arthrosc Off J ESSKA. 2008;16(6):544–8. doi:10.1007/s00167-008-0523-0.

28. Katz MA, Beck TD, Silber JS, Seldes RM, Lotke PA. Determining femoral rotational alignment in total knee arthroplasty: reliability of techniques. J Arthroplasty. 2001;16(3):301–5.
29. Kim H, Pelker RR, Gibson DH, Irving JF, Lynch JK. Rollback in posterior cruciate ligament-retaining total knee arthroplasty. A radiographic analysis. J Arthroplasty. 1997;12(5):553–61.
30. Kobayashi T, Suzuki M, Sasho T, Nakagawa K, Tsuneizumi Y, Takahashi K. Lateral laxity in flexion increases the postoperative flexion angle in cruciate-retaining total knee arthroplasty. J Arthroplasty. 2012;27(2):260–5. doi:10.1016/j.arth.2011.04.025.
31. Laskin RS, Beksac B. Computer-assisted navigation in TKA: where we are and where we are going. Clin Orthop Relat Res. 2006;452:127–31. doi:10.1097/01.blo.0000238823.78895.dc.
32. Laskin RS, Beksac B, Phongjunakorn A, Pittors K, Davis J, Shim JC, Pavlov H, Petersen M. Minimally invasive total knee replacement through a mini-midvastus incision: an outcome study. Clin Orthop Relat Res. 2004;428:74–81.
33. Lee HJ, Lee JS, Jung HJ, Song KS, Yang JJ, Park CW. Comparison of joint line position changes after primary bilateral total knee arthroplasty performed using the navigation-assisted measured gap resection or gap balancing techniques. Knee Surg Sports Traumatol Arthrosc Off J ESSKA. 2011;19(12):2027–32. doi:10.1007/s00167-011-1468-2.
34. Lombardi Jr AV, Berend KR, Aziz-Jacobo J, Davis MB. Balancing the flexion gap: relationship between tibial slope and posterior cruciate ligament release and correlation with range of motion. J Bone Joint Surg Am. 2008;90(Suppl 4):121–32. doi:10.2106/JBJS.H.00685.
35. Lombardi Jr AV, Viacava AJ, Berend KR. Rapid recovery protocols and minimally invasive surgery help achieve high knee flexion. Clin Orthop Relat Res. 2006;452:117–22. doi:10.1097/01.blo.0000238824.56024.7a.
36. Luring C, Beckmann J, Haibock P, Perlick L, Grifka J, Tingart M. Minimal invasive and computer assisted total knee replacement compared with the conventional technique: a prospective, randomised trial. Knee Surg Sports Traumatol Arthrosc Off J ESSKA. 2008;16(10):928–34. doi:10.1007/s00167-008-0582-2.
37. Maloney WJ, Schurman DJ. The effects of implant design on range of motion after total knee arthroplasty. Total condylar versus posterior stabilized total condylar designs. Clin Orthop Relat Res. 1992;278:147–52.
38. Mantas JP, Bloebaum RD, Skedros JG, Hofmann AA. Implications of reference axes used for rotational alignment of the femoral component in primary and revision knee arthroplasty. J Arthroplasty. 1992;7(4):531–5.
39. Markolf KL, Mensch JS, Amstutz HC. Stiffness and laxity of the knee--the contributions of the supporting structures. A quantitative in vitro study. J Bone Joint Surg Am. 1976;58(5):583–94.
40. Maruyama S, Yoshiya S, Matsui N, Kuroda R, Kurosaka M. Functional comparison of posterior cruciate-retaining versus posterior stabilized total knee arthroplasty. J Arthroplasty. 2004;19(3):349–53.
41. Matsumoto T, Kubo S, Muratsu H, Matsushita T, Ishida K, Kawakami Y, Oka S, Matsuzaki T, Kuroda Y, Nishida K, Akisue T, Kuroda R, Kurosaka M. Different pattern in gap balancing between the cruciate-retaining and posterior-stabilized total knee arthroplasty. Knee Surg Sports Traumatol Arthrosc Off J ESSKA. 2013;21(10):2338–45. doi:10.1007/s00167-013-2376-4.
42. Matsumoto T, Kuroda R, Kubo S, Muratsu H, Mizuno K, Kurosaka M. The intra-operative joint gap in cruciate-retaining compared with posterior-stabilised total knee replacement. J Bone Joint Surg Br. 2009;91(4):475–80. doi:10.1302/0301-620X.91B4.21862.
43. Matsumoto T, Mizuno K, Muratsu H, Tsumura N, Fukase N, Kubo S, Yoshiya S, Kurosaka M, Kuroda R. Influence of intra-operative joint gap on post-operative flexion angle in osteoarthritis patients undergoing posterior-stabilized total knee arthroplasty. Knee Surg Sports Traumatol Arthrosc Off J ESSKA. 2007;15(8):1013–8. doi:10.1007/s00167-007-0331-y.
44. Matsumoto T, Muratsu H, Kawakami Y, Takayama K, Ishida K, Matsushita T, Akisue T, Nishida K, Kuroda R, Kurosaka M. Soft-tissue balancing in total knee arthroplasty: cruciate-retaining versus posterior-stabilised, and measured-resection versus gap technique. Int Orthop. 2014;38(3):531–7. doi:10.1007/s00264-013-2133-9.

45. Matsumoto T, Muratsu H, Kubo S, Matsushita T, Ishida K, Sasaki H, Oka S, Kurosaka M, Kuroda R. Soft tissue balance using the tibia first gap technique with navigation system in cruciate-retaining total knee arthroplasty. Int Orthop. 2011;36(5):975–80. doi:10.1007/s00264-011-1377-5.
46. Matsumoto T, Muratsu H, Kubo S, Matsushita T, Kurosaka M, Kuroda R. Soft tissue tension in cruciate-retaining and posterior-stabilized total knee arthroplasty. J Arthroplasty. 2011;26(5):788–95. doi:10.1016/j.arth.2010.06.006.
47. Matsumoto T, Muratsu H, Kubo S, Matsushita T, Kurosaka M, Kuroda R. Intraoperative soft tissue balance reflects minimum 5-year midterm outcomes in cruciate-retaining and posterior-stabilized total knee arthroplasty. J Arthroplasty. 2012;27(9):1723–30. doi:10.1016/j.arth.2012.02.020.
48. Matsumoto T, Muratsu H, Kubo S, Mizuno K, Kinoshita K, Ishida K, Matsushita T, Sasaki K, Tei K, Takayama K, Sasaki H, Oka S, Kurosaka M, Kuroda R. Soft tissue balance measurement in minimal incision surgery compared to conventional total knee arthroplasty. Knee Surg Sports Traumatol Arthrosc Off J ESSKA. 2011;19(6):880–6. doi:10.1007/s00167-010-1224-z.
49. Matsumoto T, Muratsu H, Tsumura N, Mizuno K, Kuroda R, Yoshiya S, Kurosaka M. Joint gap kinematics in posterior-stabilized total knee arthroplasty measured by a new tensor with the navigation system. J Biomech Eng. 2006;128(6):867–71. doi:10.1115/1.2354201.
50. Matsumoto T, Muratsu H, Tsumura N, Mizuno K, Kurosaka M, Kuroda R. Soft tissue balance measurement in posterior-stabilized total knee arthroplasty with a navigation system. J Arthroplasty. 2009;24(3):358–64. doi:10.1016/j.arth.2008.01.001.
51. Matsumoto T, Takayama K, Muratsu H, Matsushita T, Kuroda R, Kurosaka M. Semimembranosus release reduces tibial internal rotation and flexion angle in cruciate-retaining total knee arthroplasty. J Arthroplasty. 2015;30(9):1537–41. doi:10.1016/j.arth.2015.03.039.
52. Matsuzaki T, Matsumoto T, Kubo S, Muratsu H, Matsushita T, Kawakami Y, Ishida K, Oka S, Kuroda R, Kurosaka M. Tibial internal rotation is affected by lateral laxity in cruciate-retaining total knee arthroplasty: an intraoperative kinematic study using a navigation system and offset-type tensor. Knee Surg Sports Traumatol Arthrosc Off J ESSKA. 2014;22(3):615–20. doi:10.1007/s00167-013-2627-4.
53. Matsuzaki T, Matsumoto T, Muratsu H, Kubo S, Matsushita T, Kawakami Y, Ishida K, Oka S, Kuroda R, Kurosaka M. Kinematic factors affecting postoperative knee flexion after cruciate-retaining total knee arthroplasty. Int Orthop. 2013;37(5):803–8. doi:10.1007/s00264-013-1803-y.
54. Mihalko WM, Whiteside LA, Krackow KA. Comparison of ligament-balancing techniques during total knee arthroplasty. J Bone Joint Surg Am. 2003;85-A(Suppl 4):132–5.
55. Mitsuyasu H, Matsuda S, Fukagawa S, Okazaki K, Tashiro Y, Kawahara S, Nakahara H, Iwamoto Y. Enlarged post-operative posterior condyle tightens extension gap in total knee arthroplasty. J Bone Joint Surg Br. 2011;93(9):1210–6. doi:10.1302/0301-620X.93B9.25822.
56. Moore TM, Meyers MH, Harvey Jr JP. Collateral ligament laxity of the knee. Long-term comparison between plateau fractures and normal. J Bone Joint Surg Am. 1976;58(5):594–8.
57. Morris BA, D'Lima DD, Slamin J, Kovacevic N, Arms SW, Townsend CP, Colwell Jr CW. e-Knee: evolution of the electronic knee prosthesis. Telemetry technology development. J Bone Joint Surg Am. 2001;83-A Suppl 2(Pt 1):62–6.
58. Muratsu H, Matsumoto T, Kubo S, Maruo A, Miya H, Kurosaka M, Kuroda R. Femoral component placement changes soft tissue balance in posterior-stabilized total knee arthroplasty. Clin Biomech (Bristol, Avon). 2010;25(9):926–30. doi:10.1016/j.clinbiomech.2010.06.020.
59. Muratsu H, Tsumura N, Yamaguchi M, Mizuno K, Kuroda R, Kurosaka M. Patellar eversion affects soft tissue balance in total knee arthroplasty. Trans Orthop Res. 2003;28:242.
60. Nakano N, Matsumoto T, Muratsu H, Takayama K, Kuroda R, Kurosaka M. Postoperative knee flexion angle is affected by lateral laxity in cruciate-retaining total knee arthroplasty. J Arthroplasty. 2015;31(2):401–5. doi:10.1016/j.arth.2015.09.028.

61. Niki Y, Takeda Y, Kanagawa H, Iwamoto W, Matsumoto H, Enomoto H, Toyama Y, Suda Y. Effects of four different surgical approaches on intra-operative joint gap in posterior-stabilized total knee arthroplasty. Knee Surg Sports Traumatol Arthrosc Off J ESSKA. 2011;20(10):2026–31. doi:10.1007/s00167-011-1813-5.
62. Oka S, Muratsu H, Matsumoto T, Kubo S, Maruo A, Miya H, Kuroda R, Kurosaka M. The influence of patellar position on soft tissue balance in minimal incision total knee arthroplasty. Knee Surg Sports Traumatol Arthrosc Off J ESSKA. 2011;20(6):1064–8. doi:10.1007/s00167-011-1642-6.
63. Pagnano MW, Meneghini RM, Trousdale RT. Anatomy of the extensor mechanism in reference to quadriceps-sparing TKA. Clin Orthop Relat Res. 2006;452:102–5. doi:10.1097/01.blo.0000238788.44349.0f.
64. Pang HN, Yeo SJ, Chong HC, Chin PL, Ong J, Lo NN. Computer-assisted gap balancing technique improves outcome in total knee arthroplasty, compared with conventional measured resection technique. Knee Surg Sports Traumatol Arthrosc Off J ESSKA. 2011;19(9):1496–503. doi:10.1007/s00167-011-1483-3.
65. Paxton EW, Furnes O, Namba RS, Inacio MC, Fenstad AM, Havelin LI. Comparison of the Norwegian knee arthroplasty register and a United States arthroplasty registry. J Bone Joint Surg Am. 2011;93(Suppl 3):20–30. doi:10.2106/JBJS.K.01045.
66. Poilvache PL, Insall JN, Scuderi GR, Font-Rodriguez DE. Rotational landmarks and sizing of the distal femur in total knee arthroplasty. Clin Orthop Relat Res. 1996;331:35–46.
67. Ritter MA, Faris PM, Keating EM. Posterior cruciate ligament balancing during total knee arthroplasty. J Arthroplasty. 1988;3(4):323–6.
68. Roberts VI, Mereddy PK, Donnachie NJ, Hakkalamani S. Anatomical variations in vastus medialis obliquus and its implications in minimally-invasive total knee replacement. An MRI study. J Bone Joint Surg Br. 2007;89(11):1462–5. doi:10.1302/0301-620X.89B11.18636.
69. Sambatakakis A, Attfield SF, Newton G. Quantification of soft-tissue imbalance in condylar knee arthroplasty. J Biomed Eng. 1993;15(4):339–43.
70. Schnurr C, Nessler J, Konig DP. Is referencing the posterior condyles sufficient to achieve a rectangular flexion gap in total knee arthroplasty? Int Orthop. 2009;33(6):1561–5. doi:10.1007/s00264-008-0656-2.
71. Schroer WC, Diesfeld PJ, Reedy ME, LeMarr AR. Isokinetic strength testing of minimally invasive total knee arthroplasty recovery. J Arthroplasty. 2010;25(2):274–9. doi:10.1016/j.arth.2008.09.017.
72. Seering WP, Piziali RL, Nagel DA, Schurman DJ. The function of the primary ligaments of the knee in varus-valgus and axial rotation. J Biomech. 1980;13(9):785–94.
73. Seon JK, Song EK, Park SJ, Lee DS. The use of navigation to obtain rectangular flexion and extension gaps during primary total knee arthroplasty and midterm clinical results. J Arthroplasty. 2011;26(4):582–90. doi:10.1016/j.arth.2010.04.030.
74. Sharkey PF, Hozack WJ, Rothman RH, Shastri S, Jacoby SM. Insall Award paper. Why are total knee arthroplasties failing today? Clin Orthop Relat Res. 2002;404:7–13.
75. Sugama R, Kadoya Y, Kobayashi A, Takaoka K. Preparation of the flexion gap affects the extension gap in total knee arthroplasty. J Arthroplasty. 2005;20(5):602–7. doi:10.1016/j.arth.2003.12.085.
76. Takayama K, Matsumoto T, Kubo S, Muratsu H, Ishida K, Matsushita T, Kurosaka M, Kuroda R. Influence of intra-operative joint gaps on post-operative flexion angle in posterior cruciate-retaining total knee arthroplasty. Knee Surg Sports Traumatol Arthrosc Off J ESSKA. 2011;20(3):532–7. doi:10.1007/s00167-011-1594-x.
77. Tanaka K, Muratsu H, Mizuno K, Kuroda R, Yoshiya S, Kurosaka M. Soft tissue balance measurement in anterior cruciate ligament-resected knee joint: cadaveric study as a model for cruciate-retaining total knee arthroplasty. J Orthop Sci Off J Jpn Orthop Assoc. 2007;12(2):149–53. doi:10.1007/s00776-006-1108-8.
78. Tigani D, Sabbioni G, Ben Ayad R, Filanti M, Rani N, Del Piccolo N. Comparison between two computer-assisted total knee arthroplasty: gap-balancing versus measured resection tech-

nique. Knee Surg Sports Traumatol Arthrosc Off J ESSKA. 2010;18(10):1304–10. doi:10.1007/s00167-010-1124-2.

79. Tokuhara Y, Kadoya Y, Kanekasu K, Kondo M, Kobayashi A, Takaoka K. Evaluation of the flexion gap by axial radiography of the distal femur. J Bone Joint Surg Br. 2006;88(10):1327–30. doi:10.1302/0301-620X.88B10.17793.
80. Tokuhara Y, Kadoya Y, Nakagawa S, Kobayashi A, Takaoka K. The flexion gap in normal knees. An MRI study. J Bone Joint Surg Br. 2004;86(8):1133–6.
81. Tria Jr AJ. Advancements in minimally invasive total knee arthroplasty. Orthopedics. 2003;26(8 Suppl):s859–63.
82. Tria Jr AJ, Coon TM. Minimal incision total knee arthroplasty: early experience. Clin Orthop Relat Res. 2003;416:185–90. doi:10.1097/01.blo.0000093030.56370.d9.
83. Udomkiat P, Meng BJ, Dorr LD, Wan Z. Functional comparison of posterior cruciate retention and substitution knee replacement. Clin Orthop Relat Res. 2000;378:192–201.
84. Unitt L, Sambatakakis A, Johnstone D, Briggs TW. Short-term outcome in total knee replacement after soft-tissue release and balancing. J Bone Joint Surg Br. 2008;90(2):159–65. doi:10.1302/0301-620X.90B2.19327.
85. Viskontas DG, Skrinskas TV, Johnson JA, King GJ, Winemaker MJ, Chess DG. Computer-assisted gap equalization in total knee arthroplasty. J Arthroplasty. 2007;22(3):334–42. doi:10.1016/j.arth.2006.05.018.
86. Wasielewski RC, Galat DD, Komistek RD. Correlation of compartment pressure data from an intraoperative sensing device with postoperative fluoroscopic kinematic results in TKA patients. J Biomech. 2005;38(2):333–9. doi:10.1016/j.jbiomech.2004.02.040.
87. Whiteside LA, Arima J. The anteroposterior axis for femoral rotational alignment in valgus total knee arthroplasty. Clin Orthop Relat Res. 1995;321:168–72.
88. Winemaker MJ. Perfect balance in total knee arthroplasty: the elusive compromise. J Arthroplasty. 2002;17(1):2–10.
89. Yagishita K, Muneta T, Ikeda H. Step-by-step measurements of soft tissue balancing during total knee arthroplasty for patients with varus knees. J Arthroplasty. 2003;18(3):313–20. doi:10.1054/arth.2003.50088.
90. Yamakado K, Kitaoka K, Yamada H, Hashiba K, Nakamura R, Tomita K. Influence of stability on range of motion after cruciate-retaining TKA. Arch Orthop Trauma Surg. 2003;123(1):1–4. doi:10.1007/s00402-002-0453-0.
91. Yoshino N, Watanabe N, Watanabe Y, Fukuda Y, Takai S. Measurement of joint gap load in patella everted and reset position during total knee arthroplasty. Knee Surg Sports Traumatol Arthrosc Off J ESSKA. 2009;17(5):484–90. doi:10.1007/s00167-008-0656-1.

Intraoperative Assessment with Computer Navigation

14

Gianmarco V.M. Regazzola and Myles R.J. Coolican

Contents

14.1 Introduction

Soft tissue balancing in total knee replacement (TKR) is paramount to obtain optimal stability of the joint, improve kinematics, produce equal load on each side of the prosthetic components and decrease component wear [1].

There is some variation between registry data and published literature in the prevalence of instability as a cause for revision TKR. In the Australian Orthopaedic Association National Joint Replacement Registry (AOANJRR), instability represents only 6.3% of revisions, whilst this figure is 12% in the Swedish Knee Arthroplasty Register 2015, 16% in the British National Joint Registry (NJR) and 12.4% in the Canadian Joint Replacement Registry. Case series suggest the incidence for revision for instability could be much higher – 22% in one large series [2].

Irrespective of variations in incidence of instability leading to revision, it is a scenario which both surgeon and patient wish to avoid. The clinical and economic

G.V.M. Regazzola, MD • M.R.J. Coolican, MB, BS, FRACS, FAOrthA (✉)
Sydney Orthopaedic Research Institute, 445 Victoria Avenue,
Chatswood, 2067 NSW, Australia
e-mail: myles@mylescoolican.com.au

S. Matsuda et al. (eds.), *Soft Tissue Balancing in Total Knee Arthroplasty*,
DOI 10.1007/978-3-662-54082-4_14

implications for revision surgery in TKR have been estimated. Over 55,000 revisions were performed in 2010 in the USA, with 48% of these revisions on patients under 65 years [3]. By 2030, nearly two in three TKA revision patients will be under 65 years, including almost 120,000 patients under 54 years who will likely experience device failure at least once in their lifetime [4]. Minimising or avoiding revision TKR makes clear economic sense.

Computer-assisted surgery for TKR (CAS-TKR) is well established in total knee arthroplasty. It improves accuracy of both tibial and femoral component placement and optimises coronal alignment within 3° of neutral when compared to conventional instrumentation [5–8]. Deviation in coronal alignment of more than 3° of varus or valgus has been correlated with poorer results [9]. Conversely, functional and quality-of-life outcomes are significantly better in patients with mechanical axis within 3° of neutral [10]. Furthermore, a lower revision rate has been reported in the Australian Orthopaedic Association National Joint Replacement Registry in patients under 65 years old [11]. Despite the significant improvement with alignment and survivorship that CAS affords with navigated bony cuts, soft tissue and ligament balancing in TKR continues to present a challenge.

Computer navigation does more than produce accurate bone cuts – it also plays an important role in obtaining real-time data intraoperatively on alignment, range of motion and stability, reducing malalignment and achieving a well-aligned and well-balanced TKR. The surgeon is made well aware of the deformities to be corrected before any bony cuts are made; in particular, the size of a flexion contracture is quantified – something not always visually clear particularly in the morbidly obese. The information can be utilised to minimally adjust bony cuts or implant size to achieve correction of a flexion contracture and balance the knee, with a subsequent decrease in the risk of revision and the associated economic burden.

14.2 Ligament Balancing in TKR

Most surgeons rely on tactile evaluation of the knee when addressing ligament balancing issues during TKR, checking whether the knee fully extends with trial implants in situ and confirming coronal plane stability by applying a varus and valgus stress to the knee in full extension and at different degrees of flexion. Specifically, whilst applying force to the joint, the surgeon evaluates the amount of gapping in each compartment with palpation of ligaments under tension. A relative feel of the joint determines whether the joint is 'loose', 'tight' or satisfactorily stable. Following this, soft tissue releases are performed as necessary to obtain a stable and well-balanced joint. The literature describes two techniques for ligament balancing in TKR – gap-balancing and measured resection technique.

14.2.1 Gap-Balancing Technique

The gap-balancing technique relies on ligament releases prior to and during bony cuts. Correction of fixed deformity is obtained with ligament releases whilst the limb is in the approximate correct alignment before determining femoral component rotation [12]. Gap balancing initially creates a rectangular flexion space with the plane of the tibial cut determining femoral component rotation. Following resection of the distal femur, this rectangular flexion space matches the extension space. Thus equal flexion and extension rectangular gaps are created based on the plane of the bony cuts and the tension of the ligaments. Spaces are checked with rectangular spacer blocks with or without a tensiometer in both flexion and extension.

A perpendicular tibial cut is crucial for the gap-balancing technique. A varus tibial cut will result in an internally rotated femoral component, whilst a valgus cut will result in an externally rotated femoral component [13]. In addition, an over- or under-resection of the femur can produce a mismatch between flexion and extension gaps with consequent ligament imbalance. Furthermore, integrity of the medial and lateral collateral ligaments are crucial for precise ligament balancing.

14.2.2 Measured Resection Technique

Measured resection technique relies on bony landmarks to determine femoral component rotation. Bony cuts are performed independent of soft tissue tension, and ligament balancing is addressed after trial components are implanted. The surgical landmarks to determine femoral rotation are: [14] [15]

- Anteroposterior axis (AP) – often referred to as Whiteside's line: This is a line drawn between the deepest point of the trochlear groove anteriorly and the centre of the notch posteriorly.
- Surgical transepicondylar axis (TEA): This is a line drawn from the lateral femoral epicondyle to the sulcus of the medial femoral epicondyle at the insertion of the fibres of the deep portion of the medial collateral ligament. This line is perpendicular to Whiteside's line and externally rotated to the posterior condylar axis.
- Posterior condyle axis (PCA): This is the line drawn on the most prominent points of the posterior femoral condyles, and it is internally rotated to the TEA of a mean of 3.5° (±1.2°) for males and a mean of 0.3° (±1.2°) for females.

Olcott and Scott [16] evaluated in 100 consecutive TKRs the consistency of the AP, TEA and PCA in providing a balanced and symmetric flexion space. Transepicondylar appeared to be the most accurate reference for femoral component rotation, producing a balanced symmetric flexion space in 90% of cases with a deviation of <3°. The least accurate referencing landmark was the PCA, with an accuracy of 70%, whereas AP axis was accurate in 83% of cases to within 3° of deviation from a symmetric flexion gap [16]. However, identifying the TEA can be difficult during surgery, and some authors have challenged the accuracy of these landmarks [17]. Moreover, AP and PCA axis can be inaccurate due to trochlear dysplasia, chondral wear or posterior condyle bony erosion as seen in severe varus or valgus malalignment [18, 19].

14.3 Measured Resection with CAS

Computer navigation has been shown to be an excellent tool to deliver a well-functioning and well-aligned prosthesis, improving implant survivorship and conferring greater accuracy when compared to conventional techniques. In a randomised controlled trial, Choong et al. [10] compared the alignment obtained with CAS to conventional technique and correlated alignment with knee function and quality of life. Alignment in the CAS group was more accurate with 88% within 3° of neutral when compared to 33% of the conventional group when measured using full-leg standing radiographs. There was a significant difference in alignment between CAS and conventional in an obese subgroup with the postoperative mechanical axis within 3° of neutral in 93% of the cases with CAS and 57% with conventional technique.

However, femoral rotation assessed with CT scanning did not demonstrate a significant difference between CAS and conventional alignment. In addition, outcomes are improved with more accurate surgery. Irrespective of surgical technique, patients within 3° of neutral alignment obtained significantly better IKS and SF-12 scores highlighting the importance of achieving optimal alignment. In a meta-analysis performed on 16 high-quality studies, Hetaimish and colleagues [8] reported that coronal alignment with CAS is more accurate compared to conventional. However, again there was no difference detected in femoral rotation. In summary, CAS in TKR demonstrates a statistically significant improvement in implant alignment in the coronal and sagittal planes, but not in the axial plane.

14.3.1 Surgical Technique

Patients receive a spinal anaesthesia if possible with sedation or a light general anaesthesia. Spinal anaesthesia lowers arterial and venous blood pressure, reducing blood loss if a tourniquet is not utilised. In combination with periarticular injections, it provides effective postoperative pain relief in the first 24 h and eliminates the need for intraarticular pain pumps or peripheral nerve blocks [20–22]. A tourniquet is positioned but not inflated – this reduces total blood loss and thrombosis, reduces postoperative pain and improves quadriceps recovery [23]. Examination under anaesthesia is performed to evaluate fixed flexion deformity, stability and correctibility of the coronal plane deformity as well as the integrity of the PCL.

Bi-cortical pins for computer navigation are positioned into the distal femur and proximal tibia, and after joint exposure, landmarks are registered and recorded. The surgeon evaluates the passive range of motion, alignment and stability which allows planning of the femoral and tibial cuts in order to achieve full extension, matching flexion and extension spaces whilst optimising soft tissue balancing.

Femoral cuts are performed first. The amount of bone resected from the distal femur matches the implant thickness, and it is referenced to the lesser worn femoral condyle. In some situations an extra 1–1.5 mm bone can be resected with a prodigious flexion contracture particularly when other circumstances are not favourable to correct a flexion contracture. The presence of large posterior osteophytes or a femur whose anteroposterior diameter is well above a size (but not large enough for the next size up) will assist in correcting a flexion contracture by shortening the excursion of the posterior capsule, and extra distal resection may be not necessary. Computer navigation provides this information before cuts are made. We typically make a femoral cut perpendicular to the mechanical axis at 3° degrees of flexion or as recommended by the manufacturer. Flexion of the femoral component over 3° increases the risk of fixed flexion deformity by a factor of 2.9 [24].

Rotation and sizing are determined with computer navigation – the surgeon may reference from the TEA or AP axis of PCA or he/she may choose an average of some or all. Manual sizing and rotation reference guides may also be used. Navigation displays the amount of posterior condylar bone to be resected so the surgeon may position the femoral component optimally. Following completion of femoral cuts, the thickness of bony offcuts are measured, recorded and compared to navigation data.

The tibial cut is navigated perpendicular to the tibial axis, with the depth of cut being determined by chosen reference points. For most varus knees, we utilise the apex of the lateral tibial plateau, but the reference point can be varied both medially and laterally depending on bone loss. Planned cut depth may be reviewed with a stylus. Posterior slope is matched to the manufacturer's guidance. Following removal of osteophytes and periarticular local anaesthetic injections, a trial baseplate is positioned using a size that achieves optimal coverage without overhang, and it is rotated parallel to a line between the junction of the middle and medial third of the tibial tubercle and the centre of the PCL.

With trial implants in place, alignment and extension are evaluated with navigation and laxity of the knee to varus and valgus at full extension and at 90° of flexion checked (Fig. 14.1). Typically, a knee in full extension will allow 1–1.5° of angulation into varus and into valgus (Figs. 14.2 and 14.3). In the setting where a knee

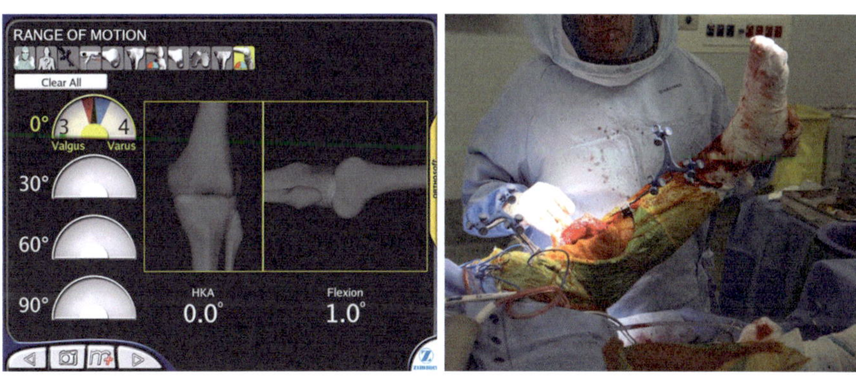

Fig. 14.1 Limb is held by the foot and elevated. There is a 1° flexion contracture with optimal alignment. Note the limb appears fully extended

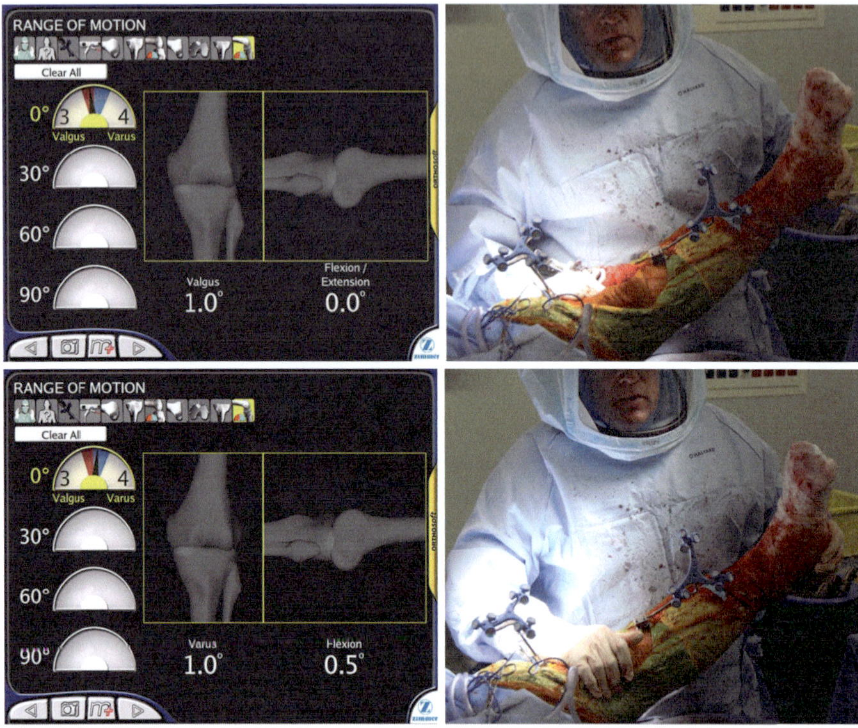

Figs. 14.2 and 14.3 Surgeon evaluates soft tissue balancing in extension applying a valgus and varus force at or close to 0° of flexion

rests in 2–3° flexion with gravity, tightening the posterior capsule whilst forcing full extension to evaluate play in full extension will artificially reduce coronal plane deviation, and comparative figures for varus/valgus play are best performed at the angle that the knee rests with gravity alone. At 90° a knee would typically rest in 3° of varus if a navigation system utilises the PCA to determine the coronal plane with 3° of varus representing 3°of external rotation of the femoral component. A varus force at 90° will deviate the knee into approximately 7° or 8° of varus and be within a degree or two of neutral when a valgus force is applied but usually stays in varus. The total excursion at 90° is in the vicinity of 6–8°, and in the author's experience, a total excursion of less than 4° at 90° flexion is associated with an excessively tight flexion space. In this setting, patients will complain of the knee feeling too tight unless ligaments are released or more bone is resected (Figs. 14.4 and 14.5). Data obtained from navigation allows correct balancing usually by pie crusting of tight structures utilising Whiteside's technique [25].

Whilst optimal balancing is often appreciated as a tactile phenomenon by ligament palpation, applying a consistent but approximately similar varus and valgus force at different degrees of flexion generates an objective and consistent measurement of the amount of play within the joint (Fig. 14.6).

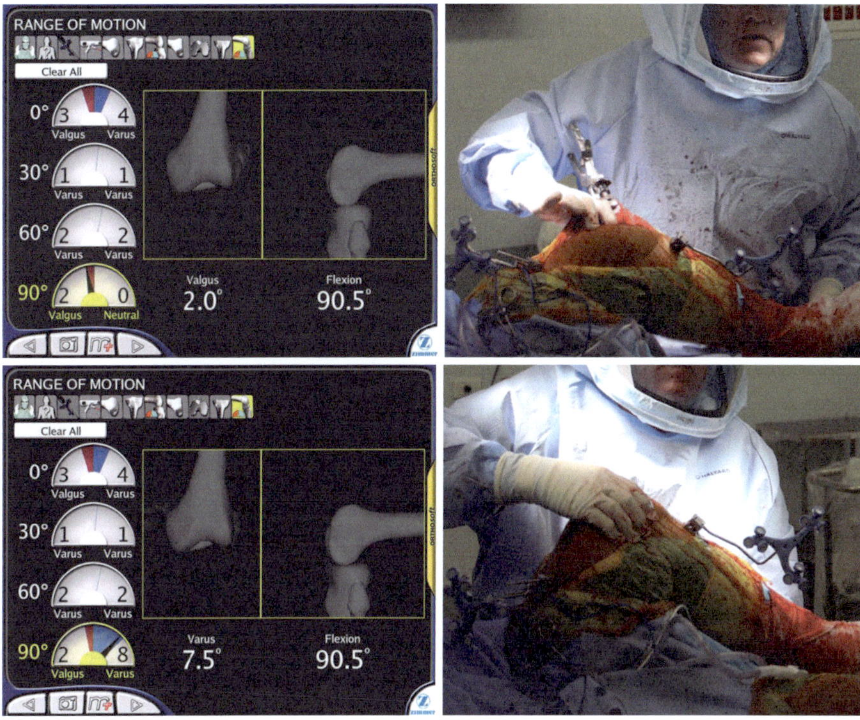

Figs. 14.4 and 14.5 Surgeon evaluates the soft tissue balancing at 90° of flexion applying a varus and valgus force

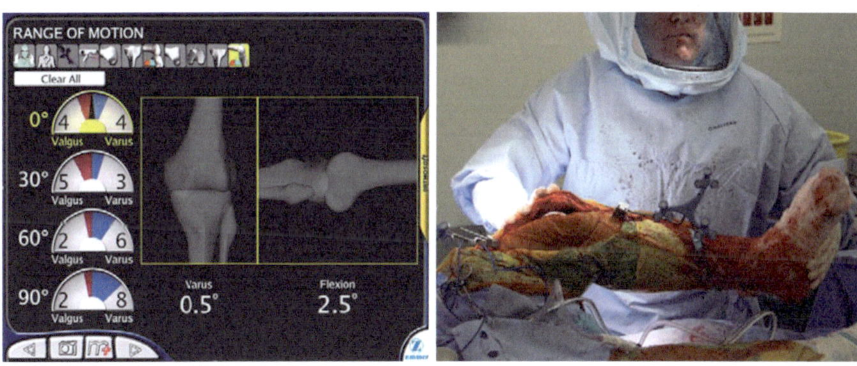

Fig. 14.6 Figures captured on the left side of the screen show the play in degrees reflecting soft tissue balancing along the arc of motion

14.3.2 Outcomes

We acknowledge correct performance of a TKR requires more than the accurate bony cuts delivered by navigation. Soft tissue balancing is paramount in the delivery of a satisfied patient and a symptom-free arthroplasty. Traditionally, surgeons manually assess soft tissue balance based upon their experience and their tactile sense that a ligament that is too tight or too loose. Whilst this technique is easily taught, it is neither measurable nor precisely reproducible from surgeon to surgeon. Several devices have been designed to measure and evaluate soft tissue tension and balancing – these include tensors, spacers and a recently introduced pressure-sensitive micro-electric instrument [3, 13, 26]. We prefer to measure laxity and balancing with navigation data and have utilised data from computer navigation for the past 10 years for real-time information on extension, flexion and joint play with gratifying results. We acknowledge that whilst computer navigation provides a reproducible and objective measurement of soft tissue balancing, the desirable and acceptable gaps in the medial and lateral compartments along the flexion arc remain yet to be determined and may be variable between patients with different degrees of ligamentous laxity.

In a case series of 90 TKRs, Saragaglia et al. [27] evaluated the role of computer navigation to predict whether soft tissue release would be required in TKR. Fully correctable deformities as shown with navigation were identified, and releases that may have been routinely performed were avoided. The incidence of medial release for genu varum was 17.6% compared with Engh's estimated incidence of greater than 50% [28].

Matsumoto et al. compared computer navigation with a ligament tensor for soft tissue balancing in 30 TKRs analysing at 0° and 90° of flexion and confirmed the accuracy of computer navigation for soft tissue assessment when compared to tensors, without a statistically significant difference between the two methods [29]. In a randomised controlled trial, Joseph et al. [30] demonstrated that computer navigation is more accurate than conventional techniques for soft tissue balancing of the mediolateral extension space, utilising navigation software as a gold standard, but not the flexion space nor between the flexion and extension spaces.

Song et al. [31] reported a comparative study of medial and lateral laxity utilising stress radiographs on 86 conventional and navigated TKRs. They found no significant difference between the groups with an average of 3.5° laxity to valgus force and 4.4° for varus at full extension in the navigated group and, respectively, 4.0° and 4.2° in the conventional group. Similarly there was no significant difference in HSS scores and final range of motion between conventional and navigated knees.

Pang et al. [32] demonstrated more precise soft tissue balancing with computer-assisted surgery than conventional balancing. They demonstrated improved function scores in the navigated group at 6 months and 2 years, lower rates of residual flexion contracture and less malalignment outliers.

14.4 Summary

The role of computer navigation in TKR is well established in the literature and is the most accurate means of obtaining desired alignment in the sagittal and coronal planes. Its role in soft tissue balancing is more recent with the use of navigation data allowing the surgeon to recognise imbalance including mid flexion instability, tightness in flexion, failure to resolve flexion contractures and persisting pathological recurvatum.

Navigation-derived information allows the surgeon a real-time assessment across the entire flexion arc, and, importantly, objective measurements enable the surgeon to then address abnormalities revealed by navigation that may otherwise compromise the patient's outcome and confirm resolution before the patient leaves the operating room.

References

1. Seon JK et al. In vivo stability of total knee arthroplasty using a navigation system. Int Orthop. 2007;31(1):45–8.
2. Sharkey PF et al. Insall award paper. Why are total knee arthroplasties failing today? Clin Orthop Relat Res. 2002;404:7–13.
3. Roche M, Elson L, Anderson C. Dynamic soft tissue balancing in total knee arthroplasty. Orthop Clin North Am. 2014;45(2):157–65.
4. Kurtz SM et al. Future young patient demand for primary and revision joint replacement: national projections from 2010 to 2030. Clin Orthop Relat Res. 2009;467(10):2606–12.
5. Blakeney WG, Khan RJ, Wall SJ. Computer-assisted techniques versus conventional guides for component alignment in total knee arthroplasty: a randomized controlled trial. J Bone Joint Surg Am. 2011;93(15):1377–84.
6. Matziolis G et al. A prospective, randomized study of computer-assisted and conventional total knee arthroplasty. Three-dimensional evaluation of implant alignment and rotation. J Bone Joint Surg Am. 2007;89(2):236–43.
7. Decking R et al. Leg axis after computer-navigated total knee arthroplasty: a prospective randomized trial comparing computer-navigated and manual implantation. J Arthroplasty. 2005;20(3):282–8.
8. Hetaimish BM et al. Meta-analysis of navigation vs conventional total knee arthroplasty. J Arthroplasty. 2012;27(6):1177–82.
9. Jeffery RS, Morris RW, Denham RA. Coronal alignment after total knee replacement. J Bone Joint Surg Br. 1991;73(5):709–14.
10. Choong PF, Dowsey MM, Stoney JD. Does accurate anatomical alignment result in better function and quality of life? Comparing conventional and computer-assisted total knee arthroplasty. J Arthroplasty. 2009;24(4):560–9.
11. de Steiger RN, Liu YL, Graves SE. Computer navigation for total knee arthroplasty reduces revision rate for patients less than sixty-five years of age. J Bone Joint Surg Am. 2015;97(8):635–42.
12. Griffin FM, Insall JN, Scuderi GR. Accuracy of soft tissue balancing in total knee arthroplasty. J Arthroplasty. 2000;15(8):970–3.
13. Dennis DA et al. Gap balancing versus measured resection technique for total knee arthroplasty. Clin Orthop Relat Res. 2010;468(1):102–7.
14. Arima J et al. Femoral rotational alignment, based on the anteroposterior axis, in total knee arthroplasty in a valgus knee. A technical note. J Bone Joint Surg Am. 1995;77(9):1331–4.
15. Berger RA et al. Determining the rotational alignment of the femoral component in total knee arthroplasty using the epicondylar axis. Clin Orthop Relat Res. 1993;286:40–7.
16. Olcott CW, Scott RD. A comparison of 4 intraoperative methods to determine femoral component rotation during total knee arthroplasty. J Arthroplasty. 2000;15(1):22–6.
17. Jerosch J et al. Interindividual reproducibility in perioperative rotational alignment of femoral components in knee prosthetic surgery using the transepicondylar axis. Knee Surg Sports Traumatol Arthrosc. 2002;10(3):194–7.

18. Poilvache PL et al. Rotational landmarks and sizing of the distal femur in total knee arthroplasty. Clin Orthop Relat Res. 1996;331:35–46.
19. Griffin FM, Insall JN, Scuderi GR. The posterior condylar angle in osteoarthritic knees. J Arthroplasty. 1998;13(7):812–5.
20. Parker DA et al. Safety of combined use of local anesthetic infiltration and reinfusion drains in total knee arthroplasty. J Arthroplasty. 2009;24(6):918–24.
21. Widmer B et al. Incidence and severity of complications due to femoral nerve blocks performed for knee surgery. Knee. 2013;20(3):181–5.
22. Widmer BJ et al. Is femoral nerve block necessary during total knee arthroplasty?: a randomized controlled trial. J Arthroplasty. 2012;27(10):1800–5.
23. Smith TO, Hing CB. Is a tourniquet beneficial in total knee replacement surgery? A meta-analysis and systematic review. Knee. 2010;17(2):141–7.
24. Lustig S et al. Sagittal placement of the femoral component in total knee arthroplasty predicts knee flexion contracture at one-year follow-up. Int Orthop. 2012;36(9):1835–9.
25. Whiteside LA. Soft tissue balancing: the knee. J Arthroplasty. 2002;17(4 Suppl 1):23–7.
26. Nodzo SR, Franceschini V, Gonzalez Della Valle A. Intraoperative load-sensing variability during cemented, posterior-stabilized total knee arthroplasty. J Arthroplasty. 2017;32(1):66–70.
27. Saragaglia D, Chaussard C, Rubens-Duval B. Navigation as a predictor of soft tissue release during 90 cases of computer-assisted total knee arthroplasty. Orthopedics. 2006;29(10 Suppl):S137–8.
28. Engh GA. The difficult knee: severe varus and valgus. Clin Orthop Relat Res. 2003;416:58–63.
29. Matsumoto T et al. Soft tissue balance measurement in posterior-stabilized total knee arthroplasty with a navigation system. J Arthroplasty. 2009;24(3):358–64.
30. Joseph J et al. The use of navigation to achieve soft tissue balance in total knee arthroplasty - a randomised clinical study. Knee. 2013;20(6):401–6.
31. Song EK et al. Comparative study of stability after total knee arthroplasties between navigation system and conventional techniques. J Arthroplasty. 2007;22(8):1107–11.
32. Pang HN et al. Computer-assisted gap balancing technique improves outcome in total knee arthroplasty, compared with conventional measured resection technique. Knee Surg Sports Traumatol Arthrosc. 2011;19(9):1496–503.

Part V

Clinical Relevance: Primary TKA

Postoperative Changes in Soft Tissue Balance

15

Hitoshi Sekiya

Contents

15.1 Introduction

The goal of total knee arthroplasty (TKA) is to achieve a stable and well-balanced knee with good alignment, with the aim of a good clinical result and patient satisfaction in the long term [1–3]. Instability due to ligament imbalance has been described as a possible preventable cause of revision TKA. Fehring et al. studied 279 revision surgeries within 5 years of their index TKA and reported 74 revision cases (27%) caused by instability [4].

H. Sekiya
Department of Orthopaedic Surgery, Shin-Kaminokawa Hospital,
Kaminokawa Town, Tochigi, Japan
e-mail: hsekiya@jichi.ac.jp

S. Matsuda et al. (eds.), *Soft Tissue Balancing in Total Knee Arthroplasty*,
DOI 10.1007/978-3-662-54082-4_15

15.2 Classical Concept of Ideal Soft Tissue Balancing in TKA

The goal of ideal soft tissue balancing remains unclear. The classical concept of TKA is to achieve equal medial and lateral rectangular gaps, as well as equal flexion and extension gaps [4, 5]. Theoretically, a rectangular gap in extension and flexion minimizes the disequilibrium of the load to the implants and provides the advantage of less damage for the surrounding soft tissue and the tibial insert. The classical concept of balancing by rectangular gaps had been advocated as the key to successful TKA [5, 6].

15.3 Intraoperative Soft Tissue Balance in TKA

However, even in normal knees, lateral and medial ligamentous laxities are not equal [7–9]. A cadaveric study using computer navigation by Van Mamme et al. [10] confirmed the typical kinematic feature of ligament function by noting 2–3° of laxity in extension, which increased to 6–8° degrees when measured in flexion, with more laxity in the lateral compartment.

The medial soft tissues are shortened more in varus knees, whereas the lateral soft tissues are lax preoperatively compared to normally aligned knees [3, 11]. To achieve a rectangular gap in extension and flexion, the medial soft tissue must be released to the level of the lateral side. However, achieving a perfect balance both in extension and flexion has been extremely difficult [12–15]. Excessive medial release to create a rectangular gap in extension has often resulted in a wide medial gap in flexion [16, 17]. Furthermore, the greater the preoperative varus deformity, the more lateral laxity that remained after TKA [18]. In recent years, many researchers have reported that a small amount of lateral laxity in TKA is not hazardous, but that it was related to a good clinical result [19, 20].

15.4 Soft Tissue Balance in TKA Over the Long Term

Thus, in TKA, a few more degrees of lateral laxity than medial laxity was thought to be acceptable intraoperatively [19, 20]. If lateral laxity compared to the medial side at TKA did not change after the surgery, more laxity should always be found at the lateral side even a long time after TKA.

Ishii et al. [21] measured coronal laxity in 71 well-functioning TKAs 5–9 years after surgery using a Telos arthrometer (Fa Telos, Medizinisch-Technische, Griesheim, Germany) with a force of 150 N with the knee flexed from 0° to 20°. The mean values of medial laxity were 4.6–4.8° and of lateral laxity were 4.0–4.5° [21]. They stated that laxity of approximately 4° was suitable in TKA for a satisfactory clinical outcome.

There have been several reports about the changes in coronal laxity in TKA at 3 months or more after the surgery [7, 18, 21–24]. All studies used a Telos arthrometer to apply the external force for valgus or varus stress to the knee. Some variations existed in the degree of the external force (70–150 N) and in the flexion angle of the knee; however, the values of lateral or medial laxity had surprising similarity [7, 18, 21–24]. From these results, postoperative coronal laxity was approximately 4° in both the medial and lateral sides, and the values did not change from 3 months to 2 years after surgery.

15.5 Possibility of Postoperative Change in Soft Tissue Balance in TKA

The lateral soft tissues are generally lax in varus-deformed knees. Due to the greater lateral laxity than medial laxity preoperatively, some amount of residual lateral laxity is inevitable even at TKA in many cases [19, 20], whereas coronal balance 3 months or after was similar in the medial and lateral sides [7, 18, 21–24]. We speculated that the intraoperative soft tissue balance would change before 3 months after the surgery.

15.6 Postoperative Change in Soft Tissue Balance in Varus-Deformed Knees

We evaluated the postoperative changes in coronal medial or lateral laxity in 71 knees with varus deformities immediately after surgery and at 3, 6, and 12 months after posterior-stabilized TKA (Table 15.1) [18]. At the time of surgery, the lateral gap was far larger than the medial gap in many cases. The medial release was terminated at the point when the medial gap reached 20 mm in extension and 90° to maintain medial stability, allowing residual lateral laxity. Coronal laxity was assessed by stress radiographs of the knees using a Telos SE arthrometer with valgus or varus forces of 7 kg at 15° of flexion. The mean medial ligamentous laxity was relatively constant postoperatively in all periods; however, the mean lateral ligamentous laxity was 8.6° immediately after surgery and decreased to 5.1° at 3 months (Table 15.1, Fig. 15.1). Based on these results, we thought that if appropriate knee alignment was achieved by the surgery, the residual lateral ligamentous laxity observed in the preoperative varus knee might be corrected spontaneously after TKA. Nakajima et al. also reported a decrease in intraoperative lateral laxity in CR TKA for varus-deformed knees at 4–6 weeks after surgery [25].

On the other hand, Ishii et al. reported no significant postoperative change in coronal laxity between under anesthesia and 6 months after surgery in both mobile cruciate ligament-retaining TKA and rotating-type cruciate-sacrificing TKA in knees with osteoarthritis (Table 15.1) [24]. Their mean lateral ligamentous laxity under anesthesia was 4.4° in cruciate-retaining TKA and 4.4° in cruciate-sacrificing TKA. These values were smaller than our values of 8.6° in posterior-stabilized TKA. However, due to the lack of data on preoperative deformity and detail regarding soft tissue balancing in Ishii et al.'s report, the reason for the difference in the values cannot be determined.

Why was the large lateral laxity that was observed immediately after surgery in the present study dramatically decreased 3 months after surgery? A change in

Table 15.1 Postoperative changes in medial laxity (=valgus laxity) and lateral laxity (=varus laxity) after TKA

Author	Year of publication	Type of implant	Preoperative knee alignment	Method of stress	Degree of knee flexion	Stress direction	Angles between the femoral and tibial components (degrees)						
							Intraoperative	3 weeks	1 month	3 months	6 months	1 year	2 years
Ishii [24]	2003	Mobile CR TKA(N:20)	NA	Tebs 150 N	0–20°	Varus Valgus	4.4 ± 2.8 2.9 ± 1.8				3.6 ± 1.5 3.0 ± 1.2		
		Mobile PS TKA (N:20)	NA	Tebs 150 N	0–20°	Varus Valgus	4.6 ± 3.8 3.8 ± 1.4				4.0 ± 1.7 3.5 ± 0.9		
Chkawa [7]	2007	Fixed PS TKA(N:131)	NA	Tebs 150 N	0°	Varus Valgus		6.0 ± 3.7 5.5 ± 3.2			5.5 ± 1.7 4.5 ± 1.7	4.7 ± 3.3 5.5 ± 2.7	
Sekiya [18]	2009	Fixed PS TKA(N:71)	15.9°± 6.5° varus	Tebs 70 N	15°	Varus Valgus	8.6 ± 3.2 3.6 ± 1.7			5.1 ± 22 4.3 ± 22	4.5 ± 2.4 4.2 ± 2.1	4.8 ± 2.2 3.9 ± 1.8	
Takeda [23]	2011	Mobile CR TKA (N:30)	NA	Tebs 150 N	20°	Varus Valgus					3.7 ± 1.2 3.5 ± 1.3	4.0 ± 1.3 3.5 ± 1.3	4.1 ± 1.7 3.5 ± 1.1
		Mobile PS TKA (N:30)	NA	Tebs 150 N	20°	Varus Valgus					4.3 ± 1.9 3.7 ± 1.3	4.3 ± 1.9 3.4 ± 1.3	4.3 ± 1.8 3.5 ± 1.1
Sekiya [22]	2011	Fixed PS TKA(N:37)	12.8°± 1.6° valgus	Tebs 70N	15°	Varus Valgus	5.5 ± 2.3 5.0 ± 2.3			4.1 ± 2.2 4.8 ± 2.6	4.2 ± 1.8 4.1 ± 2.1	3.9 ± 1.9 4.2 ± 1.5	

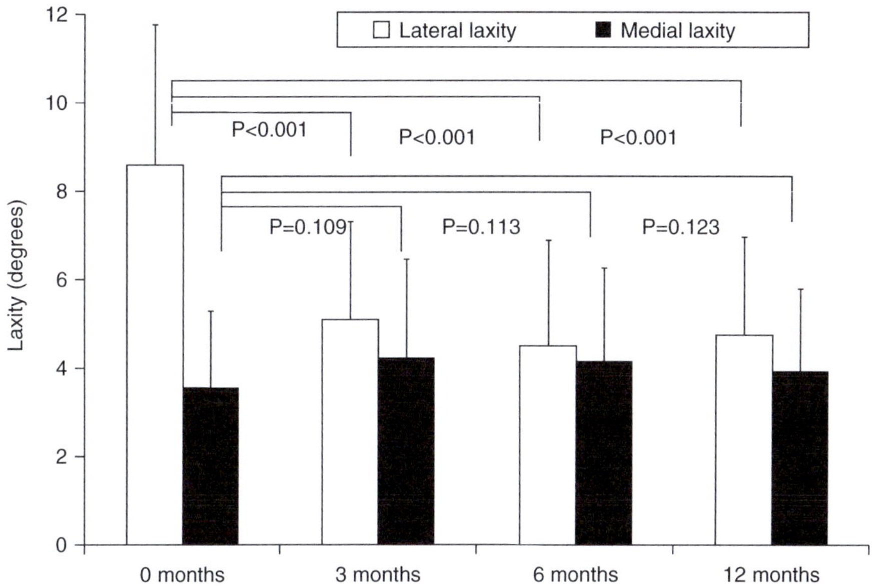

Fig. 15.1 Postoperative values of lateral laxity (=varus laxity) and medial laxity (=valgus laxity) after TKA in varus-deformed knees. The error bars represent one standard deviation. The lateral laxity is greater immediately after surgery than at 3, 6, and 12 months postoperatively

alignment due to TKA from varus to valgus would decrease the tension on the soft tissues at the lateral side of the knee. Yamamoto et al. reported approximately 10% shortening of the length of the patellar tendon in rabbits 2 weeks after stress shielding of the tendon [26]. Decreased tension at the lateral side of the knee in TKA may cause the shortening of the soft tissue observed by Yamamoto et al.

15.7 Postoperative Change in Soft Tissue Balance in Valgus-Deformed Knees

To the best of our knowledge, there have been no reports dealing with the postoperative change in the soft tissue balance in TKA for valgus-deformed knees in the English literature. We now present our original study written in Japanese [22]. We evaluated the changes in coronal laxity after TKA in 37 valgus-deformed knees (4 osteoarthritis, 33 rheumatoid arthritis, all females). Posterior-stabilized TKA (Scorpio NRG) was used in all cases. Lateral soft tissues including the iliotibial band were properly released to adjust the soft tissue balance using a Tensor device. Postoperative alignment of the knee was 1.4 ± 1.6° varus. We measured coronal valgus or varus ligamentous laxity by stress X-ray using the same method as the previous study [18] immediately after surgery and 3, 6, and 12 months thereafter. Lateral laxity decreased significantly during these periods, and medial laxity tended to decrease during these periods (Table 15.1, Fig. 15.2). Furthermore, we

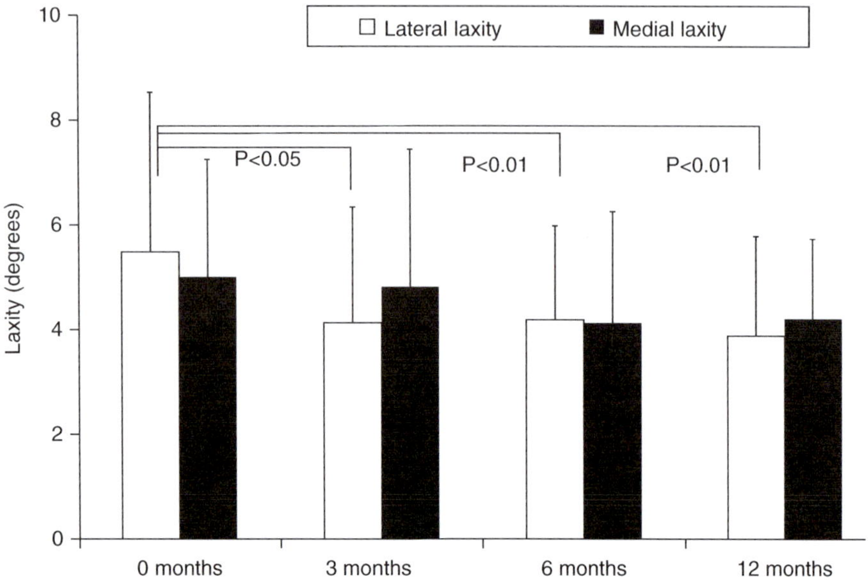

Fig. 15.2 Postoperative values of lateral laxity (=varus laxity) and medial laxity (=valgus laxity) after TKA in valgus-deformed knees. The error bars represent one standard deviation. The lateral laxity is greater immediately after surgery than at 3, 6, and 12 months postoperatively

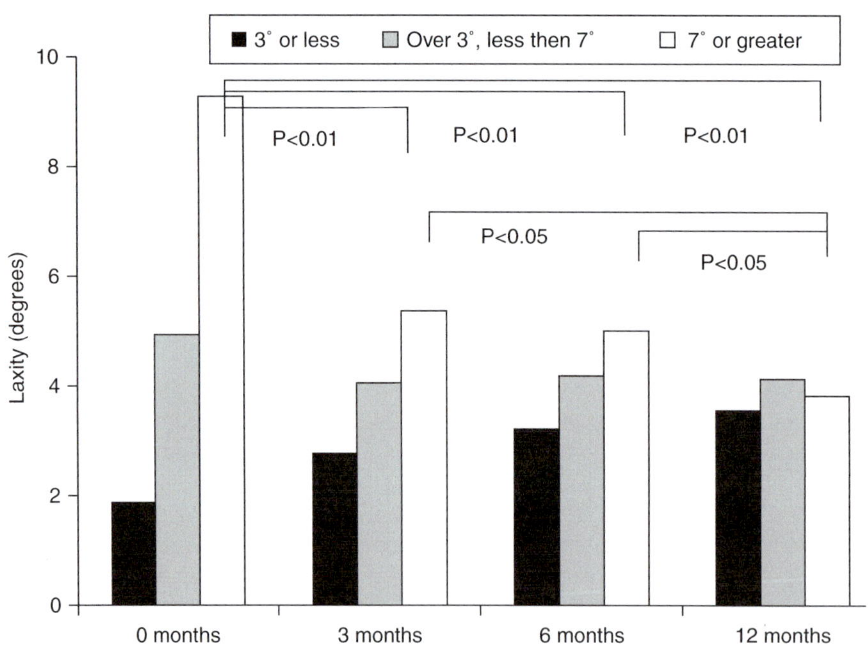

Fig. 15.3 Postoperative values of lateral laxity (=varus laxity) after TKA in valgus-deformed knees. Knees were divided by the values of laxity into three groups: 3° or less, over 3° and less than 7°, and 7° or greater. The values of the group of 7°or greater at 3, 6, and 12 months are smaller than the value immediately after surgery

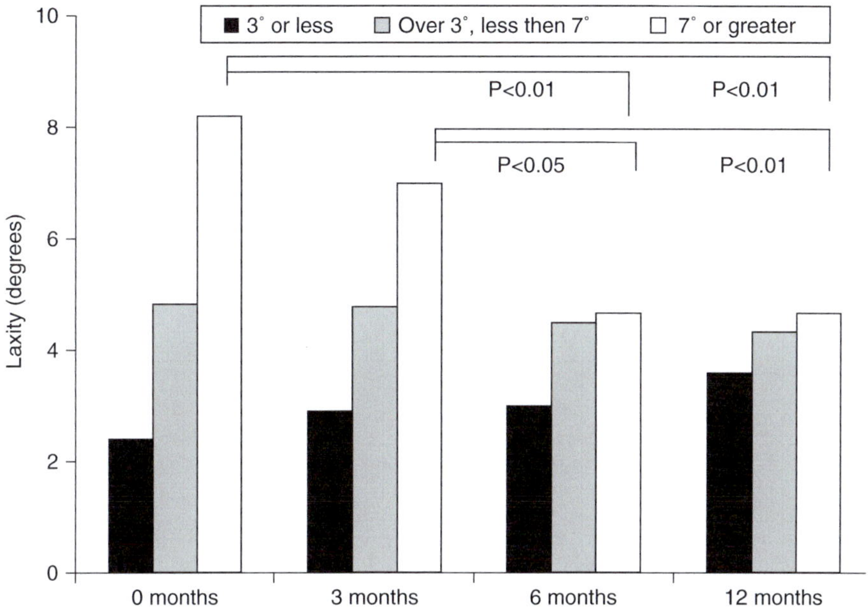

Fig. 15.4 Postoperative values of medial laxity (=valgus laxity) after TKA in valgus-deformed knees. Knees were divided by the values of laxity into three groups: 3° or less, over 3° and less than 7°, and 7° or greater. The values of the group of 7° or greater at 6 and 12 months are smaller than the value immediately after surgery

divided the cases into three groups according to the value of coronal laxity immediately after TKA: 3° or less, over 3° and less than 7°, and 7° or greater. The coronal laxity in the "3° or less" group had a tendency to increase over follow-up, and that in the "7° or greater" group had decreased (Figs. 15.3 and 15.4). Regardless of the size of the laxity immediately after surgery, medial and lateral laxity had converged to approximately 4° at 12 months after TKA. In the case of a valgus deformity with a narrow joint gap at the medial side, we released the soft tissues until the medial and lateral gaps were equal at least in extension. However, in the case of valgus deformity with a wide medial gap preoperatively, to equalize the gap at the medial and lateral sides, we had to release extensively at the lateral side. This extensive lateral release may result in failure with elevation of the joint line and being too loose at the lateral side in flexion. To prevent such a failure, we aimed for 1–2° of varus alignment from neutral at TKA, allowing a small amount of medial laxity.

15.8 Postoperative Change in Soft Tissue Balance in Flexion

Although flexion instability after TKA is a major reason for revision surgery [27], only a few studies reported flexion laxity objectively after TKA. Oh et al. [28] first reported flexion laxity at 90° after TKA. Patients were asked to sit on a radiolucent wooden chair, and radiographic examinations were performed with the knee joint flexed to 90°. Under varus and valgus loads with a force of 50 N, varus and valgus stress X-rays were taken. Mean lateral laxity, mean medial laxity, and total laxity were 4.7° ± 2.4°, 4.1 ± 2.1°, and 8.8° ± 3.5° in 61 TKAs at a mean 26.1 months after surgery. Yoshihara et al. [29] measured varus and valgus laxities at 90° under a 1.5-kg external force in 49 TKAs at a minimum of 10 years after surgery. They reported laxity of 6° ± 4° (0–20°) in varus, 4° ± 3° (0–9°) in valgus, and 10° ± 5° (0–21°) in total laxity. To the best of our knowledge, there have been no reports about the postoperative change in flexion laxity in TKA. If flexion laxity during TKA was lax laterally and tight medially, as has been reported [20, 30], flexion laxity would be spontaneously adjusted in the postoperative period, similar to the phenomenon found in extension [18]. Further studies are needed to clarify the postoperative change in flexion after TKA.

15.9 Influence of Anesthesia on Measurement of Coronal Laxity

To compare the value of coronal laxity between immediately after surgery and in the late period after surgery, the effect of anesthesia must be considered. Tsukeoka and Tsuneizumi reported the effect of anesthesia during the measurement of soft tissue in TKA [31]. They measured varus and valgus laxities without anesthesia and again immediately under spinal anesthesia. The laxity was significantly increased from 3.0° to 3.6° and from 4.7° to 5.7° in the medial and lateral sides, respectively.

The difference of approximately 1° in these studies might possibly be due to the effect of anesthesia; however, it was difficult to explain the large change in lateral laxity observed in our study of varus-deformed knees.

Methods of laxity measurement also have limitations. To elucidate the precise and detailed change in laxity, we have to measure laxity repeatedly after surgery. However, repeated external varus or valgus force with the Telos SE to the knee could interfere with soft tissue healing, especially during the early period after TKA.

15.10 Factors for Spontaneous Correction of Soft Tissue Balance After TKA

From our experience, in both varus- and valgus-deformed knees, lateral and medial soft tissue laxity observed at TKA would spontaneously correct themselves after the surgery if the appropriate alignment and appropriate soft tissue balance were achieved by the surgery [22].

From the number of revision TKAs due to instability, it is reasonable to think that spontaneous balance correction did not occur after TKA in all cases. What must we pay attention to in order to achieve spontaneous correction of soft tissue imbalance after TKA? We believe that coronal alignment and soft tissue balance are the two most important factors. In addition, complete preservation of the PCL at surgery is crucial in CR TKA. Postoperative damage or rupture of the PCL may dramatically change the soft tissue balance, especially in flexion [32, 33].

Coronal alignment after surgery is closely related to soft tissue tension surrounding the knee [34]. In the varus knee after TKA, the soft tissue at the lateral side of the knee is stretched. In contrast, in the valgus knee after TKA, the soft tissue at the medial side of the knee is stretched [34]. Many studies have addressed the impact of postoperative coronal alignment on the outcomes of TKA [35–37]. They have accepted the premise that deviation beyond a postoperative mechanical axis of 0 ± 3° is associated with worse implant survival following TKA [37–40].

Matsuda and Ito emphasized the importance of medial side stability in TKA with neutral alignment for better kinematics and stability [41]. For correcting soft tissue balance with a tight medial gap in varus knees, medial release procedures are often required [42]. However, we have to be aware that extensive release can lead to complications such as instability and neurovascular injury [43]. Aunan et al. [34] evaluated the relationship between intraoperative ligament laxity and functional outcomes 1 year after TKA in 122 CR TKA cases. They stated that medial laxity more than 2 mm in extension and 3 mm in flexion at surgery must be avoided in neutral and valgus-aligned TKAs for better outcomes. They also stated that varus-aligned TKAs seemed to be more forgiving of medial laxity [34]. As mentioned in our study, even in preoperative valgus-deformed knees, some amount of medial residual laxity could be made acceptable by achieving 1–2° of varus alignment at TKA [22]. However, extreme medial laxity could not be spontaneously corrected after surgery. Under such conditions, we have to use a medial soft tissue advancement or tightening procedure or select a more constrained prosthesis to acquire stability.

15.11 Future Directions

Thus, spontaneous soft tissue correction occurs after TKA in many instances. However, thinking about revision TKA due to instability, it is quite reasonable to think of the limitations of spontaneous correction. The final clinical outcomes of TKA were generally excellent in most previous studies of postoperative laxity in TKA [7, 18, 21–23]. To elucidate the limitations, we have to clarify the postoperative changes in soft tissue balance in the cases of revision TKA due to instability. From the data of the failed cases, we could get valuable factors to prevent postoperative instability.

Many studies used a stress radiograph with a Telos arthrometer [7, 18, 21–24]; however, the method was not suitable for repeated measurements, especially in the early period after surgery, for fear of damaging the soft tissue in the repair phase. Furthermore, the angle of knee flexion was limited by this method.

Recent advances of technology have resulted in the development of a sensor-embedded tibial insert or component [44, 45]. Using these devices for in vivo analysis of contact stress during daily activities after TKA could be done over the full range of motion. Because of the high cost of such electronic devices, it is not realistic to use them in every TKA case. However, with such devices the precise and detailed changes in soft tissue balance after TKA can be identified.

References

1. Dorr LD, Boiardo RA. Technical considerations in total knee arthroplasty. Clin Orthop Relat Res. 1986;205:5–11.
2. Insall J, Tria AJ, Scott WN. The total condylar knee prosthesis: the first 5 years. Clin Orthop Relat Res. 1979;145:68–77.
3. Insall JN, Binazzi R, Soudry M, Mestriner LA. Total knee arthroplasty. Clin Orthop Relat Res. 1985;192:13–22.
4. Fehring TK, Odum S, Griffin WL, Mason JB, Nadaud M. Early failures in total knee arthroplasty. Clin Orthop Relat Res. 2001;392:315–8.
5. Sharkey PF, Hozack WJ, Rothman RH, Shastri S, Jacoby SM. Insall Award paper. Why are total knee arthroplasties failing today? Clin Orthop Relat Res. 2002;404:7–13.
6. Unitt L, Sambatakakis A, Johnstone D, Briggs TW. Short-term outcome in total knee replacement after soft-tissue release and balancing. J Bone Joint Surg. 2008;90(2):159–65.
7. Ohkawa S, Soda K, Nishikawa K, Otsubo S, Okuhara A, Tajiri T, et al. Relationship of intraoperative balance and postoperative stability in TKA (in Japanese). Jpn J Replacement Arthroplasty. 2007;37:100–1.
8. Tokuhara Y, Kadoya Y, Nakagawa S, Kobayashi A, Takaoka K. The flexion gap in normal knees. An MRI study. J Bone Joint Surg. 2004;86(8):1133–6.
9. Markolf KL, Mensch JS, Amstutz HC. Stiffness and laxity of the knee--the contributions of the supporting structures. A quantitative in vitro study. J Bone Joint Surg Am. 1976;58(5):583–94.
10. Van Damme G, Defoort K, Ducoulombier Y, Van Glabbeek F, Bellemans J, Victor J. What should the surgeon aim for when performing computer-assisted total knee arthroplasty? J Bone Joint Surg Am. 2005;87(Suppl 2):52–8.
11. Matsumoto T, Muratsu H, Kubo S, Matsushita T, Kurosaka M, Kuroda R. The influence of preoperative deformity on intraoperative soft tissue balance in posterior-stabilized total knee arthroplasty. J Arthroplasty. 2011;26(8):1291–8.
12. Griffin FM, Insall JN, Scuderi GR. Accuracy of soft tissue balancing in total knee arthroplasty. J Arthroplasty. 2000;15(8):970–3.
13. Mullaji AB, Shetty GM. Surgical technique: computer-assisted sliding medial condylar osteotomy to achieve gap balance in varus knees during TKA. Clin Orthop Relat Res. 2013;471(5):1484–91.
14. Okamoto S, Okazaki K, Mitsuyasu H, Matsuda S, Mizu-Uchi H, Hamai S, et al. Extension gap needs more than 1-mm laxity after implantation to avoid post-operative flexion contracture in total knee arthroplasty. Knee surgery, sports traumatology, arthroscopy : official journal of the ESSKA. 2014;22(12):3174–80.
15. Yagishita K, Muneta T, Yamamoto H, Shinomiya K. The relationship between postoperative ligament balance and preoperative varus deformity in total knee arthroplasty. Bull Hosp Joint Dis. 2001;60(1):23–8.
16. Matsueda M, Gengerke TR, Murphy M, Lew WD, Gustilo RB. Soft tissue release in total knee arthroplasty. Cadaver study using knees without deformities. Clin Orthop Relat Res. 1999;366:264–73.
17. Yagishita K, Muneta T, Ikeda H. Step-by-step measurements of soft tissue balancing during total knee arthroplasty for patients with varus knees. J Arthroplasty. 2003;18(3):313–20.
18. Sekiya H, Takatoku K, Takada H, Sasanuma H, Sugimoto N. Postoperative lateral ligamentous laxity diminishes with time after TKA in the varus knee. Clin Orthop Relat Res. 2009;467(6):1582–6.
19. Okazaki K, Miura H, Matsuda S, Takeuchi N, Mawatari T, Hashizume M, et al. Asymmetry of mediolateral laxity of the normal knee. J Orthop Sci Off J Japanese Orthop Assoc. 2006;11(3):264–6.
20. Sasanuma H, Sekiya H, Takatoku K, Takada H, Sugimoto N. Evaluation of soft-tissue balance during total knee arthroplasty. J Orthop Surg (Hong Kong). 2010;18(1):26–30.

21. Ishii Y, Matsuda Y, Ishii R, Sakata S, Omori G. Coronal laxity in extension in vivo after total knee arthroplasty. J Orthop Sci Off J Japanese Orthop Assoc. 2003;8(4):538–42.
22. Sekiya H, Takatoku K, Takada H, Sugimoto N, Hoshino Y. Postoperative changes of coronal laxity after total knee arthroplasty in valgus knee (in Japanese). J Phys Med. 2011;22(4):411–5.
23. Takeda M, Ishii Y, Noguchi H, Matsuda Y, Sato J. Changes in varus-valgus laxity after total knee arthroplasty over time. Knee Surg Sports Traumatol Arthrosc Off J ESSKA. 2012;20(10):1988–93.
24. Ishii Y, Matsuda Y, Noguchi H, Kiga H. Effect of soft tissue tension on measurements of coronal laxity in mobile-bearing total knee arthroplasty. J Orthop Sci Off J Jpn Orthop Assoc. 2005;10(5):496–500.
25. Nakajima A, Aoki Y, Murakami M, Nakagawa K. Changes in joint gap balances between intra- and postoperation in total knee arthroplasty. Adv Orthop. 2014;2014:790806.
26. Yamamoto N, Ohno K, Hayashi K, Kuriyama H, Yasuda K, Kaneda K. Effects of stress shielding on the mechanical properties of rabbit patellar tendon. J Biomech Eng. 1993;115(1):23–8.
27. Cottino U, Sculco PK, Sierra RJ, Abdel MP. Instability after total knee arthroplasty. Orthop Clin North Am. 2016;47(2):311–6.
28. Oh CS, Song EK, Seon JK, Ahn YS. The effect of flexion balance on functional outcomes in cruciate-retaining total knee arthroplasty. Arch Orthop Trauma Surg. 2015;135(3):401–6.
29. Yoshihara Y, Arai Y, Nakagawa S, Inoue H, Ueshima K, Fujiwara H, et al. Assessing coronal laxity in extension and flexion at a minimum of 10 years after primary total knee arthroplasty. Knee Surg Sports Traumatol Arthrosc Off J ESSKA. 2016;24(8):2512–6.
30. Nagai K, Muratsu H, Matsumoto T, Miya H, Kuroda R, Kurosaka M. Soft tissue balance changes depending on joint distraction force in total knee arthroplasty. J Arthroplasty. 2014;29(3):520–4.
31. Tsukeoka T, Tsuneizumi Y. Varus and valgus stress tests after total knee arthroplasty with and without anesthesia. Arch Orthop Trauma Surg. 2016;136(3):407–11.
32. Pagnano MW, Hanssen AD, Lewallen DG, Stuart MJ. Flexion instability after primary posterior cruciate retaining total knee arthroplasty. Clin Orthop Relat Res. 1998;356:39–46.
33. Matsuda S, Miura H, Nagamine R, Urabe K, Matsunobu T, Iwamoto Y. Knee stability in posterior cruciate ligament retaining total knee arthroplasty. Clin Orthop Relat Res. 1999;366:169–73.
34. Aunan E, Kibsgard TJ, Diep LM, Rohrl SM. Intraoperative ligament laxity influences functional outcome 1 year after total knee arthroplasty. Knee Surg Sports Traumatol Arthrosc Off J ESSKA. 2015;23(6):1684–92.
35. Jeffery RS, Morris RW, Denham RA. Coronal alignment after total knee replacement. J Bone Joint Surg. 1991;73(5):709–14.
36. Ritter MA, Faris PM, Keating EM, Meding JB. Postoperative alignment of total knee replacement. Its effect on survival. Clin Orthop Relat Res. 1994;299:153–6.
37. Sikorski JM. Alignment in total knee replacement. J Bone Joint Surg. 2008;90(9):1121–7.
38. Bauwens K, Matthes G, Wich M, Gebhard F, Hanson B, Ekkernkamp A, et al. Navigated total knee replacement. A meta-analysis. J Bone Joint Surg Am. 2007;89(2):261–9.
39. Bonutti PM, Dethmers D, Ulrich SD, Seyler TM, Mont MA. Computer navigation-assisted versus minimally invasive TKA: benefits and drawbacks. Clin Orthop Relat Res. 2008;466(11):2756–62.
40. Ensini A, Catani F, Leardini A, Romagnoli M, Giannini S. Alignments and clinical results in conventional and navigated total knee arthroplasty. Clin Orthop Relat Res. 2007;457:156–62.
41. Matsuda S, Ito H. Ligament balancing in total knee arthroplasty? Medial stabilizing technique. Asia-Pacific J Sports Med Arthroscopy, Rehabil Tech. 2015;2:108–13.
42. Whiteside LA. Soft tissue balancing: the knee. J Arthroplasty. 2002;17(4 Suppl 1):23–7.

43. Hunt NC, Ghosh KM, Athwal KK, Longstaff LM, Amis AA, Deehan DJ. Lack of evidence to support present medial release methods in total knee arthroplasty. Knee Surg Sports Traumatol Arthrosc Off J ESSKA. 2014;22(12):3100–12.
44. Gustke KA, Golladay GJ, Roche MW, Elson LC, Anderson CR. A new method for defining balance: promising short-term clinical outcomes of sensor-guided TKA. J Arthroplasty. 2014;29(5):955–60.
45. Zhao D, Banks SA, D'Lima DD, Colwell Jr CW, Fregly BJ. In vivo medial and lateral tibial loads during dynamic and high flexion activities. J Orthop Res Off Pub Orthop Res Soc. 2007;25(5):593–602.

Intraoperative Soft-Tissue Balance and Clinical Results (ROM, Function)

16

Eun-Kyoo Song, Jong-Keun Seon, Young-Joo Shin, and Hong-Ahn Lim

Contents

16.1 Introduction

A good outcome in total knee arthroplasty (TKA) depends on many factors: joint alignment, range of motion (ROM), patella tracking, and ligament stability [1]. If correct soft-tissue balancing is not achieved after TKA, the patient may initially suffer instability of joint, pain, and swelling after surgery and experience gait disturbance due to giving way, and as it increases risk of wear and aseptic loosening in long-term follow-up, it is considered the most important process. However, achieving accurate soft-tissue balancing is not an easy goal in TKA. Generally, well intraoperative balance affects good postoperative gap balance. Some studies report that the more intraoperative flexion laxity, the better

E.-K. Song, MD (✉) • J.-K. Seon, MD • Y.-J. Shin, MD • H.-A. Lim, MD
Department of Orthopaedic Surgery, Kyoto University Department of Orthopaedic Surgery, Kyoto, Japan

Department of Orthopedic Surgery, Center for Joint Disease, Chonnam National University Bitgoeul Hospital, Gwangju, Korea
e-mail: eksong@jnu.ac.kr

S. Matsuda et al. (eds.), *Soft Tissue Balancing in Total Knee Arthroplasty*,
DOI 10.1007/978-3-662-54082-4_16

postoperative ROM [2]. But the best method for obtaining appropriate soft-tissue balance and better ROM remains controversial, with dispute focusing on the cut-off value of flexion laxity [3, 4].

Soft-tissue release, serving to correct imbalances, is performed until the flexion and extension gap appear symmetrical and balanced. A knee is considered perfectly balanced when the flexion and extension gaps are perfectly rectangular, and all the measurements are equal [1]. As a general guideline, 1–2 mm of balanced varus-valgus plays in the prosthetic knee is reasonable goal. Regardless of the type of deformity being corrected, stability should be checked after each stage of soft-tissue release because over-release can lead to excessive coronal plane instability and requires conversion to a constrained prosthesis [4]. We can say that soft-tissue balancing is consisted of various factors, including flexion and extension gap balancing, mediolateral (ML) balancing, and patellofemoral (PF) balancing.

16.2 Flexion and Extension Gap Balancing

Flexion and extension gap balancing is influenced by appropriate bony resection, sizing and rotation of the femoral component, appropriate ligament balancing, and posterior cruciate ligament (PCL) resection. Among them, excessive bony resection of the proximal femur or wrong size of the femoral implant is the major cause of extension and flexion gap imbalance [5]. Testing for soft-tissue balancing during TKA was introduced by Insall, who used spacer blocks and laminar spreaders intraoperatively to assess the extension and flexion gaps in varus and valgus stress [6]. Also, another method with the trial component has been introduced to check the gap of flexion and extension. Temporary trial method uses trial insert of appropriate thickness after bony resection and makes extension and flexion of the knee to see if the gap is right; one of the typical methods is POLO (pullout, lift off) test that decides flexion gap in cruciate-retaining (CR)-type implant introduced by Scott [7] (Fig. 16.1). In resection of PCL, Mihalko reported increased flexion gap more than 5.2 mm at average, and also Cho et al. reported increase in both flexion and extension gap, with flexion gap 2.8 mm more than extension gap [5, 8].

Despite advanced accuracy in bony alignment with the development of surgical instruments, such as the computer-assisted navigation system, obtaining an accurate intraoperative soft-tissue balance remains difficult, especially for young surgeons, as experienced surgeons traditionally address soft-tissue balance through "subjective feel." Therefore, various offset-type tensor has been developed for use during TKA, which enables soft-tissue balance assessment throughout range of motion (ROM) in the physiological knee after TKA (Fig. 16.2), with reduced PF joint and with the femoral component in place [9]. Therefore, clinical relevance using such intraoperative tensor device is being reported nowadays (discussed in next section).

Attifield et al. reported that knees balanced in full extension and in flexion ($< \pm 2°$) showed a significant improvement in proprioception ($p < 0.0005$), and soft-tissue balance in both flexion and extension is important to allow satisfactory postoperative

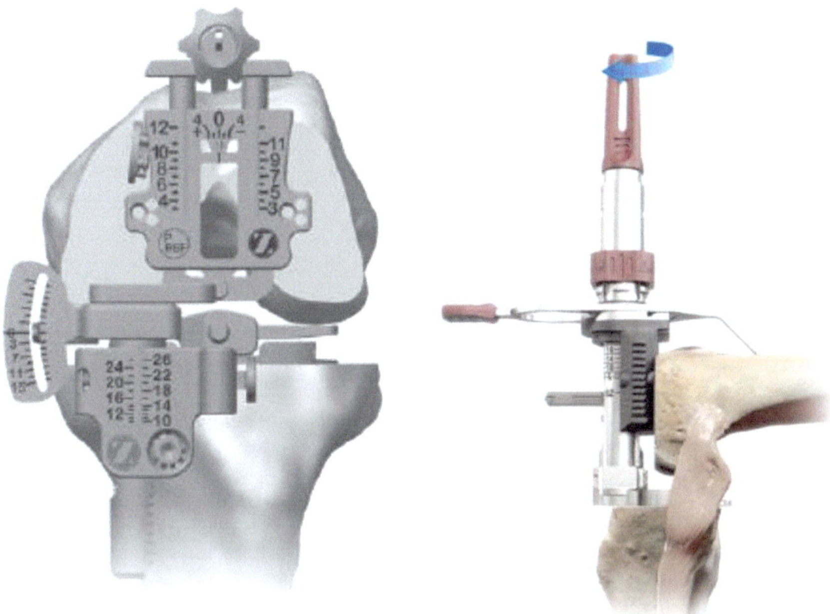

Fig. 16.1 Offset-type sensor used in total knee arthroplasty, which enables soft-tissue balance assessment. *Left*; Fuzion (Zimmer, Warsaw, USA), *Right*; Attune (Depuy Synthes, Warsaw, USA)

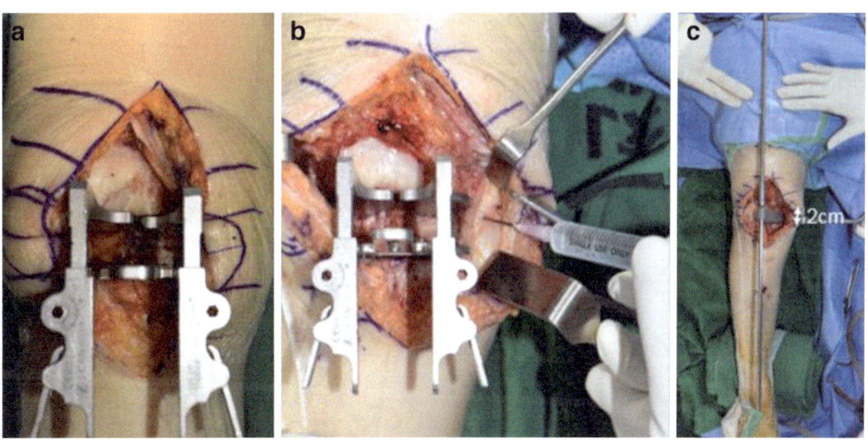

Fig. 16.2 Gap balancing technique. (**a**) Extension gap balancing using tensioner. Smaller medial gap was found with tightness. (**b**) Needle-assisted medial collateral ligament (MCL) release using an 18 gauge needle. (**c**) Medial and lateral balance and good alignment were acquired after MCL release

proprioception of the knee [10]. Pang et al. reported the TKA group with computer-assisted gap balancing technique had less occurrence of flexion contracture in 2 years after the surgery, less outlier number (anterior tibial translation >5 mm), and less functional score than conventional measured resection technique [11]. Lampe et al. studied clinical outcomes within the first year after computer-navigated total knee arthroplasty (TKA) and reported that higher flexion-extension gap equality values led to statistically significant better KSS-F and KSS-K scores at 1 year [12]. Furthermore, Matsumoto et al. argued that in achieving equalized rectangular gaps at extension and flexion, CR TKA using the gap technique with navigation system is more effective than measured technique, but it does not directly reflect 2-year post-operative clinical outcomes [9].

However, it has been often reported that computer navigation offers little advantage over experienced surgeon judgment in achieving soft-tissue balance in knee replacement. Joseph et al. reported that balancing the mediolateral extension gap in navigated group was superior to non-navigated group ($p = 0.001$), but no significant difference was found between the two groups in balancing the mediolateral flexion gap or in achieving equal flexion and extension gaps [13]. Widmer et al. reported alignment and component position can be precisely measured intraoperatively with navigation, but intrinsic patient factors remain dominant in determining the clinical outcome at 1 year. Therefore, he reported that intraoperative computer navigation parameters (coronal alignment, ligament balance, range of motion, external tibiofemoral rotation) are predictors of function 1 year after total knee arthroplasty [14].

16.3 Mediolateral Gap Balancing

Mediolateral (ML) balancing is one of the most influential factors in TKA. ML balancing is known to have wider range of tolerance than alignment of lower extremity, but it should be strict [5]. Especially, in PCL substituting type, precise ML balancing is very crucial to knee stability and also influences ROM. Matsuda et al. reported that ROM decreased about 11° when ML balancing is off more than 2° [15].

Most of osteoarthritis patients show some degree of varus deformity, regardless of bone defect. If arthritis progresses in medial side, medial joint capsule and medial collateral ligament (MCL) contracts, which is accompanied by lateral collateral ligament elongate along with flexion contracture in most cases. The ideal goal of ML gap balancing is the balance of bilateral collateral ligaments with 4–7° valgus of tibiofemoral alignment, and it should not be overcorrected. In balancing ligament, osteophyte must be thoroughly removed first, then, releasing the side with contracture is more preferable than reefing elongated ligament of the other side. Liebs et al. reported that pain becomes severe when medial gap is 1.5 mm wider or more than lateral gap in extension [16]. Okazaki et al. argues that lateral gap is greater than medial gap, and this is a compensation mechanism of dynamic stability by iliotibial band [17]. However, Yoon et al. reported the gaps in patella eversion demonstrated smaller gaps both in knee extension and flexion position compared to the gaps of patella reduction position. The amount of decreased gaps was more definite in knee flexion position. Therefore, the intraoperative patellar positioning has influence on the measurement of the joint gap. Keeping the patella in reduced position is important during gap balancing [18].

16.3.1 Medial Release

As for varus deformity, release is mostly conducted in tibia, and if the ligament tissue is released in the form of sleeve, it is scarred into a thick connective tissue after the surgery, which poses little difficulty to its function, whereas transverse incision poses a lot of difficulty in function and should not be performed. Medial release is first conducted on medial semimembranosus tendon, at last as argued by some operators, or not at all or partially by others. Most of the operators gradually release superficial medial collateral ligament (MCL) until lower extremity alignment returns. Clayton recommended the superficial MCL release to be conducted up to 5–6 cm before semimembranosus [19]. However, Insall et al. argued that it must be conducted in 7–8 cm to fulfill wanted goals [20]. Matsumoto et al. argued that semimembranosus release does not influence clinical outcome but reduces tibial internal rotation and flexion angle in cruciate-retaining total knee arthroplasty [21]. Also, Ahn argued that in severe varus knee, bony resection of proximal medial tibia can be considered as an alternative technique in order to decrease total operation time and to obtain medial-lateral, soft-tissue balance in deep flexion, rather than medial soft-tissue release [22].

Whiteside reported that release of the posterior part of superficial MCL is useful for extension contracture and releasing anterior part of MCL is effective for flexion tightness [23]. Burkart et al. conducted TKA with 12 cadaveric specimens and found that the medial parapatellar arthrotomy and ACL and PCL sectioning did not result in medial or lateral gap length. The release of the anterior fibers of the deep MCL as part of the surgical exposure increased the medial gap [24]. Also, pie crust can be conducted on superficial MCL with multiple pinning or 18 gauge needle, which must be conducted in moderate or intermediate tightness. Meneghini et al. argued pie crust method should be carefully performed, and with wrong technique, stroma of collateral ligament may rupture in joint line, which is worse than avulsion of distal part [25].

If medial gap loosening occurs in flexion after medial release, surgeon should inspect if there are external rotation of femoral component, varus resection of tibia, and whole damage of medial MCL component. If there is no specific abnormality in such inspection, small medial gap laxity in flexion is acceptable. Insall argued that large medial gap is not clinically big problem and takes time for scarring adhesion [20]. Alternative for medial release is "shift and resect" by Dixon which places a small trial in lateral side and makes more posteromedial marginal bone resection. This procedure can have same effect of MCL release [26].

16.3.2 Lateral Release

Valgus deformity of knee joint is not as common as varus deformity. Therefore, operators are not used to the surgery, and it is very difficult to release complex contracture of lateral soft tissue and ligament. Unless it is valgus deformity, general TKA rarely requires lateral release, but if insertion of thick PE is necessary due to excessive medial looseness, lateral side must be released to balance the knee. In such case, lateral collateral ligament or popliteus tendon may be released, and it is important that how much and how release is conducted. Kesman et al. evaluated influence of popliteus tendon resection during posterior stabilized TKA surgery and found that resection of popliteus tendon does not have great influence in static balance during flexion and extension [27]. However, in such cases, ML ligament release is too excessive, and it may require constrained prosthetics, which requires delicate attention.

16.3.3 Intraoperative Mediolateral Gap Check Device

Although advances in navigation system in TKA have improved the incidence of alignment outliers, spatial distance measurements do not quantify soft tissue stability or degrees of ligament tension. Recently, the development of integrated microelectronics and sensors into the knee trials (device that shows the force applied on mediolateral and anteroposterior part of the insert with attached sensor in digital number) during surgery allows surgeons to evaluate and act on real-time data regarding implant position, rotation, alignment, and soft-tissue balance through a full range of motion (Fig. 16.3). Gustke argued that ensuring soft-tissue balance by using intraoperative sensors during TKR may improve satisfaction [27]. Meneghini et al. measured intraoperative ligament balance with force-sensing implant trials and studied if an optimal "target" balance exists. Intraoperative force sensing has potential in providing real-time objective data to optimize TKA outcomes. These data support some early outcomes may improve by balancing TKAs within 60 lb. mediolateral force difference [28]. Jacob et al. previously reported that symmetrical medial and lateral compressive forces did not improve patient satisfaction, but recreating greater forces in the medial compartment much like that of the native knee may yield improved patient-reported outcomes and increased patient satisfaction. The current results further suggest that recreating greater medial compartment forces may have the greatest effect on more demanding activities [29].

Also, it recently is becoming a great help in anatomical and mechanical study related to prosthetics design using force-sensing implant trial. Manning et al. found that rotational stress in mid-flexion demonstrated the greatest mismatch in intercompartmental forces in cadaveric study using CR single-radius-type implant. They also argued that contact point position over the tibial sensor demonstrated paradoxical roll-forward with knee flexion and concluded that traditional balancing

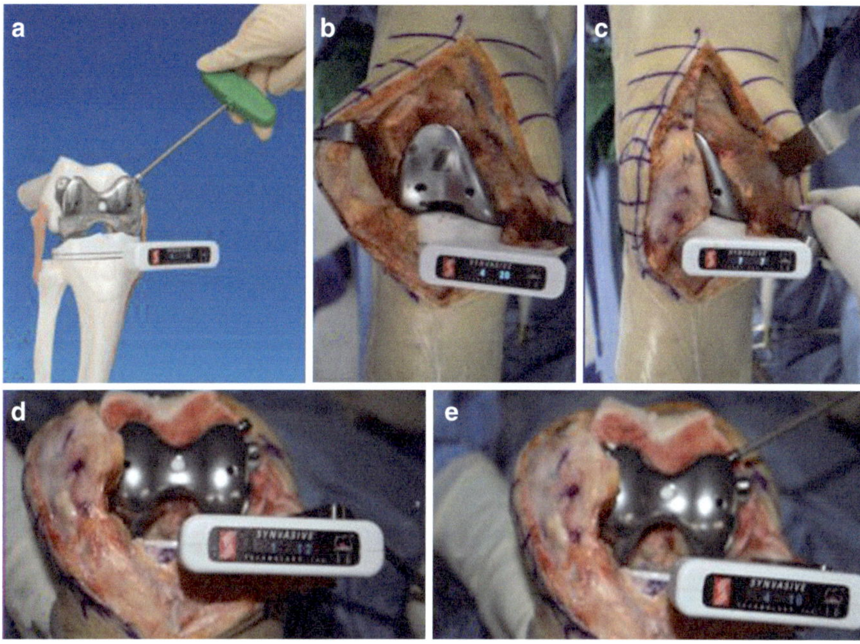

Fig. 16.3 Soft-tissue balancing by using intraoperative sensor. (**a**) eLIBRA (Synvasive Technology, Inc., Reno, Nevada). (**b**) Tibial insert assembly into the joint space with lateral transfer of the patella. The different force was found in medial and lateral joint. (**c**) Extension gap balancing by pie crust technique. Medial and lateral stability was acquired. (**d**) Flexion gap balancing with 90° flexion of knee joint. (**e**) The optimal external rotation of femoral component to achieve equal medial and lateral tension

techniques may not reliably equate to uniform laxity or contact forces across the tibiofemoral joint through a range of flexion and that the role of intraoperative sensor aids the final balancing of the knee [30].

16.4 Patellofemoral Balancing

Patellofemoral (PF) balancing is not only related to function and pain relief but also long-term survival of TKA. If alignment is not perfect, it may induce pain in anterior part of the knee, limit joint motion, induce anxiety, increase load to patella, induce patella fracture, quadriceps tendon and patella tendon rupture, and abrasion and dissociation of patella prosthetics. Lauglin et al. reported that risk of wear from cold flow increases with patellar mal-tracking. However, unlike such general understanding [31], Bindelglass argued that when using all-polyethylene patellar component, clinical result, or, in other words, pain, range of motion, and frequency of dissociation, did not differ though the movement of PF is abnormal [32].

Heesterbeek et al. argued that femoral component rotation has little correlation to abnormal postoperative patella position, but preoperative malalignment results in a higher risk at a postoperatively displaced patella [33, 34]. Balanced gap technique can safely be used without an increased risk for patella malposition.

As for surgical approach, subvastus or midvastus approach that does not involve quadriceps tendon is known to be good for patellofemoral alignment. Femoral implant size is also important, and if it is too big, it tenses lateral ligament, serving as a cause of malalignment, and articulation with patella prosthetics becomes inappropriate if it is too small. Most of patellofemoral malalignment is based on malrotated femoral and tibial component. External rotation of both components is preferable, but if external rotation is too much, it would not only bring wear of prosthetics faster but also cause the patient to have toe-in gait. Location of prosthetics is also relevant; femoral prosthesis is aligned to lateral edge of resected bone as much as possible, and tibial prosthetics must be placed in lateral for better alignment. However, laterally located patella component deteriorates the alignment.

16.5 Summary

In summary, the optimal ligament balance for good clinical outcomes undergoing TKA remains unclear. Although there are some debates whether intraoperative soft-tissue balances have direct correlation with good clinical outcomes and long survival of TKA, balanced flexion and extension is essential for good outcome in TKA and that increased medial laxity might be related to inferior clinical results.

References

1. Meloni MC, Hoedemaeker RW, Violante B, Mazzola C. Soft tissue balancing in total knee arthroplasty. Joints. 2014;2(1):37–40.
2. Sugitani K, Arai Y, Takamiya H, Terauchi R, Nakagawa S, Ueshima K, Kubo T. Factors affecting range of motion after total knee arthroplasty in patients with more than 120 degrees of preoperative flexion angle. Int Orthop. 2015;39(8):1535–40.
3. Hino K, Ishimaru M, Iseki Y, Watanabe S, Onishi Y, Miura H. Mid-flexion laxity is greater after posterior-stabilised total knee replacement than with cruciate-retaining procedures: a computer navigation study. Bone Joint J. 2013;95-B(4):493–7.
4. Campbell's operative orthopaedics. 12th ed. Philadelphia: Mosby/Elsevier; 2013. p. 407.
5. Cho WS, editor. Knee joint arthroplasty. Berlin Heidelberg: Springer; 2014.
6. Griffin FM, Insall JN, Scuderi GR. Accuracy of soft tissue balancing in total knee arthroplasty. J Arthroplasty. 2000;15:970–3.
7. Scott RD, Chmell MJ. Balancing the posterior cruciate ligament during cruciate-retaining fixed and mobile-bearing total knee arthroplasty: description of the pull-out lift-off and slide-back tests. J Arthroplasty. 2008;23(4):605–8.
8. Mihalko WM, Miller C, Krackow KA. Total knee arthroplasty ligament balancing and gap kinematics with posterior cruciate ligament retention and sacrifice. Am J Orthop (Belle Mead NJ). 2000;29(8):610–6.
9. Matsumoto T, Muratsu H, Kawakami Y, Takayama K, Ishida K, Matsushita T, Akisue T, Nishida K, Kuroda R, Kurosaka M. Soft-tissue balancing in total knee arthroplasty:

cruciate-retaining versus posterior-stabilised, and measured-resection versus gap technique. Int Orthop. 2014;38(3):531–7.
10. Attfield SF, Wilton TJ, Pratt DJ, Sambatakakis A. Soft-tissue balance and recovery of proprioception after total knee replacement. J Bone Joint Surg Br. 1996;78(4):540–5.
11. Pang HN, Yeo SJ, Chong HC, Chin PL, Ong J, Lo NN. Computer-assisted gap balancing technique improves outcome in total knee arthroplasty, compared with conventional measured resection technique. Knee Surg Sports Traumatol Arthrosc. 2011;19(9):1496–503.
12. Lampe F, Marques CJ, Fiedler F, Sufi-Siavach A, Matziolis G. Do well-balanced primary TKA patients achieve better outcomes within the first year after surgery? Orthopedics. 2016;39(3 Suppl):S6–S12.
13. Joseph J, Simpson PM, Whitehouse SL, English HW, Donnelly WJ. The use of navigation to achieve soft tissue balance in total knee arthroplasty – a randomised clinical study. Knee. 2013;20(6):401–6.
14. Widmer BJ, Scholes CJ, Lustig S, Conrad L, Oussedik SI, Parker DA. Intraoperative computer navigation parameters are poor predictors of function 1 year after total knee arthroplasty. J Arthroplasty. 2013;28(1):56–61.
15. Matsuda Y, Ishii Y, Noguchi H, Ishii R. Varus-valgus balance and range of movement after total knee arthroplasty. J Bone Joint Surg Br. 2005;87(6):804–8.
16. Liebs TR, Kloos SA, Herzberg W, Rüther W, Hassenpflug J. The significance of an asymmetric extension gap on routine radiographs after total knee replacement: a new sign and its clinical significance. Bone Joint J. 2013;95-B(4):472–7.
17. Okazaki K, Miura H, Matsuda S, Takeuchi N, Mawatari T, Hashizume M, Iwamoto Y. Asymmetry of mediolateral laxity of the normal knee. J Orthop Sci. 2006; 11(3):264–6.
18. Yoon JR, Oh KJ, Wang JH, Yang JH. Does patella position influence ligament balancing in total knee arthroplasty? Knee Surg Sports Traumatol Arthrosc. 2015;23(7):2012–8.
19. Clayton ML, Thompson TR, Mack RP. Correction of alignment deformities during total knee arthroplasties: staged soft-tissue releases. Clin Orthop Relat Res. 1986;202:117–24.
20. Scott WN, editors. Insall & Scott Surgery of the Knee. 5th ed. Philadelphia: Churchill livingstone/Elsevier; 2012.
21. Matsumoto T, Takayama K, Muratsu H, Matsushita T, Kuroda R, Kurosaka M. Semimembranosus release reduces tibial internal rotation and flexion angle in cruciate-retaining total knee arthroplasty. J Arthroplasty. 2015;30(9):1537–41.
22. Ahn JH, Back YW. Comparative study of two techniques for ligament balancing in total knee arthroplasty for severe varus knee: medial soft tissue release vs. bony resection of proximal medial tibia. Knee Surg Relat Res. 2013;25(1):13–8.
23. Whiteside LA. Soft tissue balancing: the knee. J Arthroplasty. 2002;17(4 Suppl 1):23–7.
24. Burkhart TA, Perry KI, Dobbin E, Howard J, Lanting B. Effect of Soft Tissue Releases on Joint Space Opening in Total Knee Arthroplasty. J Arthroplasty. 2016. pii: S0883–5403(16)30163–2.
25. Meneghini RM, Daluga AT, Sturgis LA, Lieberman JR. Is the pie-crusting technique safe for MCL release in varus deformity correction in total knee arthroplasty? J Arthroplasty. 2013;28(8):1306–9.
26. Dixon MC, Parsch D, Brown RR, Scott RD. The correction of severe varus deformity in total knee arthroplasty by tibial component downsizing and resection of uncapped proximal medial bone. J Arthroplasty. 2004;19(1):19–22.
27. Kesman TJ, Kaufman KR, Trousdale RT. Popliteus tendon resection during total knee arthroplasty: an observational report. Clin Orthop Relat Res. 2011;469(1):76–81.
28. Gustke KA, Golladay GJ, Roche MW, Jerry GJ, Elson LC, Anderson CR. Increased satisfaction after total knee replacement using sensor-guided technology. bone Joint J. 2014 Oct;96-B(10):1333–8.
29. Meneghini RM, Ziemba-Davis MM, Lovro LR, Ireland PH, Damer BM. Can intraoperative sensors determine the "Target" ligament balance? Early outcomes in total knee arthroplasty J Arthroplasty. 2016;31(10):2181–7.

30. Jacobs CA, Christensen CP, Karthikeyan T. Greater medial compartment forces during total knee arthroplasty associated with improved patient satisfaction and ability to navigate stairs. J Arthroplasty. 2016;31(9 Suppl):87–90.
31. Manning WA, Ghosh K, Blain A, Longstaff L, Deehan DJ. Tibiofemoral forces for the native and post-arthroplasty knee: relationship to maximal laxity through a functional arc of motion. Knee Surg Sports Traumatol Arthrosc. 2016. [Epub ahead of print].
32. Laughlin RT, Werries BA, Verhulst SJ, Hayes JM. Patellar tilt in total knee arthroplasty. Am J Orthop (Belle Mead NJ). 1996;25(4):300–4.
33. Bindelglass DF, Cohen JL, Dorr LD. Patellar tilt and subluxation in total knee arthroplasty. Relationship to pain, fixation, and design. Clin Orthop Relat Res. 1993;286:103–9.
34. Heesterbeek PJ, Keijsers NL, Wymenga AB. Femoral component rotation after balanced gap total knee replacement is not a predictor for postoperative patella position. Knee Surg Sports Traumatol Arthrosc. 2011;19(7):1131–6.

Soft Tissue Balance, Kinematics, and Patient Satisfaction

17

Shuichi Matsuda

Contents

Improving postoperative patient satisfaction is a major goal in total knee arthroplasty (TKA). Studies have reported that many factors affect patient satisfaction, including pre- and postoperative condition as well as mental health. From a biomechanical standpoint, the status of knee kinematics is a key issue impacting both postoperative knee function and satisfaction. Near-normal kinematics might help patients forget they had knee surgery, while abnormal knee kinematics can cause post-TKA discomfort. Also, knee kinematics can affect postoperative range of motion (ROM), which is another major factor influencing patient satisfaction. Postoperative knee kinematics are determined by soft tissue balance, alignment, and implant design (Fig. 17.1).

In this chapter, clinical and biomechanical studies are introduced to discuss the relationship among soft tissue balance, kinematics, and clinical symptoms, including patient satisfaction.

S. Matsuda
Department of Orthopaedic Surgery, Kyoto University, Kyoto, Japan
e-mail: smat522@kuhp.kyoto-u.ac.jp

S. Matsuda et al. (eds.), *Soft Tissue Balancing in Total Knee Arthroplasty*,
DOI 10.1007/978-3-662-54082-4_17

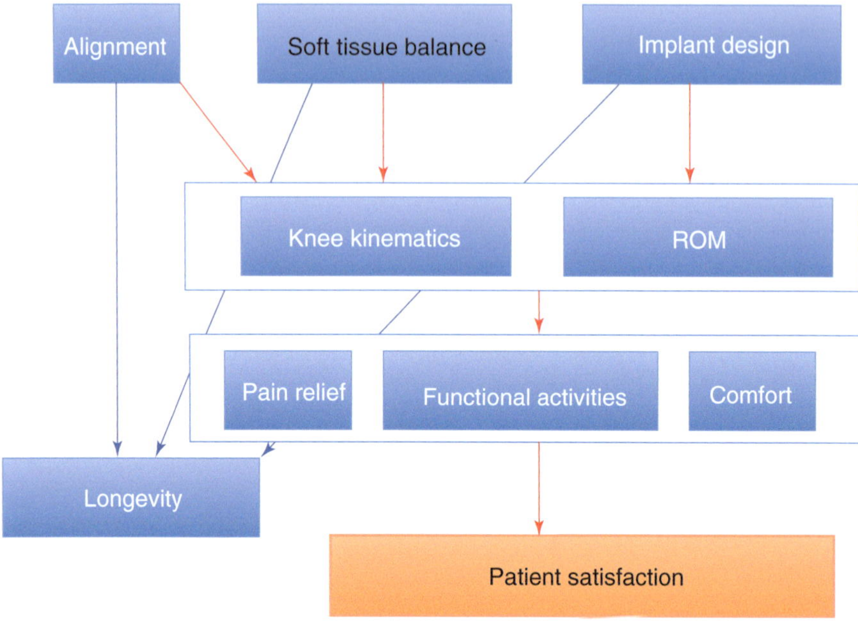

Fig. 17.1 Factors affecting clinical results after total knee arthroplasty

17.1 Intraoperative Soft Tissue Balance and Patient Symptoms

Intraoperative soft tissue balance is related to postoperative knee kinematics, which affect patient symptoms. Also, knee kinematics affect ROM, which can be significantly related to patient satisfaction and knee function [1]. In this chapter we first review studies on extension and flexion gaps and then discuss medial-lateral gap balancing (Table 17.1).

17.1.1 Extension Gap

The degree of extension gap necessary to avoid postoperative flexion contracture remains unclear [16]. Few studies have evaluated the relationship between intraoperative soft tissue tension and postoperative extension angle [17]. Usually, varus osteoarthritic knees show a smaller extension gap at the medial side than the lateral side. Therefore, we previously evaluated the effect of a medial extension gap on postoperative flexion contracture by evaluating the intraoperative extension gap in 75 knees with varus deformity undergoing TKA with the NexGen LPS (Zimmer, Warsaw, IN, USA) [2]. The extension gap was measured in the presence of a femoral component using a tension device applying a distraction force of 178 N. A "component gap" was defined as the distance calculated by subtracting the selected thickness of the tibial component, including the polyethylene liner,

Table 17.1 The effect of gap and medial-lateral balance on clinical results

	Gap	Medial-lateral balance
Extension	*Tight gap: flexion contracture* More than 1 mm was necessary to avoid flexion contracture [2]. *Loose gap: uncertain* A 2–3mm medial gap can be acceptable based on normal knee laxity [3] and clinical study [4].	*Medial-opening imbalance: possibly symptomatic* More than 1.5 mm of imbalance was related to pain [5]. *Lateral-opening imbalance: uncertain* No studies have shown that a large lateral gap is symptomatic. 2–3° of imbalance can be acceptable based on normal knee laxity [3].
Flexion	*Tight gap: decreasing flexion angle* [6–9] *Loose gap: variable results* A 2.5mm larger gap than extension was related to higher JFS in LCS [10]. A 3.0mm larger gap than extension was related to lower function score in CR [11]. Very large flexion gap causes symptomatic knees [12].	*Medial-opening imbalance: possibly symptomatic* ≥3° of imbalance was related to dissatisfaction in CS [13]. *Lateral -opening imbalance: positive effect on flexion angle* [7, 14, 15]

from the measured gap. The postoperative extension angle was measured by radiography. Flexion contracture was defined when the angle between the anatomical axis of the distal femur and the proximal tibia exceeded 5°. The knees with >1 mm medial component gap showed no flexion contracture at 1 year after surgery. Nagai et al. also reported that the postoperative active knee extension angle was positively correlated with the medial compartment gap at 0° [18]. These studies suggest that achieving an adequate medial extension gap is very important to avoid flexion contracture.

How loosely can the knee be left in extension? First and foremost, the patient should not feel any instability. Thus one possible benchmark is the stability of normal knees. We previously measured knee laxity in normal knees by stress radiography and found that the medial opening angle was 2.4° when a valgus stress of 147 N was applied [3]. Ishii et al. reported that excellent clinical results were achieved after TKA in patients with 3–4° of valgus laxity [4]. On the basis of these studies, 2–4° laxity does not lead to feelings of instability in patients who have undergone TKA. Therefore, we suggest that medial extension laxity should be 1–3 mm to avoid flexion contracture and subjective instability (note: 1° medial laxity equals approximately 1.05 mm when the transverse diameter of the tibia is 80 mm).

17.1.2 Flexion Gap

Many studies have evaluated the relationship between the intraoperative flexion gap and postoperative flexion angle. A clinical study by Takayama et al. indicated that flexion gap tightness decreases range of motion after cruciate-retaining (CR) TKA [6]. Nakano et al. evaluated the lateral and medial flexion gaps separately and found that the lateral compartment gap at 90° of flexion was positively correlated with postoperative knee flexion angle in knees after CR-TKA [7]. Hasegawa et al. reported that increased medial-lateral laxity from 90° to 120° showed a positive correlation with the postoperative flexion angle in posterior-stabilized (PS) TKA [8]. Other studies focused on deep knee flexion. For instance, Niki et al. divided patients who had undergone posterior-stabilized (PS) TKA into those who could achieve Seiza sitting (Japanese-style very deep knee flexion) and those who failed to and found that the gap length at 135° of flexion was significantly larger in the former group than the latter [9]. Watanabe also reported that in PS-TKA knees between 135° and 0° of extension, larger gap differences were associated with larger postoperative flexion angles [19]. In these studies, gaps were measured without patellar eversion so the assessments might have been affected by quadriceps tightness in deep knee flexion.

The effect of the flexion gap on postoperative symptoms has also been evaluated. Lampe et al. reported that larger flexion gaps (more than 2.9 mm) led to statistically lower Knee Society function scores and knee scores at 1 year after CR-TKA [11]. In CR-TKA, a large flexion gap results in function loss of the posterior cruciate ligament (PCL), which possibly worsens clinical results. In PCL-sacrificing TKA, the surgeon can control the flexion gap using the gap-balanced technique. In a study of knees with low-contact stress prostheses, Ismailidis et al. compared one group in which the flexion gap was intentionally 2.5 mm larger than the extension gap with another group in which these gaps were equal. They found that the former group achieved good ROM and showed a significantly higher Forgotten Joint Score-12 [10]. In normal knees, knee laxity in flexion is slightly larger than in extension, by about 1–2 mm [20]. One biomechanical study demonstrated that when the flexion gap was 2 mm greater than the extension gap, tibial forces were decreased in deep knee flexion [21].

Based on these clinical and biomechanical studies and normal knee evaluations, we should definitely avoid tighter gaps in knee flexion than extension to achieve good range of motion, and about 2 mm greater laxity in flexion can result in more normal feeling. But care should be taken to avoid excessively large flexion gaps because some patients with flexion instability after PS-TKA may present with pain, especially while negotiating stairs, as well as recurrent joint effusions, both of which can be causes of revision surgery [12].

17.1.3 Medial-Lateral Balancing

17.1.3.1 In Knee Extension

First, we discuss ligament balance in osteoarthritic knees. We previously investigated knee laxity in osteoarthritic knees during TKA [22]. In that study, the extension gap was measured after the distal part of the femur and the proximal part of the tibia were resected. The patients were divided into mild, moderate, and severe varus groups, based on preoperative hip-knee-ankle angles of <10°, 10–20°, and >20°, respectively. Measurements were made after removing osteophytes with a distraction force of 178 N. The results showed greater lateral soft tissue laxity with increasing severity of knee deformities. However, the medial side did not contract with increasing varus deformity. These results suggest that release on the medial side is unnecessary to create a space for implant replacement, even in severely deformed knees. However, gap imbalance increased up to 5 mm with increasing knee deformity. Therefore, we should determine the answer to this question: "How much of an imbalance can be tolerated in knee extension?"

As for intraoperative gap measurement, Lampe et al. reported that higher medial-lateral gap inequality (more than 2 mm) in both extension and flexion did not worsen Knee Society function or knee scores at 1 year after CR knee [11]. In postoperative stress radiograph evaluation, Nakahara et al. reported that varus laxities (5.9 ± 2.7°) or valgus laxities (5.0 ± 1.6°) under static stress in extension were not related to patient-reported outcomes after well-aligned PS-TKA [23]. Liebs et al. evaluated postoperative radiographs of gap imbalance (without any stress) and found that patients with an asymmetric medial opening extension gap of ≥ 1.5 mm had significantly higher pain scores at 3 and 6 months' follow-up, whereas a gap on the lateral side was associated with less pain [5]. Our study of normal knees showed 2.5° greater laxity on the lateral side than the medial side [3]. The results of these studies suggest that in knee extension, a couple of degrees of ligament imbalance, especially in lateral opening imbalance, can be tolerated from the standpoint of knee symptoms.

17.1.3.2 Knee Flexion

Many clinical and cadaveric studies have shown that in normal knees, soft tissue is laxer on the lateral side than the medial side in knee flexion [3, 20, 24]. Corroborating this, an MRI study by Tokuhara et al. showed that the lateral side was 4.6 mm laxer than the medial side [25].

We evaluated the effect of looseness in knee flexion on clinical outcome in 50 patients after TKA with a cruciate-sacrificed design (Kyocera Bisurface Knee) [13]. Stress radiographs were taken with a lateral traction force of 50 N applied perpendicular to the lower leg at 80° knee flexion. We measured the angle between a line tangential to the femoral condyles and a line through the tibial joint surface. Patient satisfaction, symptoms, and knee function according to the new Knee Society scoring system were compared between the knees with ≥3° medial flexion laxity (medial loose group) and knees with <3° medial flexion laxity (medial tight group). The scores of the medial loose and tight groups were 22 and 30 (out of 40) for satisfaction, 16 and 20 (out of 25) for symptoms, and 19 and 24 (out of 30) for standard activities, respectively. These results show that the knees with a medial opening imbalance had worse clinical outcomes after CS-TKA. Another clinical study by Seon et al. reported no difference between knees with rectangular and non-rectangular flexion gaps with respect to knee score [26].

Regarding knee flexion angle, Niki et al. compared a group of patients who achieved Seiza sitting with those who failed and found no significant differences in gap inclination between PS knees [9]. On the other hand, some studies reported the importance of a certain amount of lateral laxity (i.e., lateral opening imbalance) for achieving a good flexion angle. Nakano et al. showed that the lateral opening imbalance at 90° of flexion was positively correlated with postoperative knee flexion angle in CR-TKA [7]. Kobayashi et al. reported that lateral laxity during knee flexion was related to good range of motion [14].

Thus, to date, few clinical studies have indicated that it is important to achieve a medial-lateral flexion gap in order to improve clinical results. A certain amount of lateral laxity can improve knee flexion, but medial laxity will lead to inferior clinical results. It is important to recognize that medial opening and lateral opening imbalances are quite different in terms of the effect on clinical results. We believe that a certain degree of lateral laxity in flexion is close to the normal condition and is also related to better range of motion.

17.2 Soft Tissue Balance and Kinematics

Soft tissue balance and the articular geometry of the implant are two major factors determining knee kinematics after total knee arthroplasty. However, not many studies have evaluated the effects of soft tissue conditions on knee kinematics (Table 17.2).

Some studies have evaluated the effects of gap and balance on knee motion in the anterior-posterior and rotational directions. Watanabe et al. reported that following PS-TKA, the gap difference in knee flexion at 135° minus 0° was correlated with the total posterior translation of the lateral femoral condyle and femoral external rotation during squatting, and these knees had larger flexion angles [19]. This study suggested that to achieve near-normal kinematics in PS-TKA, a tight flexion gap should be avoided. In CR-TKA, the situation is slightly different because a loose flexion gap results in PCL dysfunction. Fujimoto et al. divided patients with CR-TKA into two groups according to their 90° minus 0° component gap changes: the wide flexion gap group was defined by a change of >3 mm, while the narrow flexion gap group was defined by a change of <3 mm. The authors found that under non-weight-bearing conditions, the wide flexion gap group showed significant anterior displacement of the medial femoral condyle compared with the narrow flexion

Table 17.2 The effect of gap and medial-lateral balance on knee kinematics

	Gap	Medial-lateral balance
Extension	No studies have evaluated the effect of extension gap alone on knee kinematics.	No correlation between ligament balance and lift-off [12, 27].
Flexion	Large gap difference was related to paradoxical motion in CR [14]. Larger gap difference between extension and flexion was related to near-normal kinematics in PS [8].	A greater medial flexion gap caused larger anterior translation [28]. Lateral opening imbalance was related to near-normal kinematics [26].

gap group [15]. Another clinical study also found that worse clinical scores were associated with larger flexion gaps in CR knees [11].

What are the effects of medial-lateral balance? Matsuzaki et al. evaluated intraoperative knee kinematics using navigation and found that varus ligament balance at 90° of flexion was positively correlated with tibial internal rotation at 60° and 90° of flexion, and the lateral compartment gap was positively correlated with tibial internal rotation at 60°, 90°, and 120° of knee flexion in CR knees [28]. This is one of the reasons why a large lateral flexion gap is related to good range of motion, as shown in clinical studies [7, 8, 14]. Our fluoroscopic analysis showed that a greater medial flexion gap caused larger anterior translation in knee flexion in CS-TKA [29], but lateral static instability at knee flexion did not cause any abnormal motion. CS-TKA controls AP stability via a curved articular surface and joint gap tightness, without a post-cam mechanism. Therefore, achieving an adequate flexion gap in CS-TKA is more important than in PS-TKA in order to achieve proper AP stability in flexion.

Knee motion in the coronal direction is also clinically important. Because joint laxity theoretically increases the risk of lift-off motion, we focus on that motion here. Since lift-off motion of the femoral component possibly increases wear of the articular surface [27], it should be avoided after TKA. Hamai et al. [30] used fluoroscopic stress radiography to evaluate the effect of post-CR-TKA static knee instability on dynamic lift-off motion and found that neither static varus-valgus laxity nor differences in laxity (i.e., imbalance) influenced lift-off motion. Nakahara et al. reported that no correlations were found between femoral condylar lift-off during walking and varus-valgus laxities under static stress in extension after well-aligned PS-TKA [23]. We also evaluated the effects of alignment and ligament balance on lift-off motion using computer simulations, which have recently been validated in the field of TKA [31–37], with KneeSIM software (LifeMOD/KneeSIM 2010; LifeModeler Inc., San Clemente, CA, USA). Our results showed that lift-off motion occurred with 5° varus alignment or with a combination of 2° varus deformity and 2 mm lateral laxity [38]. However, no lift-off motion was detected in knees with neutral to 1° varus malalignment, even when the knees had 5 mm lateral laxity. These findings show that alignment is also very important in terms of its impact on knee kinematics. Therefore, tolerance of ligament imbalance will be different depending on knee alignment.

Recently, knee alignment has been recognized as an important factor determining ligament balance. Bellemans [39] et al. reported that the incidence of a natural limb alignment of ≥3° varus, which is termed constitutional varus, is approximately 32% in men and 17% in women. They suggest that aiming for neutral alignment can result in overcorrection in some patients and report that patients with slight undercorrection have better function and pain scores than those with neutral alignment [40]. Their cadaver study showed that restoration of constitutional alignment in TKA led to more physiological strain in the collateral ligaments [41]. However, there is no definitive way to determine the degree of constitutional varus in a patient, and the "safe zone" of varus alignment is unknown. Some clinical studies have reported that undercorrection does not worsen clinical results [42] and that design modification can prevent wear problems even with malalignment [43–45]. Nevertheless, concerns about tibial collapse in varus alignment remain [46–48]. Howell et al. propose kinematic alignment [49, 50] as a way to maximally utilize ligamentous function. Better functional results were reported with kinematically aligned TKA than with mechanically aligned TKA [51]. Kinematically aligned TKA aims to reproduce the pre-osteoarthritic joint surface and does not align to any axis that is used in the mechanical axis method. However, the precise pre-osteoarthritic morphology cannot be determined, and this technique incurs the risk of coronal malalignment, especially in patients with severe constitutional varus.

Although these two new ideas have some unresolved problems [52], they suggest the very interesting idea that postoperative knee function can be improved by preserving ligamentous tension rather than sticking to the mechanical alignment.

17.3 Knee Kinematics and Clinical Results, Including Patient Satisfaction

How knee kinematics affect clinical symptoms is very important question that has been addressed by very few studies. Nakahara et al. reported that no correlations were found between femoral condylar lift-off during walking and patient-reported outcomes after well-aligned PS-TKA [23]. Small amounts of lift-off may not cause any clinical symptoms.

Some studies have focused on tibial internal rotation, which is seen in normal knees. Nishio et al. divided patients into a medial pivot group ($n = 20$) and a non-medial pivot group ($n = 20$) based on a kinematic pattern using intraoperative kinematics. Functional activities, patient satisfaction, and the knee flexion angle in the medial pivot group were significantly better than those in the non-medial pivot group [53]. Lützner performed fluoroscopic analysis immediately after wound closure in CR-TKA. They found that patients whose rotational mismatch between the femoral and tibial components was more than 10° showed less femoral external rotation as well as worse functional scores [54]. These studies suggest that tibial internal rotation in knee flexion is important for achieving good ROM, function, and satisfaction.

17.4 Summary

On the basis of the available clinical and biomechanical studies, we can suggest these principles:

1. To avoid flexion contracture, the extension gap should not be tight.
2. The flexion gap can be controlled with the gap-balanced technique in PS-TKA. Good clinical results are achieved with a flexion gap that is 2 mm larger than the extension gap, but very large flexion gaps can result in unwanted symptoms. In CR-TKA, the flexion gap is primarily controlled by the PCL. Care

should be taken to properly tension the PCL because a larger flexion gap (i.e., PCL deficiency) worsens clinical results.

3. Lateral opening ligament imbalance does not cause any symptoms or lift-off motion, but medial opening imbalance can cause adverse symptoms.
4. In knee flexion, a certain amount of lateral laxity is necessary to achieve near-normal kinematics, which are related to good ROM, function, and patient satisfaction. Medial opening imbalance can cause anterior movement of the femoral component in CS-TKA, producing unwanted symptoms.

References

1. Matsuda S, Kawahara S, Okazaki K, Tashiro Y, Iwamoto Y. Postoperative alignment and ROM affect patient satisfaction after TKA. Clin Orthop Relat Res. 2013;471:127–33.
2. Okamoto S, Okazaki K, Mitsuyasu H, Matsuda S, Mizu-Uchi H, Hamai S, Tashiro Y, Iwamoto Y. Extension gap needs more than 1-mm laxity after implantation to avoid post-operative flexion contracture in total knee arthroplasty. Knee Surg Sports Traumatol Arthrosc. 2014;22:3174–80.
3. Okazaki K, Miura H, Matsuda S, Takeuchi N, Mawatari T, Hashizume M, Iwamoto Y. Asymmetry of mediolateral laxity of the normal knee. J Orthop Sci. 2006;11:264–6.
4. Ishii Y, Matsuda Y, Noguchi H, Kiga H. Effect of soft tissue tension on measurements of coronal laxity in mobile-bearing total knee arthroplasty. J Orthop Sci. 2005;10:496–500.
5. Liebs TR, Kloos SA, Herzberg W, Ruther W, Hassenpflug J. The significance of an asymmetric extension gap on routine radiographs after total knee replacement: a new sign and its clinical significance. Bone Joint J. 2013;95-B:472–7.
6. Takayama K, Matsumoto T, Kubo S, Muratsu H, Ishida K, Matsushita T, Kurosaka M, Kuroda R. Influence of intra-operative joint gaps on post-operative flexion angle in posterior cruciate-retaining total knee arthroplasty. Knee Surg Sports Traumatol Arthrosc. 2012;20:532–7.
7. Nakano N, Matsumoto T, Muratsu H, Takayama K, Kuroda R, Kurosaka M. Postoperative knee flexion angle is affected by lateral laxity in cruciate-retaining total knee arthroplasty. J Arthroplasty. 2016;31:401–5.
8. Hasegawa M, Takagita H, Sudo A. Prediction of post-operative range of motion using intra-operative soft tissue balance in total knee arthroplasty with navigation. Comput Aided Surg. 2015;20:47–51.
9. Niki Y, Takeda Y, Harato K, Suda Y. Factors affecting the achievement of Japanese-style deep knee flexion after total knee arthroplasty using posterior-stabilized prosthesis with high-flex knee design. J Orthop Sci. 2015,20:1012–8.
10. Ismailidis P, Kuster MS, Jost B, Giesinger K, Behrend H. Clinical outcome of increased flexion gap after total knee arthroplasty. Can controlled gap imbalance improve knee flexion? Knee Surg Sports Traumatol Arthrosc. 2016 Feb 4. [Epub ahead of print].
11. Lampe F, Marques CJ, Fiedler F, Sufi-Siavach A, Matziolis G. Do well-balanced primary TKA patients achieve better outcomes within the first year after surgery? Orthopedics. 2016;39:S6–S12.
12. Deshmane PP, Rathod PA, Deshmukh AJ, Rodriguez JA, Scuderi GR. Symptomatic flexion instability in posterior stabilized primary total knee arthroplasty. Orthopedics. 2014;37:e768–74.
13. Matsuda S. Knee stability and implant design of total knee arthroplasty. Paper presented at: 1st Congress of APKASS; April 14–15, 2014; Nara.
14. Kobayashi T, Suzuki M, Sasho T, Nakagawa K, Tsuneizumi Y, Takahashi K. Lateral laxity in flexion increases the postoperative flexion angle in cruciate-retaining total knee arthroplasty. J Arthroplasty. 2012;27:260–5.

15. Fujimoto E, Sasashige Y, Tomita T, Sasaki H, Touten Y, Fujiwara Y, Ochi M. Intra-operative gaps affect outcome and postoperative kinematics in vivo following cruciate-retaining total knee arthroplasty. Int Orthop. 2016;40:41–9.
16. Mitsuyasu H, Matsuda S, Miura H, Okazaki K, Fukagawa S, Iwamoto Y. Flexion contracture persists if the contracture is more than 15 degrees at 3 months after total knee arthroplasty. J Arthroplasty. 2011;26:639–43.
17. Asano H, Muneta T, Sekiya I. Soft tissue tension in extension in total knee arthroplasty affects postoperative knee extension and stability. Knee Surg Sports Traumatol Arthrosc. 2008;16:999–1003.
18. Nagai K, Muratsu H, Matsumoto T, Takahara S, Kuroda R, Kurosaka M. Influence of intraoperative soft tissue balance on postoperative active knee extension in posterior-stabilized total knee arthroplasty. J Arthroplasty. 2015;30:1155–9.
19. Watanabe T, Muneta T, Sekiya I, Banks SA. Intraoperative joint gaps and mediolateral balance affect postoperative knee kinematics in posterior-stabilized total knee arthroplasty. Knee. 2015;22:527–34.
20. Ghosh KM, Merican AM, Iranpour F, Deehan DJ, Amis AA. Length-change patterns of the collateral ligaments after total knee arthroplasty. Knee Surg Sports Traumatol Arthrosc. 2012;20:1349–56.
21. Jeffcote B, Nicholls R, Schirm A, Kuster MS. The variation in medial and lateral collateral ligament strain and tibiofemoral forces following changes in the flexion and extension gaps in total knee replacement. A laboratory experiment using cadaver knees. J Bone Joint Surg Br. 2007;89:1528–33.
22. Okamoto S, Okazaki K, Mitsuyasu H, Matsuda S, Iwamoto Y. Lateral soft tissue laxity increases but medial laxity does not contract with varus deformity in total knee arthroplasty. Clin Orthop Relat Res. 2013;471:1334–42.
23. Nakahara H, Okazaki K, Hamai S, Okamoto S, Kuwashima U, Higaki H, Iwamoto Y. Does knee stability in the coronal plane in extension affect function and outcome after total knee arthroplasty? Knee Surg Sports Traumatol Arthrosc. 2015;23:1693–8.
24. Nowakowski AM, Majewski M, Muller-Gerbl M, Valderrabano V. Measurement of knee joint gaps without bone resection: "physiologic" extension and flexion gaps in total knee arthroplasty are asymmetric and unequal and anterior and posterior cruciate ligament resections produce different gap changes. J Orthop Res. 2012;30:522–7.
25. Tokuhara Y, Kadoya Y, Nakagawa S, Kobayashi A, Takaoka K. The flexion gap in normal knees. An MRI study. J Bone Joint Surg Br. 2004;86:1133–6.
26. Seon JK, Song EK, Park SJ, Lee DS. The use of navigation to obtain rectangular flexion and extension gaps during primary total knee arthroplasty and midterm clinical results. J Arthroplasty. 2011;26:582–90.
27. Jennings LM, Bell CI, Ingham E, Komistek RD, Stone MH, Fisher J. The influence of femoral condylar lift-off on the wear of artificial knee joints. Proc Inst Mech Eng H. 2007;221:305–14.
28. Matsuzaki T, Matsumoto T, Kubo S, Muratsu H, Matsushita T, Kawakami Y, Ishida K, Oka S, Kuroda R, Kurosaka M. Tibial internal rotation is affected by lateral laxity in cruciate-retaining total knee arthroplasty: an intraoperative kinematic study using a navigation system and offset-type tensor. Knee Surg Sports Traumatol Arthrosc. 2014;22:615–20.
29. Nakamura S, Ito H, Yoshitomi H, Kuriyama S, Komistek RD, Matsuda S. Analysis of the flexion gap on in vivo knee kinematics using fluoroscopy. J Arthroplasty. 2015;30:1237–42.
30. Hamai S, Miura H, Okazaki K, Shimoto T, Higaki H, Iwamoto Y. No influence of coronal laxity and alignment on lift-off after well-balanced and aligned total knee arthroplasty. Knee Surg Sports Traumatol Arthrosc. 2014;22:1799–804.
31. Morra EA, Rosca M, Greenwald JF, Greenwald AS. The influence of contemporary knee design on high flexion: a kinematic comparison with the normal knee. J Bone Joint Surg Am. 2008;90(Suppl 4):195–201.

32. Colwell Jr CW, Chen PC, D'Lima D. Extensor malalignment arising from femoral component malrotation in knee arthroplasty: effect of rotating-bearing. Clin Biomech (Bristol, Avon). 2011;26:52–7.
33. Mizu-uchi H, Colwell Jr CW, Matsuda S, Flores-Hernandez C, Iwamoto Y, D'Lima DD. Effect of total knee arthroplasty implant position on flexion angle before implant-bone impingement. J Arthroplasty. 2011;26:721–7.
34. Mihalko WM, Williams JL. Total knee arthroplasty kinematics may be assessed using computer modeling: a feasibility study. Orthopedics. 2012;35:40–4.
35. Mizu-Uchi H, Colwell Jr CW, Fukagawa S, Matsuda S, Iwamoto Y, D'Lima DD. The importance of bony impingement in restricting flexion after total knee arthroplasty: computer simulation model with clinical correlation. J Arthroplasty. 2012;27:1710–6.
36. Morra EA, Heim CS, Greenwald AS. Preclinical computational models: predictors of tibial insert damage patterns in total knee arthroplasty: AAOS exhibit selection. J Bone Joint Surg Am. 2012;94:e137(131–5).
37. Kuriyama S, Ishikawa M, Furu M, Ito H, Matsuda S. Malrotated tibial component increases medial collateral ligament tension in total knee arthroplasty. J Orthop Res. 2014;32:1658–66.
38. Matsuda S. Computer simulation in TKA. Paper presented at: 2014 ICJR Pan Pacific Congress; July 16–19, 2014; Kona.
39. Bellemans J, Colyn W, Vandenneucker H, Victor J. The Chitranjan Ranawat award: is neutral mechanical alignment normal for all patients? The concept of constitutional varus. Clin Orthop Relat Res. 2012;470:45–53.
40. Vanlommel L, Vanlommel J, Claes S, Bellemans J. Slight undercorrection following total knee arthroplasty results in superior clinical outcomes in varus knees. Knee Surg Sports Traumatol Arthrosc. 2013;21:2325–30.
41. Delport H, Labey L, Innocenti B, De Corte R, Vander Sloten J, Bellemans J. Restoration of constitutional alignment in TKA leads to more physiological strains in the collateral ligaments. Knee Surg Sports Traumatol Arthrosc. 2015;23(8):2159–69.
42. Parratte S, Pagnano MW, Trousdale RT, Berry DJ. Effect of postoperative mechanical axis alignment on the fifteen-year survival of modern, cemented total knee replacements. J Bone Joint Surg Am. 2010;92:2143–9.
43. Nishikawa K, Okazaki K, Matsuda S, Tashiro Y, Kawahara S, Nakahara H, Okamoto S, Shimoto T, Higaki H, Iwamoto Y. Improved design decreases wear in total knee arthroplasty with varus malalignment. Knee Surg Sports Traumatol Arthrosc. 2014;22:2635–40.
44. Matsuda S, Miura H, Nagamine R, Urabe K, Harimaya K, Matsunobu T, Iwamoto Y. Changes in knee alignment after total knee arthroplasty. J Arthroplasty. 1999;14:566–70.
45. Matsuda S, Whiteside LA, White SE. The effect of varus tilt on contact stresses in total knee arthroplasty: a biomechanical study. Orthopedics. 1999;22:303–7.
46. Fang DM, Ritter MA, Davis KE. Coronal alignment in total knee arthroplasty: just how important is it? J Arthroplasty. 2009;24:39–43.
47. Wong J, Steklov N, Patil S, Flores-Hernandez C, Kester M, Colwell Jr CW, D'Lima DD. Predicting the effect of tray malalignment on risk for bone damage and implant subsidence after total knee arthroplasty. J Orthop Res. 2011;29:347–53.
48. Halder A, Kutzner I, Graichen F, Heinlein B, Beier A, Bergmann G. Influence of limb alignment on mediolateral loading in total knee replacement: in vivo measurements in five patients. J Bone Joint Surg Am. 2012;94:1023–9.
49. Howell SM, Kuznik K, Hull ML, Siston RA. Results of an initial experience with custom-fit positioning total knee arthroplasty in a series of 48 patients. Orthopedics. 2008;31:857–63.
50. Howell SM, Papadopoulos S, Kuznik KT, Hull ML. Accurate alignment and high function after kinematically aligned TKA performed with generic instruments. Knee Surg Sports Traumatol Arthrosc. 2013;21:2271–80.

51. Dossett HG, Estrada NA, Swartz GJ, LeFevre GW, Kwasman BG. A randomised controlled trial of kinematically and mechanically aligned total knee replacements: two-year clinical results. Bone Joint J. 2014;96-B:907–13.
52. Ishikawa M, Kuriyama S, Ito H, Furu M, Nakamura S, Matsuda S. Kinematic alignment produces near-normal knee motion but increases contact stress after total knee arthroplasty: a case study on a single implant design. Knee. 2015;22:206–12.
53. Nishio Y, Onodera T, Kasahara Y, Takahashi D, Iwasaki N, Majima T. Intraoperative medial pivot affects deep knee flexion angle and patient-reported outcomes after total knee arthroplasty. J Arthroplasty. 2014;29:702–6.
54. Lutzner J, Kirschner S, Gunther KP, Harman MK. Patients with no functional improvement after total knee arthroplasty show different kinematics. Int Orthop. 2012;36:1841–7.

Part VI

Patella

Surgical Techniques to Avoid Patellar Maltracking in Total Knee Arthroplasty

18

Kelly Vince

Contents

K. Vince, MD FRCS(C)
Department of Orthopedic Surgery, Whangarei Hospital, Northland District Health Board, Whangarei, New Zealand
e-mail: kellyvince@mac.com

S. Matsuda et al. (eds.), *Soft Tissue Balancing in Total Knee Arthroplasty*,
DOI 10.1007/978-3-662-54082-4_18

18.1 Simplified Mechanics of Patellar Tracking

"The shortest distance between two points is a straight line." That concept explains many problems with tracking of the extensor mechanism, a linear construct that is under large tensile load and that angulates in the sagittal and frontal planes. The usual way to straighten a linear structure is to load both ends with opposing forces (tension) and eliminate all other forces, much like an archer who has drawn his bow and then releases fingers from the arrow (Fig. 18.1). This is similar to active knee extension. By contrast, the extensor must maintain a turning point at the patella in the frontal plane despite very high loads, much like the rigging of a yacht where lines under significant tension must angulate around pulleys or "turning blocks" (Fig. 18.2). The patella angulates in two planes at the femoral "trochlea," a word that originates from Greek and Latin references to a "pulley."

Knee extensor mechanics are usually analyzed as two separate systems: extensor power [1] and patellar tracking [2, 3] (Fig. 18.3a, b). Tracking, or the path of the patella in the frontal plane, including planar changes due to knee flexion, accommodates valgus knee alignment characterized by the "Q" angle (Fig. 18.3b). Reductive analyses like extensor power and "Q angle" are useful simplifications, but the real knee extensor tracks in three dimensions through a multitude of knee flexion angles, tethered to the tibia that rotates in two planes (flexion-extension and internal-external rotation) under the femur.

The phrase "patellar tracking" is misleading, as the behavior of this sesamoid bone cannot be understood in isolation from the entire limb. Tracking concerns the

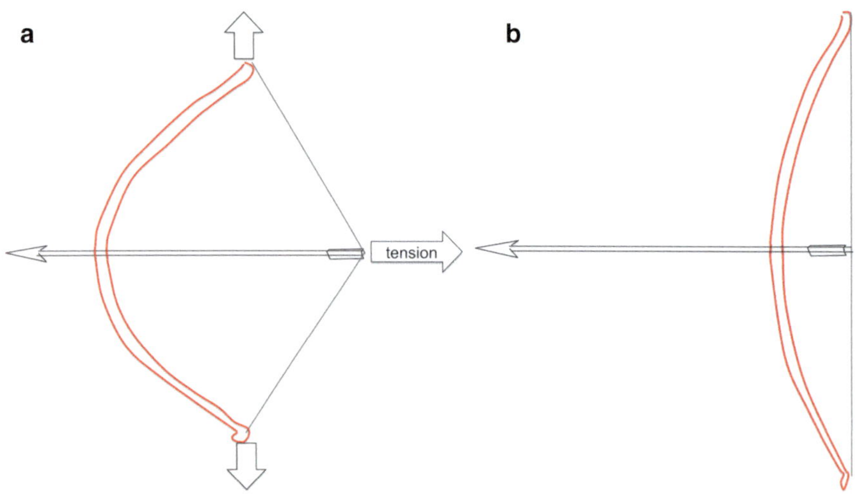

Fig. 18.1 (**a**) In some ways the extensor mechanism under load is like a drawn bow: When the energy in the bow is released, the ends spring apart and the bow string assumes the shortest distance between the two points at either end of the bow. The extensor straightens in the sagittal plane to extend the knee joint but it must still cope with angulation in the frontal plane due to the "Q" angle. (**b**) "The straight line" of the bow string propels the arrow forcefully. The patello-femoral joint converts quadriceps contraction to rotation or extension of the knee joint. The loads are significant and if the complex mechanism for guiding the extensor around the turning point at the knee fails, the patella will seek the shortest path and dislocate

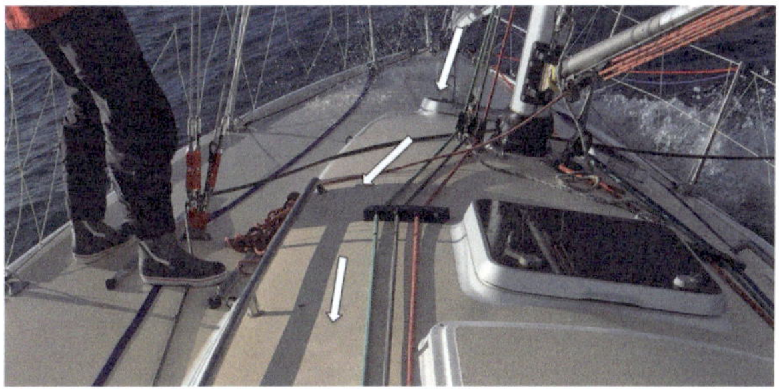

Fig. 18.2 The running rigging on a sailing boat are under hundreds of kilograms of load. Sometimes they must be angulated such as at the bottom of the mast or along the deck as indicated by the path of 3 arrows. The pulleys that accomplish this function like the lateral facet of the patellofemoral joint

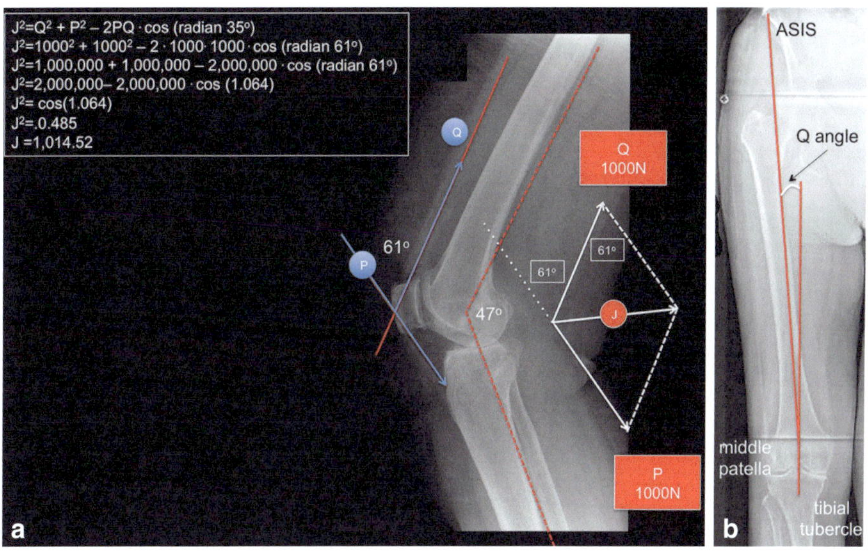

Fig. 18.3 (**a**) Usual biomechanical analysis of extensor function quantifies the joint reaction forces (*J*) based on the angle of knee flexion and the magnitude of force vectors representing the patellar tendon pull (*P*) and the quadriceps pull (*Q*). The direction and magnitude of J are solved with the parallelogram law of forces using the law of cosines: J2=P2+Q2-2PQ × COS angle between P and Q. This is only part of the story of patellar behaviour. (**b**) shows the frontal plane depiction of "Q" angle, defined as the angle subtended by lines from ASIS (anterior-superior iliac spine) to the centre of the patella, with the line of the patellar tendon. This analysis changes as the knee flexes and one plane (frontal) becomes two planes (of the tibia and the femur)

entire extensor, comprised of the origin of the quadriceps muscle, the muscle itself, the quadriceps tendon, the osseous patella, the patellar tendon, the tibial tubercle, limb alignment, and the dynamic translation and rotation of these parts in three dimensions. In an arthroplasty, by contrast with the native knee, the rotational position of implants and altered rotational dynamics of the tibia under the femur are additional variables a surgeon must consider (Fig. 18.4).

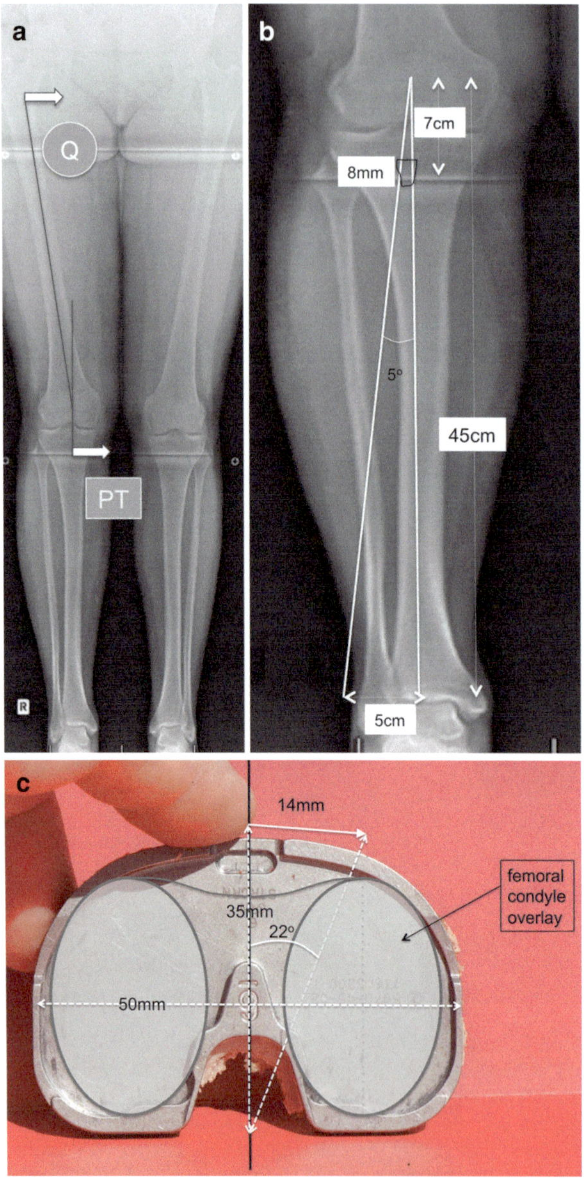

Fig. 18.4 (**a**) A straighter "Q" angle should enhance the tendency for the patella to track centrally, by eliminating the laterally directed vector of the extensor. This can theoretically be accomplished by moving the proximal (Q) or the distal vectors (PT) medially. The former is theoretically possible but difficult (see text). (**b**) Tibial component rotation around the "y" axis is more likely to increase the Q angle than an increase in valgus alignment. For example, if valgus is increased by a clinically undesirable 5 degrees, the talus would be displaced 5 cm laterally but the tubercle about one tenth of that distance. (Tangent 5°=3.38= displacement/45 cm. Internal rotation of the tibial component will have a more direct effect on displacement of the tubercle. (**c**) Assuming a tibial component size of 50 mm medial to lateral and anteroposterior of 35 mm, internal rotation of 22° would displace the tubercle about 14 mm, just across the center of the lateral femoral condyle, so that a patella with a centrally placed dome would tend to articulate outside the trochlear groove. Berger et al. allowed up to 18° degrees of internal rotation as consistent with good function

18.2 What Is Tracking?

Extensor tracking describes all contact of the patellar and femoral articular surfaces from full extension to maximum flexion, with or without prosthetic resurfacing. How the extensor tracks affects knee function, patient comfort, and component wear. The extensor mechanism can be conceived as a flexible linear structure under dynamic loads. Tracking describes its physical relationship with a rigid but articulated "track," formed by the femoral trochlea in extension and then by the distal intercondylar geometry as knee flexion proceeds.

18.3 Orientation of the Extensor: A Dynamic Structure

The orientation of the extensor is determined by the origin of the quadriceps muscle and its direction of pull proximally, the patella interacting with the trochlear groove, and the location of the tibial tubercle. Tensile load on a pliant extensor mechanism that is angled in valgus at the knee moves the (unrestrained) patella laterally. Straightening the pull of the extensor on the patella will enhance tracking. In most knees, maneuvers that move the proximal or distal vectors medially will align the quadriceps origin, the patella, and the tibial tubercle (Fig. 18.4a–c). These force vectors could theoretically be changed by modifications to the attachment of the extensor to the skeleton, but the anatomically complicated quadriceps origins are difficult to modify. Preferential vastus medialis strengthening [4] and medial surgical advancement are more practical interventions [5]. The tibial tubercle is probably the most significant structure in this equation. While the tubercle can be repositioned surgically, it is more commonly malpositioned inadvertently by the rotational position of the tibial component.

18.4 The Trochlear Track

In contrast to the supple and dynamic extensor, which controls the patella, the trochlear groove is structural and static. Tracking will improve if the groove can be located where the patellar is driven by knee function. Because the patella moves laterally when loaded, anything that positions the prosthetic trochlear groove laterally is beneficial. In a somewhat frivolous analogy, the patella is a willful teenager, determined to go where it wants. The trochlear groove must be established in that place to contain it. In another analogy, centralizing the patella in the trochlear groove is a process of conciliation: reducing lateral excursions of the patella and simultaneously positioning the femoral trochlea in a more lateral position.

18.5 Maltracking

Maltracking is the converse of a matched trajectory of the extensor with the structure of the trochlea [6–8]. Maltracking can be described as incremental subluxation in millimeters of translation or degrees of tilt [9]. Complete escape from the trochlear groove is a qualitative change—dislocation. Then, the medial-patellofemoral ligament will have ruptured, and the patella can only return to the front of the knee with extension of the joint (Fig. 18.5). As the patella dislocates laterally, part of the quadriceps muscle vector creates a *valgus moment* on the tibia-femoral joint, exacerbating tibia-femoral instability (Fig. 18.6). If the extensor migrates behind the axis of knee flexion, it can temporarily and aberrantly function as a knee flexor (Fig. 18.6).

Clinical problems that result directly from patellar maltracking include knee instability [10–12], buckling, pain, patellar fractures, patellar component loosening

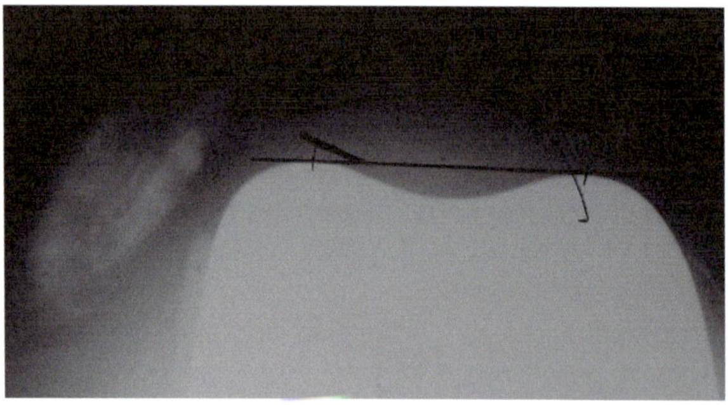

Fig. 18.5 Complete dislocation of a resurfaced patella in 45° of flexion. This patella will only be relocated as the knee extends fully, if at all. (Markings are from research protocol to measure "tilt" and "translation")

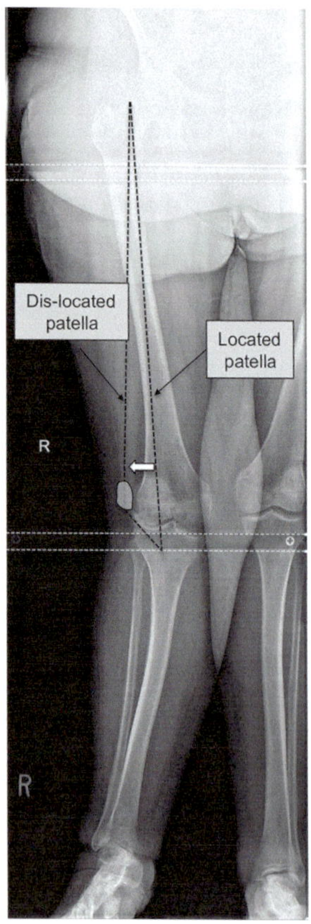

Fig. 18.6 In this arthritic knee with valgus deformity, the Q angle has "straightened" itself and the patella rides over the lateral femoral condyle, not in the trochlear groove. With the patella dislocated, the Q angle is in varus, the patella articulates with the lateral side of the femur and the extensor has become a valgus deforming force

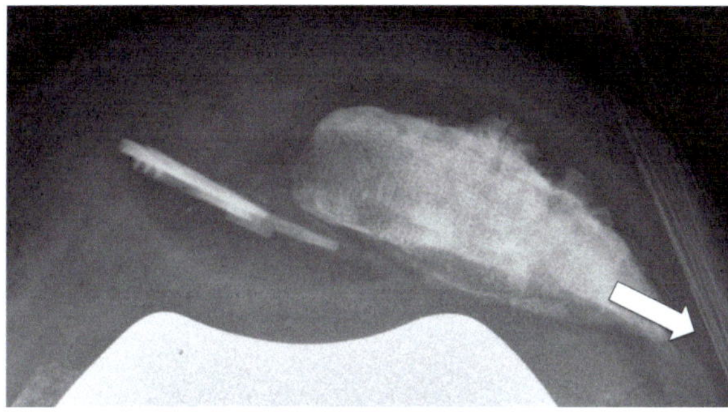

Fig. 18.7 Many problems result from mal-tracking. In this case of maltracking, the patellar prosthesis cannot escape from the highly conforming trochlear groove. As the extensor dislocates, bone and prosthesis part company: patellar component loosening is caused by maltracking

(Fig. 18.7), patellar component breakage, and wear [8]. Indirect problems associated with the same mechanics include stiffness [13].

18.6 Tracking Is Difficult Because of Valgus Knee Alignment

Extensor tracking might conceivably be improved in an arthroplasty by eliminating frontal plane angulation, except that some degree of anatomic tibial-femoral valgus (even in conjunction with an overall mechanical varus [14, 15]) is desirable. While ideal alignment has reemerged as a topic for discussion [16, 17], a valgus tibial-femoral angle decreases the energy consumption of human gait by decreasing medial-lateral oscillations of the human center of gravity with each step [18]. Despite current debates, most surgeons believe that some degree of valgus alignment also decreases medial load and aseptic loosening [19].

18.7 What Are the Forces on the Patella?

The patella-femoral joint experiences high anterior to posterior compression when the quadriceps contracts to extend the knee, to maintain a given flexion angle, or to slow the rate of flexion. Patellofemoral forces increase with flexion and diminish almost to zero in full knee extension [1]. The patella, sitting between the anterior femur and the extensor mechanism, displaces the quadriceps and patellar tendons anteriorly by a distance equal to its thickness, even in full extension, as a means to increase the moment arm in terminal extension. The extensor is never completely straight in the sagittal or frontal planes in most knees.

The magnitude of the lateral vector on the patella increases directly with the load generated by the quadriceps. The more forcefully the quadriceps contracts, the greater the force tending to straighten the extensor in both planes. Muscle action drives both desired knee extension and undesired lateral patellar subluxation. Extension power will be lost if the patella escapes laterally, out of the groove. Tension in the medial patella-femoral ligament (MPFL) resists lateral patellar dislocation, and the lateral trochlear ridge exerts compression medially against the lateral patellar facet to oppose patellar subluxation and keep the patella in front of the knee (Fig. 18.8a). Given the obliquity of the native lateral facet joint, much of this constraining force is shear. Part of the vector will be compression that forces the patella anteriorly in opposition to

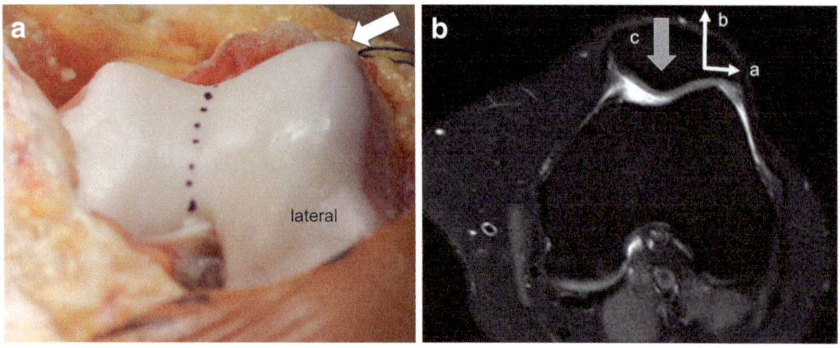

Fig. 18.8 (**a**) Intra-operative photograph at time of patello-femoral arthroplasty. The anteroposterior axis has been marked with dots. The prominent lateral trochlear ridge is indicated by the arrow. This is an anatomic mechanism opposing lateral patellar dislocation. (**b**) MRI of knee. As the patella begins to translate laterally with flexion (*vector a*) the shape of the lateral trochlear ridge forces it anteriorly. (*vector b*) This tendency is opposed by the patello-femoral joint reaction force (*vector c*) which maintains the patella in the groove

patella-femoral compression (Fig. 18.8b). In the words of Kapandji: "…the force of the quadriceps, directed obliquely superiorly and *slightly laterally*, is turned into a *strictly vertical force*" [3]. We fail to appreciate this interplay when extensor function is separated into extensor power and patellar tracking for analysis. A comparison of patellofemoral imaging with the extensor loaded and unloaded illustrates the potent effect of muscle contraction on a extensor tracking [20].

18.8 Rotational Mechanisms that Centralize the Native Patella

When the knee is fully extended, the patella sits proximal to and above the femoral trochlear groove. Even under conditions where maltracking is imminent, the problem will not be apparent in this position. As the knee flexes, the patella descends toward the groove, which is wider and flatter proximally, much like the opening of a funnel viewed in cross section. With further flexion, the patella is "captured" and descends into a conforming articulation, first in the trochlear groove and then between the distal femoral condyles, from which it cannot easily escape. In conditions of patella-femoral dysplasia, the confining lateral trochlear ridge may not easily guide and then restrain the patella, which can dislocate. Only with the patella in the groove can the quadriceps forcefully extend the knee joint.

Particular rotational phenomena aid patellar tracking at the extremes of flexion and extension. First, the "screw-home" mechanism locks the joint in full extension, diminishing quadriceps activity during standing. This involves external rotation of the tibia relative to the femur in terminal extension, displacing the patella laterally above the trochlear groove and seemingly increasing the risk of maltracking. The popliteus muscle however "unscrews" the mechanism prior to initiating flexion, rotating the tibia internally before the patella descends into the trochlear groove.

Secondly, femoral "rollback" describes the track of the femoral condyle on the tibial plateau anterior to posterior as flexion progresses. Though originally described as a symmetric path on both tibial condyles [21], more rollback occurs on the lateral tibial plateau. The tibia and its tubercle effectively rotate internally under the femoral condyles in deep flexion as the lateral femoral condyle progresses posteriorly on the tibia [22]. This draws the patella medially into the groove. Neither the asymmetric rollback [23] nor the popliteus-driven [24] screw-home mechanism is reliably replicated by arthroplasty surgery, leaving the replaced knee at an increased risk of patellar maltracking.

18.9 Arthroplasty Component Positioning to Avoid Maltracking

18.9.1 Depicting Component Position

Physical space can be depicted on three axes: X (medial to lateral), Y (proximal to distal), and Z (anterior to posterior). The position of objects, including knee arthroplasty components, can be defined as deviations from a neutral position in terms of translation (millimeters) and rotation (degrees) on these three axes, accounting for the frequent reference to "6 degrees of freedom" [25]. For example, rotation of a component around the "z" axis is commonly described as "varus" or "valgus" depending on the direction of rotation. Rotation around the vertical or "y" axis is reported as "internal" or "external" rotation, and translation on the "x" axis is described as "medial" or "lateral" (Fig. 18.9). Each choice can be described as beneficial, detrimental, or noncontributory to patellar tracking (Table 18.1).

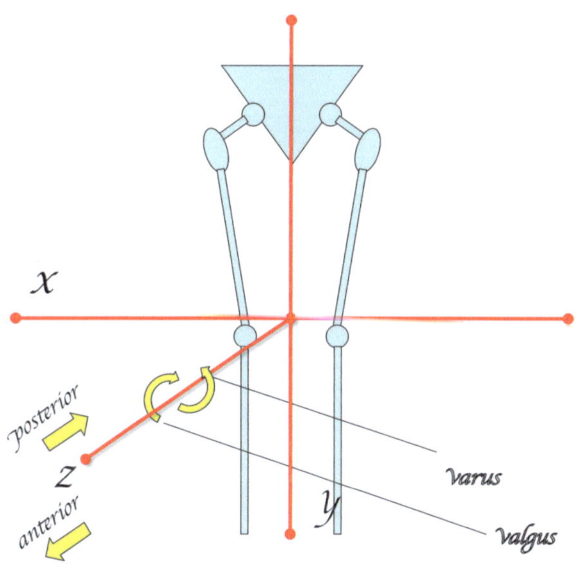

Fig. 18.9 Component position can be depicted on three axes: x (medial-lateral) y (proximal-distal) and z (anterior-posterior). Component position can be defined as deviations from the central or neutral position in terms of translation (measured as distance) and rotation (measured in degrees). This accounts for 6 degrees of freedom. The bi-directionality of each vector doubles those options. Accordingly, varus and valgus can be described as counter-clock wise and clockwise rotation respectively around the z axis. Anterior and posterior as translation on the z axis

Table 18.1 "Six-degrees of freedom" for positioning of objects in three dimensions. The far left column refers to the three axes: "X" horizontal or medial-lateral, "Y" inferior-superior or vertical and "Z" anterior-posterior, or at right angles to the plane formed by the intersection of "X" and "Y". Physical motion can be described as "translation" indicating a new location without re-orientation and measured as length or distance and "rotation" indicating a reorientation and measured in "degrees". The second and third columns describe three degrees of freedom; translation on each of the three axes. Because translation is bidirectional, there are a total of 6 translational directions possible. The third column has common clinical terms used to describe these motions.

Columns 4 and 5 refer to rotation about each of the three axes. Rotation is possible in two directions on each axis. Column five includes the common clinical descriptions for each rotation.

The numbers 1 through 6 in the third and fourth columns describe the degrees of freedom. The areas shaded in gray are of less importance to patellar tracking

	TRANSLATE		ROTATE	
X	1	Medial	2	Flex
		Lateral		Extend
Y	3	Superior	4	Internal
		Inferior		External
Z	5	Anterior	6	Varus
		Posterior		Valgus

Six degrees of freedom, each expressible in two directions and applied to both tibial and femoral components, give a multitude of permutations. The addition of a patellar component and soft tissue techniques create more choices. Only some options enhance patellar tracking, but the ones that do are critically important. Choices that straighten the pull of the extensor mechanism, i.e., less valgus, or that lateralize the structural patellar track enhance tracking. We can consider each of the degrees of freedom for all components as a comprehensive assessment of how to avoid maltracking.

18.9.2 Position of the Femoral Component

18.9.2.1 Mechanical Axis Implications

For most techniques of knee arthroplasty, the tibial component position is predetermined, either at right angles to the tibial axis (classic alignment) or to reproduce proximal tibial geometry (anatomic and kinematic alignments) [26]. Control of knee alignment is generally a function of the angular (rotational) position of the femoral component around the "z" axis. A decreased valgus mechanical axis of the knee straightens the extensor mechanism pull by reducing the Q angle. Decreased knee valgus also straightens the track. Assuming that the summed vectors of all parts of the quadriceps originate close to the center of the femoral head, a straight or "neutral mechanical axis" of the limb (collinear centers of femoral head, knee, and ankle) means that the mechanical alignment of the extensor mechanism (center of femoral head to articular center of the patella to the tibial tubercle) and the mechanical alignment of the extensor track (center of femoral head to center of trochlear groove to center of the knee) are both straight lines, at least in the fully extended knee. This would effectively resolve problems of patellar tracking.

However, most modeling of quadriceps pull follows from the anatomical origins of parts of the muscle on the femoral shaft, which has a valgus angle with the tibia (Fig. 18.10a). The optimal varus-valgus angulation of the femoral component

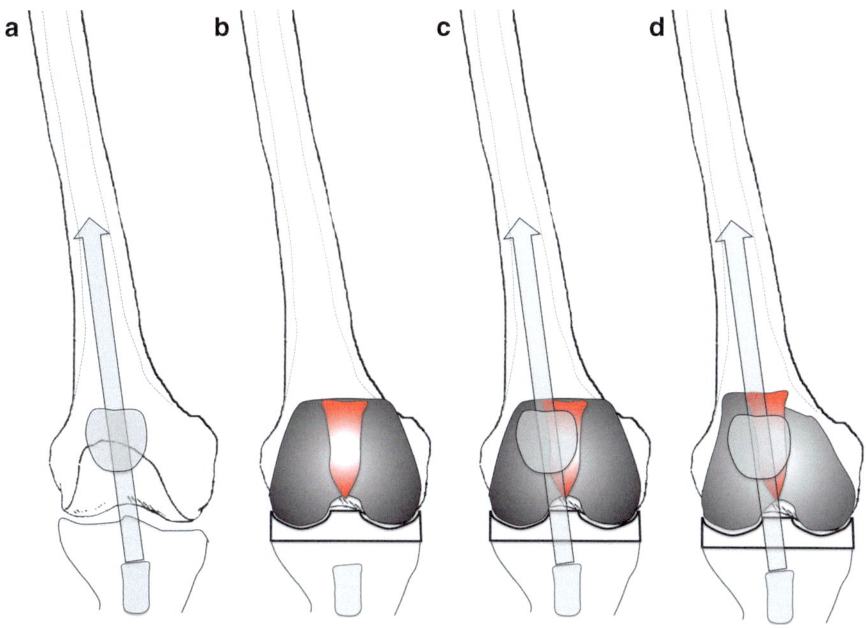

Fig. 18.10 (**a**) Schematic diagram of distal femur and direction of travel of patella, parallel with the trochlear groove in early flexion. The groove is oriented in valgus parallel with the distal femoral shaft. (**b**) TKA with a symmetric (non right or left sided) femoral implant and classic alignment tibial component at right angles to the tibial axis. The trochlear groove (shaded red) is oriented at right angles to the distal articular surface, not the femoral shaft. (**c**) The path of the patella is not parallel with the trochlear groove, and the patella will enter the lateral side of the groove on the initiation of flexion. Any additional factors that favor lateral tracking could result in dislocation. At a minimum, tracking would not be smooth. (**d**) Asymmetric, right and left specific femoral component that includes a trochlear groove oriented in more valgus, implanted with classic alignment, replicating the anatomic direction of the groove. Congruent tracking has been restored. This would be the best overal alignment for patellar tracking with current femoral component designs. (**e**) Symmetric femoral component in "anatomic" alignment: tibial component replicating normal varus and greater distal valgus alignment for overall valgus knee alignment. (**f**) This means that the femoral component has been rotated several more degrees around the "z" axis, away from the orientation of the track. This would be the worst scenario for patellar tracking with the greatest divergence between the prosthetic and anatomic patellar tracks. (**g**) A specific right sided femoral component with valgus in the trochlear groove, implanted with anatomic technique. (**h**) The standard anatomic prosthesis is still not in as much valgus as the native knee. Components would have to be designed specifically for anatomic alignment to replicate the orientation of the anatomic groove

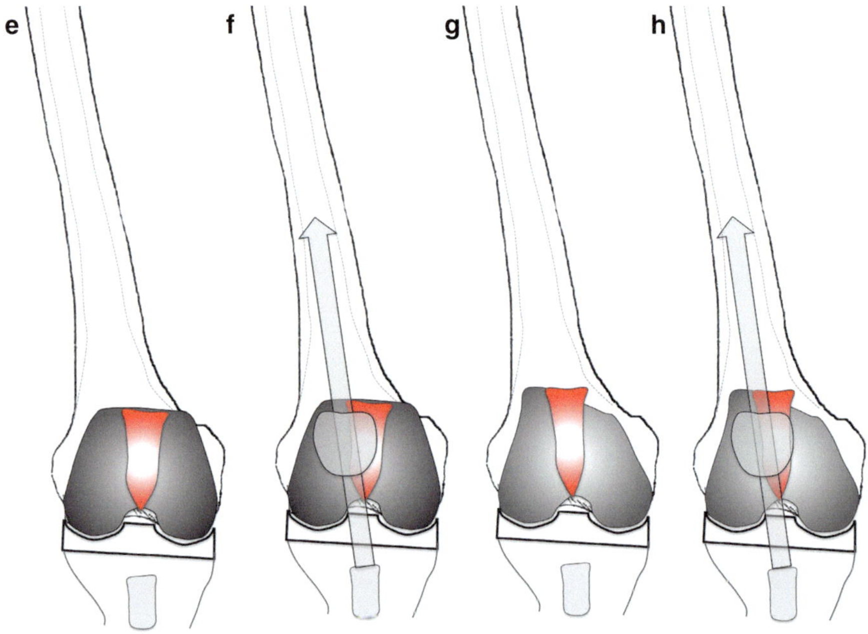

Fig. 18.10 (continued)

depends on the planned relative positions of the tibial and femoral components plus the design of the femoral prosthesis.

Until right and left femoral components were introduced, the prosthetic trochlear groove was oriented at right angles to its distal articular surface (Fig. 18.10b). If a femoral component was oriented at right angles to the mechanical axis of the femur (classic alignment with the goal of a neutral mechanical axis), this means that the proximal lateral edge of the trochlear ridge was positioned more medially than the normal knee, risking difficulties in "capturing" the patella as it descends along this track with flexion (Fig. 18.10c). As the patella descends the trochlear groove with this geometry, it will be likely to dislocate if it initially tracks lateral to the proximal lateral trochlear ridge. Asymmetric (right and left sided) femoral components should include a trochlear groove that is angled in valgus, resembling the normal patellar track (Fig. 18.10d). Some prostheses have been modified along gender lines to have a trochlear groove that is even more angulated in valgus [27]. While many of these gender-driven changes have not proven substantive [28], they do highlight anatomical observations with implications for patellar tracking in the native human knee.

18.9.2.2 Knee Alignment Options: Classic Versus Anatomic

The majority of arthroplasties today and for the last several decades have been implanted with "classic alignment": a tibial component at right angles to the axis of the tibia and a femoral component oriented in valgus that determines the mechanical angle of the limb. This is based on the belief that varus positioning of the tibial component is associated with higher rates of aseptic loosening, a conclusion that has been challenged in recent years. Classic alignment means that the femoral component would be *rotated around the "z" axis* close to right angles with the line from the center of femoral head to the center of the knee, depending on the alignment the surgeon planned.

18.9.2.3 Femur Rotation Around the "z" Axis: Varus-Valgus Alignment

Assuming some degree of valgus angulation between the femur and tibia to reduce loosening, do different combinations of femoral and tibial *component* angulation, all of which might add up to the same overall tibial-femoral alignment, affect patellar tracking? As a femoral component is placed in more valgus, the proximal trochlear groove is rotated medially, away from the lateral position where it is more likely to capture the descending patella as the knee flexes. As "anatomic" alignment of a TKA, with anatomically inspired varus placement of the tibial component, requires even greater femoral valgus component position to achieve the same overall valgus alignment, this technique would position a prosthetic groove further medially—a disadvantage to patellar tracking (Fig. 18.10e, f). The same conclusion applies to recently introduced "kinematic alignment" where components are placed to replicate the articular surfaces of the patient's own knee joint [29].

The adverse orientation of the prosthetic trochlear groove with anatomic alignment could be improved if femoral implants were designed specifically for implantation in higher degrees of valgus, if the trochlear groove itself was designed with more valgus (Fig. 18.10g, h). The final verdict with respect to the best rotational positioning of the femoral component on the "z" axis, (varus-valgus) to enhance tracking, is that patellar tracking with contemporary right- and left-sided femoral components is theoretically maximized with a neutral or slightly varus mechanical limb axis and classic alignment technique.

18.9.2.4 Femoral Component Translation Along the "x" Axis: Medial-Lateral Position

Femoral component size is determined primarily to reconstruct the anteroposterior dimension of the femur and avoid undue tension on the collateral ligaments in flexion, with consequent stiffness. A femoral component that is larger AP than the native condyles will stretch the collateral ligaments during flexion. Consequently, many appropriately sized femoral components will be smaller from medial to lateral than the native bone, because they were selected to match the AP dimension. This creates options for medial-lateral placement or translation along the "x" axis. This is most common in male patients where the ratio of AP to ML indicates generally wider distal femurs. A femoral component placed laterally, against the lateral cortex, reduces the valgus angle of the patellar track (Fig. 18.11). Rhoads and colleagues confirmed the advantage of lateral femoral component position for patellar tracking in a cadaver study [30, 31]. Their study, cited again later, highlights the value of positioning the groove where the patella must be, rather than trying to constrain the patella against forces favoring dislocation.

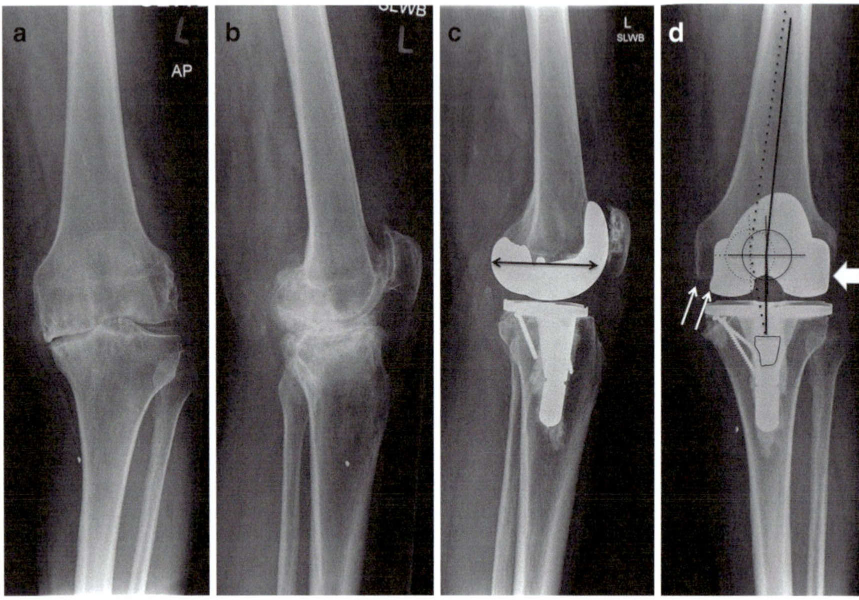

Fig. 18.11 (**a**) Single Leg weight bearing, antero-posterior (*AP*) left knee radiograph showing osteoarthritis and varus deformity. The ratio of medial-lateral to AP dimension shows a relatively wide femur, characteristic of a male femur. There is a medial tibial defect from arthritic deterioration. (**b**) Lateral radiograph showing osteoarthritis and the AP dimension. (**c**) Lateral radiograph post TKA. The AP dimension has been restored by two he prosthesis. (**d**) AP radiograph post TKA. The AP/ML ratio of the implant is greater than the male anatomy. This is the correct prosthesis size even though it does not replicate the medial-lateral dimension. This creates choice-lateral placement of the femoral component brings the trochlear groove more lateral, closer to where the patella will track

18.9.2.5 Femur Rotation Around the "y" Axis: Internal-External Rotation

Practical guides for the rotational position of the femoral component include the trans-epicondylar axis [32] and the "anteroposterior" axis or "Whiteside's" line [33, 34]. Over more than two decades, numerous investigations have evaluated and sometimes questioned the accuracy and reproducibility of these landmarks. To date, no superior alternative has emerged. Moreland previously described the necessity of external femoral component rotation relative to the posterior articular surfaces, when the tibia is resected at right angles to its long axis instead of anatomically in varus. His highly lucid discussion focused on symmetry of the flexion gap however and not patellar tracking [26] (Fig. 18.12).

In a study predating the description of the "anteroposterior axis," Anouchi, Whiteside, and colleagues identified benefits of an external rotation position of the femoral component and a deleterious effect of internal rotation when compared with femoral components that are rotated identically to the native posterior articular condyles [35]. They noted that internal and external rotation had effects on collateral ligament tension in flexion but not extension and discounted the effect of

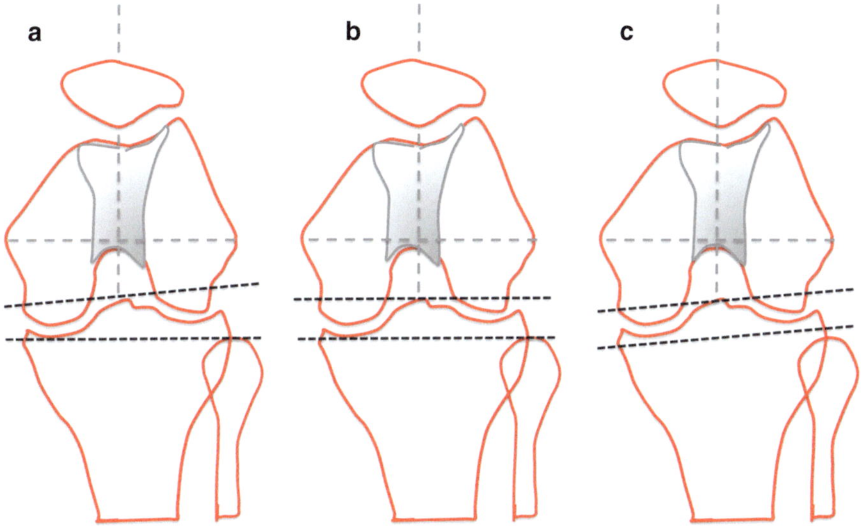

Fig. 18.12 (**a–c**) Redrawn from Moreland 1988. (**a**) Schematic depiction of the flexed knee joint and theoretical bone resection. In this case the tibia has been resected at the typical "neutral" or 90° to the axis of the tibia and the femoral component has been rotated to the same orientation to the native posterior condyles. This creates a larger flexion gap on the lateral side, with lateral laxity and perhaps instability on the lateral side in flexion. As the femur rotates externally to contact the lateral tibia, the origin of the quadriceps on the femur also rotates externally, favoring lateral tracking. This approach is of historical interest and is not recommended. (**b**) "Classic Alignment" The tibia again resected at right angles to the long axis of the tibia but now the femoral component is externally rotated to create a more symmetric flexion gap. The femoral component is rotated either to the "*Trans-epicondylar axis*" (*horizontal dashed gray line*) or the "anteroposterior" axis (vertical dashed gray line). (**c**) "Anatomic" and more recent "Kinematic alignment". Proximal tibia is resected parallel to its articular surface and femoral component is rotated to its posterior condylar articular surface. This creates a parallel flexion gap

rotation on the position or height of the femoral groove: "in weight bearing flexion the patellar groove is unchanged but the ligament balance is altered." They did not discuss the relative external rotation of the femur and with it the external rotation of the origins of the quadriceps muscle that result from internally rotating the femoral component. This would be expected to pull the patella more laterally.

They clearly identified one of the most potent ill effects of internal rotation of a femoral component: "the internally rotated specimens rotated into valgus in flexion." This means that the tibial tubercle moved laterally, and with it the patella, as flexion proceeds on an internally rotated femoral component. The shortest distance from the tibial tubercle to the origin of the quadriceps rapidly travels outside the trochlear groove. At the critical moment when the patella reaches the opening of the trochlear groove, the straight line from the tubercle to the origin of the quadriceps can lie outside of the lateral trochlear ridge, depending on the degree of internal femoral component rotation (Fig. 18.13). This occurs concurrent in knee flexion with dramatic increases in the patellofemoral compressive forces that favor posterior displacement of the patella. The result can be disastrous. Accordingly, to keep

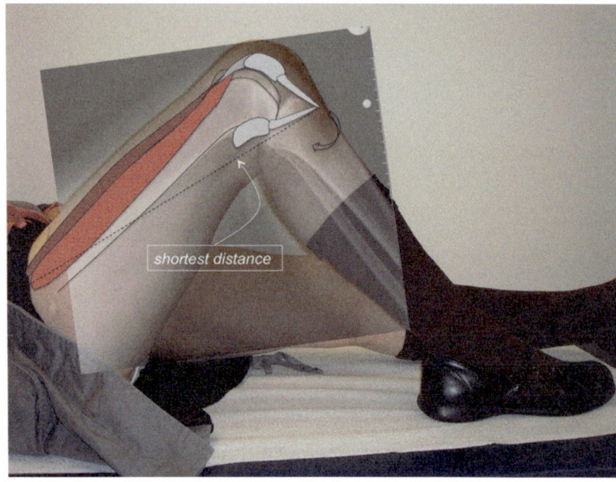

Fig. 18.13 The internally rotated femoral component forces the tibia and knee into valgus with flexion, displacing the tubercle laterally. The internally rotated tibial component displaces the tubercle laterally increasing the Q angle. The combination of the two makes it possible for the patella to escape from the trochlear groove and assume the shortest distance between two points: dislocation

the tibial tubercle of the flexed knee under the distal femoral condyles and the patella between those condyles, the femoral component should be externally rotated on the "y" axis relative to the native posterior condyles, a position approximated by the anteroposterior or "Whiteside's" line and the trans-epicondylar axis. This applies to "classic alignment" strategies as argued by Moreland. These recommendations and component designs might require modification, if more anatomic positioning of components was adopted.

18.9.2.6 Femoral Component Position Summary: What Works and What Does Not

In summary, patellar tracking is enhanced by translating the femoral component laterally along the "x" axis and externally rotating the femoral component to the trans-epicondylar axis or the anteroposterior line on the "y" axis. Balancing the advantages of valgus alignment as a means to reduce load and loosening against the improvements to patellar tracking with less valgus determine the ideal compromise for rotation of the femoral component on the "z" axis.

The other positioning options for femoral components affect arthroplasty durability and function but have little impact on patellar tracking. Rotation of the femoral component on the "x" axis (flexion-extension position) may tighten the flexion gap (flexed) or create an anterior femoral notch (extended) but should not affect tracking. Translation of the femoral component proximally or distally on the "y" axis influences gap balance and the position of the joint line. It is a maneuver that may help correction of fixed flexion contractures [36]. Translation of the component on the "z" axis tightens the flexion gap if the component is moved posteriorly and at the same time creates an anterior notch. Anterior displacement of the component will increase the dimensions of the flexion gap and risk flexion instability unless accompanied by compensatory maneuvers plus it creates a prominent femoral flange that may restrict flexion, with a subtle effect on tracking. None of these remaining options could be manipulated independently to improve tracking.

18.9.3 Position of the Tibial Component

There are few variations in tibial component position that affect tracking, but the rotational position on the "y" axis (internal and external rotation) is probably the single most important factor to ensure central patellar tracking. Every degree of internal rotation of the tibial component displaces the tibial tubercle a corresponding distance laterally. A laterally positioned tubercle may lie directly beneath the lateral femoral condyle rather than the intercondylar groove. If the patella rides on the lateral condyle, rather than the trochlea, in early flexion, it is likely to slide right off the lateral side with further flexion and compression. This effect can spin the tibia laterally under the femur to the extent that flexion gap tightness and articular conformity permit. If the gap is relatively tight, the tendency to dislocate might manifest as painful inability to bend. Internal rotation of the tibial component is a frequent finding in stiff arthroplasties [13].

One of the earliest studies to associate internal tibial rotation with patellar tracking problems also introduced a CT scan protocol to quantify rotational position [37]. This study demonstrated an additive effect of combined femoral and tibial component malrotation, with more severe patellofemoral complications arising from larger amounts of combined malrotation. This study observed the best function when tibial component rotation was oriented to the extensor, specifically the tubercle. Numerous techniques have since been proposed to orient the rotational position of the tibial component. Most are hypothetical, based on replicating some landmark on the tibial articular surface that does not necessarily correspond to arthroplasty function [38]. The so-called "free-floating" technique is misguided and inaccurate [39], assuming that passive motion of the knee in an anesthetized patient will somehow direct the component to the correct location.

Anatomic landmarks are useful if they are oriented to the extensor mechanism and link the patella to the intercondylar groove [40]. Rotating the component to the medial third of the tubercle has been a guiding principle in successful arthroplasty for several decades [41]. For many years, surgeons were preoccupied with maximizing coverage of the proximal tibia, to distribute load and combat high rates of tibial component loosening. While loosening was never correlated with degree of coverage, this goal persisted. In an earlier era of prostheses with flat articular polyethylene, the internally rotated component often had little effect on patellar tracking as the tubercle lined up under the trochlear groove in response to the pull of the extensor. As more conforming articular geometry was introduced to decrease wear and improve stability, the internally rotated component obliged lateral displacement of the tubercle and confounded tracking. Anatomically designed right and left tibial components enable surgeons to maximize both coverage and rotation.

The other positioning variables for the tibial component do not affect tracking substantively. Translation on the "x" and "z" axes is rarely feasible, as tibial components are provided in a range of sizes that ultimately match the proximal anatomy and provide the desired "coverage." Rotation on the "x" axis, commonly referred to as tibial slope, influences the degree of flexion but not tracking. Translation on the "y" axis only reflects the amount of tibial bone resected, which must be replaced with polyethylene to avoid recurvatum. Rotation on the "z" axis epitomizes the difference between classical and anatomic alignment techniques discussed above.

18.9.4 Patella

The native patella may or may not be resurfaced in a successful knee arthroplasty. When replaced, most contemporary implant systems provide a rotationally symmetric or dome-shaped prosthesis. This avoids complications that have occurred with more anatomic implants due to the difficulty of accurately positioning them rotationally. The dome-shaped implant does not resemble the native patella, which has a prominent ridge from inferior to superior and is elliptically shaped with a longer medial to lateral axis. These observations can be used to improve tracking by translating a dome to the medial patella border, on the "x" axis [42]. Translating the patella either anteriorly or posteriorly on the "z" axis, accomplished by resecting more or less bone, affects tension in the peri-patellar tissues. "Overstuffing" the PF joint, by displacing the component posteriorly, makes the knee tighter and stiffer. Superior or inferior displacement (translation on the "y" axis) is rarely feasible given the shapes of the bone and the implant.

18.9.5 Surgical Approach and Lateral Patellar Retinacular Release

It was hoped that more anatomic surgical approaches might improve patellar tracking [9]. No compelling studies support one surgical approach over another with respect to extensor mechanism tracking. The subvastus approach probably allows a more accurate assessment of patellar tracking with the medial tendon intact and so avoids unnecessary releases [43]. Patients with pathologic tracking prior to arthroplasty may require proximal soft tissue realignment. This will be difficult with surgical approaches like the subvastus, which do not divide the quadriceps tendon longitudinally, a necessary prelude to advancement of the vastus medialis. Deflation of the tourniquet appears to give a more realistic appraisal of patellar tracking and tension in the lateral retinaculum [44]. When a release seems necessary due to lateral subluxation intraoperatively, most surgeons critically reevaluate the rotation of tibial and femoral components.

Lateral patellar retinacular release was performed frequently and considered the mainstay of patellar tracking, with older implant designs, in an era when the importance of rotational positioning of the tibial and femoral components was not appreciated. Many older implants had prominent anterior femoral contours with straight trochlear grooves. Other older designs that have tried to confine patellae in highly conforming trochlear grooves performed poorly (Fig. 18.14), emphasizing the superiority of modifying the forces that direct the patella, by straightening the pull of the extensor and positioning a "patellar friendly" trochlear groove where the

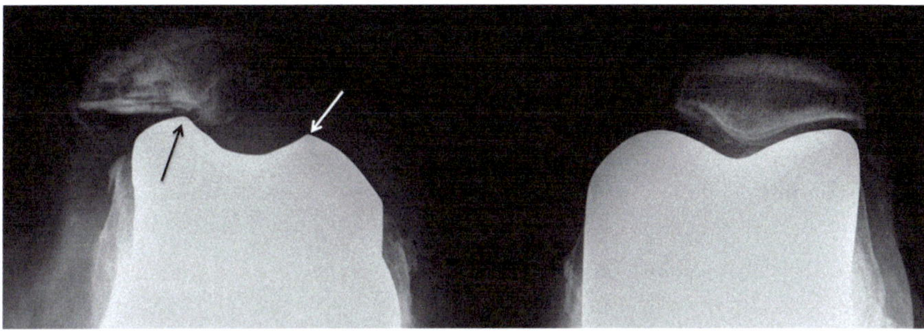

Fig. 18.14 Some older knee prostheses include highly conforming non-anatomically shaped trochlear grooves. The goal is to control patellar tracking, with additional benefit of uniform loading of matching patellar and trochlear curves. This designs ends with sharp edges on both side of the groove (*arrows*). If the extensor mechanism and trochlear groove are both perfectly aligned, with no changes during flexion and extension, this might be advantageous. However, if the patellar is constrained in the groove despite a strong lateral vector there is likely to be binding with pain and poor motion. If the patella enters the groove laterally in early flexion, it is likely to track outside the groove as seen in this case. The contralateral arthroplasty has a patellar "friendly" design and functions well in this case with an unresurfaced patella

patella needs to articulate, rather than fighting these forces with constraint or soft tissue modification.

Rhoads and colleagues commented in their cadaver study that "the high lateral ridge on the femoral component effectively prevents patellar dislocation but may produce abnormally high stresses on the patellar implant, especially if the implant is medially displaced or internally rotated. This could lead to accelerated wear or loosening of the patellar component" [30]. It probably also causes pain and, consequently, poor motion. In general, attempts to physically constrain the patella with component shape are unsuccessful. The dynamics of knee motion means that a patella driven toward dislocation will either be locked painfully in a constrained groove or snap up and over a sharp or elevated lateral trochlear ridge to dislocate. The extensor under load seeks the shortest distance between two points—ideally that track will pass through the femoral trochlear groove.

References

1. Nordin M, Frankel VH. Basic biomechanics of the musculoskeletal system. Philadelphia: Lippincott Williams & Wilkins; 2001.
2. Kapandji IA. The physiology of the joints. New York: Churchill Livingstone. 2015.
3. Kapandji IA, Honoré LH. The physiology of the joints: annotated diagrams of the mechanics of the human joints. Vol. 2, lower limb. Edinburgh: E. & S. Livingstone; 1970.
4. Souza DR, Gross MT. Comparison of vastus medialis obliquus: vastus lateralis muscle integrated electromyographic ratios between healthy subjects and patients with patellofemoral pain. Phys Ther. 1991;71(4):310–6. discussion 7–20.
5. Insall J, Bullough PG, Burstein AH. Proximal "tube" realignment of the patella for chondromalacia patellae. Clin Orthop. 1979;144:63–9.

6. Spitzer A, Vince K. Patellar considerations in total knee arthroplasty. In: Scuderi GR, editor. The Patella. 1st ed. New York: Springer; 1995. p. 309–31.
7. Vince KG, McPherson EJ. The patella in total knee arthroplasty. Orthop Clin North Am. 1992;23(4):675–86.
8. Malo M, Vince KG. The unstable patella after total knee arthroplasty: etiology, prevention, and management. J Am Acad Orthop Surg. 2003;11(5):364–71.
9. Bindelglass DF, Vince KG. Patellar tilt and subluxation following subvastus and parapatellar approach in total knee arthroplasty. Implication for surgical technique. J Arthroplasty. 1996;11(5):507–11.
10. Vince K. The instabilities: you rock, it rolls. Bone Joint J Orthop Proc Suppl. 2013;95(Supp 22):95.
11. Vince KG. Diagnosis and management of patients with instability of the knee. Instr Course Lect. 2012;61:515–24.
12. Vince K, Malo M. Instability in total knee arthroplasty. In: Berry DJ, Trousdale RT, Dennis DA, Paprosky W, editors. Revision total hip and knee arthroplasty. Philadelphia: Lippincott, Williams and Wilkins; 2006.
13. Bedard M, Vince KG, Redfern J, Collen SR. Internal rotation of the tibial component is frequent in stiff total knee arthroplasty. Clin Orthop Relat Res. 2011;469(8):2346–55.
14. Bellemans J, Colyn W, Vandenneucker H, Victor J. The Chitranjan Ranawat award: is neutral mechanical alignment normal for all patients? The concept of constitutional varus. Clin Orthop Relat Res. 2012;470(1):45–53.
15. Moreland JR, Bassett LW, Hanker GJ. Radiographic analysis of the axial alignment of the lower extremity. J Bone Joint Surg Am. 1987;69(5):745–9.
16. Parratte S, Pagnano MW, Trousdale RT, Berry DJ. Effect of postoperative mechanical axis alignment on the fifteen-year survival of modern, cemented total knee replacements. J Bone Joint Surg Am Vol. 2010;92(12):2143–9.
17. Howell SM, Papadopoulos S, Kuznik K, Ghaly LR, Hull ML. Does varus alignment adversely affect implant survival and function six years after kinematically aligned total knee arthroplasty? Int Orthop. 2015;39(11):2117–24.
18. Saunders JB, Inman VT, Eberhart HD. The major determinants in normal and pathological gait. J Bone Joint Surg Am Vol. 1953;35-A(3):543–58.
19. Lotke PA, Ecker ML. Influence of positioning of prosthesis in total knee replacement. J Bone Joint Surg Am. 1977;59(1):77–9.
20. Baldini A, Anderson JA, Cerulli-Mariani P, Kalyvas J, Pavlov H, Sculco TP. Patellofemoral evaluation after total knee arthroplasty. Validation of a new weight-bearing axial radiographic view. J Bone Joint Surg Am. 2007;89(8):1810–7.
21. Gunston FH. Polycentric knee arthroplasty. Prosthetic simulation of normal knee movement. J Bone Joint Surg Br. 1971;53(2):272–7.
22. Pinskerova V, Johal P, Nakagawa S, Sosna A, Williams A, Gedroyc W, et al. Does the femur roll-back with flexion? J Bone Joint Surg Br. 2004;86(6):925–31.
23. Bertin KC, Komistek RD, Dennis DA, Hoff WA, Anderson DT, Langer T. In vivo determination of posterior femoral rollback for subjects having a NexGen posterior cruciate-retaining total knee arthroplasty. J Arthroplasty. 2002;17(8):1040–8.
24. Kesman TJ, Kaufman KR, Trousdale RT. Popliteus tendon resection during total knee arthroplasty: an observational report. Clin Orthop Relat Res. 2011;469(1):76–81.
25. Lin F, Makhsous M, Chang AH, Hendrix RW, Zhang LQ. In vivo and noninvasive six degrees of freedom patellar tracking during voluntary knee movement. Clin Biomech (Bristol, Avon). 2003;18(5):401–9.
26. Moreland JR. Mechanisms of failure in total knee arthroplasty. Clin Orthop. 1988;226:49–64.
27. Singh H, Mittal V, Nadkarni B, Agarwal S, Gulati D. Gender-specific high-flexion knee prosthesis in Indian women: a prospective randomised study. J Orthop Surg (Hong Kong). 2012;20(2):153–6.

28. Greene KA. Gender-specific design in total knee arthroplasty. J Arthroplasty. 2007;22(7 Suppl 3):27–31.
29. Howell SM, Howell SJ, Kuznik KT, Cohen J, Hull ML. Does a kinematically aligned total knee arthroplasty restore function without failure regardless of alignment category? Clin Orthop Relat Res. 2013;471(3):1000–7.
30. Rhoads DD, Noble PC, Reuben JD, Tullos HS. The effect of femoral component position on the kinematics of total knee arthroplasty. Clin Orthop. 1993;286:122–9.
31. Rhoads DD, Noble PC, Reuben JD, Mahoney OM, Tullos HS. The effect of femoral component position on patellar tracking after total knee arthroplasty. Clin Orthop. 1990;260:43–51.
32. Berger RA, Rubash HE, Seel MJ, Thompson WH, Crossett LS. Determining the rotational alignment of the femoral component in total knee arthroplasty using the epicondylar axis. Clin Orthop. 1993;286:40–7.
33. Whiteside LA, Arima J. The anteroposterior axis for femoral rotational alignment in valgus total knee arthroplasty. Clin Orthop. 1995;321:168–72.
34. Arima J, Whiteside LA, McCarthy DS, White SE. Femoral rotational alignment, based on the anteroposterior axis, in total knee arthroplasty in a valgus knee. A technical note. J Bone Joint Surg Am. 1995;77(9):1331–4.
35. Anouchi YS, Whiteside LA, Kaiser AD, Milliano MT. The effects of axial rotational alignment of the femoral component on knee stability and patellar tracking in total knee arthroplasty demonstrated on autopsy specimens. Clin Orthop. 1993;287:170–7.
36. Kim SH, Lim JW, Jung HJ, Lee HJ. Influence of soft tissue balancing and distal femoral resection on flexion contracture in navigated total knee arthroplasty. Knee Surg Sports Traumatol Arthrosc. 2016;24:3747–50.
37. Berger RA, Crossett LS, Jacobs JJ, Rubash HE. Malrotation causing patellofemoral complications after total knee arthroplasty. Clin Orthop Relat Res. 1998;356:144–53.
38. Cobb JP, Dixon H, Dandachli W, Iranpour F. The anatomical tibial axis: reliable rotational orientation in knee replacement. J Bone Joint Surg Br. 2008;90(8):1032–8.
39. Ikeuchi M, Yamanaka N, Okanoue Y, Ueta E, Tani T. Determining the rotational alignment of the tibial component at total knee replacement: a comparison of two techniques. J Bone Joint Surg Br. 2007;89(1):45–9.
40. Baldini A, Indelli PF, De Luca L, Mariani PC, Marcucci M. Rotational alignment of the tibial component in total knee arthroplasty: the anterior tibial cortex is a reliable landmark. Joints. 2013;1(4):155–60.
41. Insall J. Total knee arthroplasty. In: Insall J, editor. Surgery of the knee. New York: Churchill Livingstone; 1984. p. 1478–552.
42. Lewonowski K, Dorr LD, McPherson EJ, Huber G, Wan Z. Medialization of the patella in total knee arthroplasty. J Arthroplasty. 1997;12(2):161–7.
43. Ogata K, Ishinishi T, Hara M. Evaluation of patellar retinacular tension during total knee arthroplasty. Special emphasis on lateral retinacular release. J Arthroplasty. 1997;12(6):651–6.
44. Komatsu T, Ishibashi Y, Otsuka H, Nagao A, Toh S. The effect of surgical approaches and tourniquet application on patellofemoral tracking in total knee arthroplasty. J Arthroplasty. 2003;18(3):308–12.

Part VII

Trouble Shooting

Trouble Shooting: Intraoperative MCL Injury

19

Carlos Eduardo Silveira Franciozi, Rogério Teixeira de Carvalho, Yasuo Itami, and Marcus Vinicius Malheiros Luzo

Contents

19.1 Introduction

The medial collateral ligament (MCL) of the knee is the primary static restraint against valgus stress in 30° of flexion and assists in knee rotation and coronal stability [1]. The MCL is composed of two layers: the longitudinal fibers of the superficial portion and the short fibers of the deep part that keeps close relation with articular capsule and medial meniscus. The MCL plays an important role in the tibiofemoral kinematics during the gait. The anterior and posterior fibers present a reciprocal function keeping the knee stable during the stance phase [2]. In the osteoarthritic knee, the MCL can be compromised due to contracture (stiff knee, severe varus deformity) and elongation (severe valgus deformity, rheumatoid diseases) and sometimes partially damaged due to osteophytes that can cause structural alterations in relation to the original anatomy [3].

C.E.S. Franciozi, PhD, MD (✉) • R.T. de Carvalho, MD • M.V.M. Luzo, PhD, MD
Federal University of São Paulo, São Paulo, Brazil
e-mail: cacarlos66@hotmail.com; rtcarv@terra.com.br; smluzo@uol.com.br

Y. Itami, PhD, MD
Osaka Medical College, Takatsuki, Japan
e-mail: yasuo801115@gmail.com

S. Matsuda et al. (eds.), *Soft Tissue Balancing in Total Knee Arthroplasty*,
DOI 10.1007/978-3-662-54082-4_19

Biomechanical studies have shown important joint opening in extension and flexion after the MCL is transected [4, 5].

Total knee arthroplasty (TKA) is one surgical option to relieve pain and improve the function in the osteoarthritic knee. One of the goals in TKA is to obtain symmetric and balanced flexion and extension gaps. The status of the MCL is important for a stable and well-balanced knee. However, this ligament can be inadvertently damaged during TKA surgery causing a ligament unbalancing and compromising knee stability in flexion and extension. Imbalance can produce instability and a maldistribution of the tibiofemoral contact forces, which generates an overload of one compartment, thus accelerating wear process with component loosening affecting the survivorship of the prosthetic joint [3, 6–19].

The most common patient's complaint after MCL lesion is instability in the coronal plane that can affect the gait pattern [10]. The unstable knee after TKA can cause symptoms like swelling, giving way in mid-flexion and extension, and functional disability. If intraoperative MCL injury diagnosis is neglected, instability may compromise the surgery. The incidence rate of the intraoperative MCL injury during TKA has been reported from 0.3 to 2.7% [3, 7–9, 11, 13, 15, 16, 18]. Clinical diagnosis and proper management are crucial to achieve good functional results. There are controversies about which options for treatment can be performed in different scenarios related to the intraoperative MCL injury in TKA to get optimal clinical outcomes.

19.2 Lesion Type and Cause

There are different types of intraoperative MCL lesion and causes. Table 19.1 displays this information.

19.3 Intraoperative Findings

Intraoperative MCL injury diagnosis can sometimes be neglected. It is imperative to know what signs to expect from this kind of lesion in order to recognize it, as it can sometimes present as a hidden injury. A sudden unexpected medial laxity is a common reported finding [9, 16]. A sudden excessive exposure or unstable forward movement of the tibia is also an indicative of intraoperative MCL damage [15]. Also, it can be recognized as a medial laxity when there was no preoperative medial instability or during ligament balance with trial components or, more uncommon, after the final implants were cemented into place [3, 13]. Occasionally, a popping sound can be heard, and increased laxity at 30° and 90° can be confirmed in some MCL tibial avulsions [13].

Table 19.1 Lesion type and cause

Lesion type	Frequency*	Cause	Reference
Femoral avulsion	1/48	–	[8]
	1/16	Osteopenic patient	[3]
Mid-substance	24/48	–	[8]
	1/8	Transection with saw during tibial cut	[9]
	7/7	Unknown, possibly due to saw during tibial cut, sharp instrumentation used for subperiosteal tibial MCL elevation, or medial meniscus excision	[11]
	28/37	During tibial resection or femoral posterior condyle resection	[13]
	12/16	Saw blade during tibial cut or sharp instrument used for subperiosteal elevation	[3]
	11/15	–	[15]
	22/23	–	[16]
	9/9	–	[18]
	1/1	–	[19]
Tibial avulsion	20/48	–	[8]
	7/8	From hyperflexion to extension with the trial component not perfectly placed	[9]
	15/15	During medial soft tissue release at the tibia using narrow osteotome	[12]
	9/37	During hyperflexion for exposition	[13]
	3/16	Medially placed retractors or sharp instrument used for subperiosteal elevation	[3]
	1/23	–	[16]
Stretching	2/7	–	[11]

* *Frequency: specific lesion type/total number of MCL lesions for each reference*

19.4 Treatment Types

There is a myriad of different treatments according to MCL lesion type. Table 19.2 displays this information.

All treatment types seem to achieve successful results, with exception to primary repair. However, primary repair had more failures than other treatments only on the study of Lee and Lotke (2011), while it had also successful results in other studies [3, 8, 11, 13, 16, 18].

Repair types include end-to-end suture, modified Becker technique, end-to-end interrupted suture, interrupted nonabsorbable braided suture, modified Kessler end-to-end stitch, and modified Becker stitch [3, 8, 9, 11, 15, 18].

Regarding what surgical step order repair should be applied, it can be made with the trial components in place in order to maintain proper tension [15, 18].

Table 19.2 Treatment types

Treatment type	Failure rate*	Peculiarity	Reference
Femoral reinsertion	0/1	Screw and washer	[8]
	0/1	Screw and washer	[3]
Tibial reinsertion	0/20	Screw and washer and/or suture anchors and/or sutures to the bone	[8]
	0/2	Suture anchors on the medial tibial plateau level added to bicortical screw ligament fixation	[9]
	0/9	Staples	[13]
	0/3	Suture anchor. Preoperative valgus excluded	[3]
Primary repair	2/3	–	[13]
	0/10	–	[16]
	0/9	–	[18]
Primary repair + cast	2/4	4 weeks casting	[13]
Primary repair + bracing	0/47	6 weeks bracing	[8]
	0/2	4 weeks bracing	[11]
	0/12	6 weeks bracing. Preoperative valgus excluded	[3]
Repair + increase tibial insert thickness (larger insert than the trial)	0/3	The only failure occurred in a patient that poly-insert thickness was not increased in comparison to the trial	[9]
Repair + augmentation	0/5	Augmentation with quadriceps free graft	[11]
	0/11	Augmentation with polyester synthetic ligament fibers. 2 weeks bracing	[15]
Hamstrings reconstruction	0/1	Anatomical reconstruction sMCL + POL. 6 weeks bracing	[19]
	not reported	Technical note. Reconstruction of the sMCL. 4 weeks bracing	[7]
Constrained prosthesis	0/23	Constrained varus/valgus design (not hinged)	[13]
	0/8	Constrained varus/valgus design (not hinged)	[16]
Primary repair + constrained prosthesis	0/3	Constrained varus/valgus design (not hinged)	[9]
	0/7	Constrained varus/valgus design (not hinged)	[13]
	0/3	Constrained varus/valgus design (not hinged)	[16]
Increase tibial insert thickness (augmented 2–4 mm in relation to trial)	0/15	All lesions were tibial avulsions	[12]
No treatment	0/2	–	[16]

**Failure rate: just related to instability*

Also, the sutures can be placed at the ligament before cementing, while the final tension and knots will be made after component cementing and final polyethylene insert in place [8]. However, it is also described the MCL repair before the trial components, so the thickness of the tibial polyethylene spacer used in each patient is determined after the ligament has been repaired, with the goal of balancing the knee in flexion and extension, as would be done in any knee arthroplasty [3].

Lee and Lotke (2011) evaluated both nonconstrained and constrained designs suggesting the use of constrained designs has better outcomes in MCL iatrogenic injuries [13]. However, Siqueira et al. [16] evaluated repair, constrained designs, repair added to constrained design, and no treatment. They found no difference between those treatment types [16].

Currently, there is no gold standard treatment for intraoperative MCL injuries during TKA. All options seem to achieve successful results. However, constrained prosthesis appears to be safer. Nonetheless, these implants may have several disadvantages as they may place more stress on the cement bone–implant interfaces, be associated with increased wear, sacrifice more bone stock, and complicate future revisions if needed. Also, they are more expensive and technically more demanding. Thus, the use of constrained implants in general is discouraged when less constrained options are available that can adequately restore knee stability [15]. Repairs seem to have adequate results, but they can be more reliable if associated to additional procedures such as increasing the tibial thickness insert, augmentation (autograft or synthetic material), and association to a constrained prosthesis. This last combination provides additional stability and also probably lessens the resultant forces on the post, ultimately lessening the stress on the cement bone–implant interface (Figs. 19.1, 19.2, and 19.3).

19.5 Tips to Prevent Iatrogenic MCL Injury

- Careful placement of retractors and meticulous care in soft tissue handling and bony resections.
- Early removal of medial osteophytes to relieve tension on the MCL.
- Use thin saw for posterior medial cut in the femur, mainly for small knees in female patients.
- Put a retractor between medial femoral condyle and MCL origin in the femur to protect against saw blade oscillation excursion during posterior and medial femoral cut.
- Put a retractor between medial tibial plateau and MCL in the tibia to protect against saw blade during tibial cut.
- Use a curved osteotome and external rotation of the tibia to release MCL on the tibia more in mid-coronal plane at the level of the joint line than in proximal to distal direction.

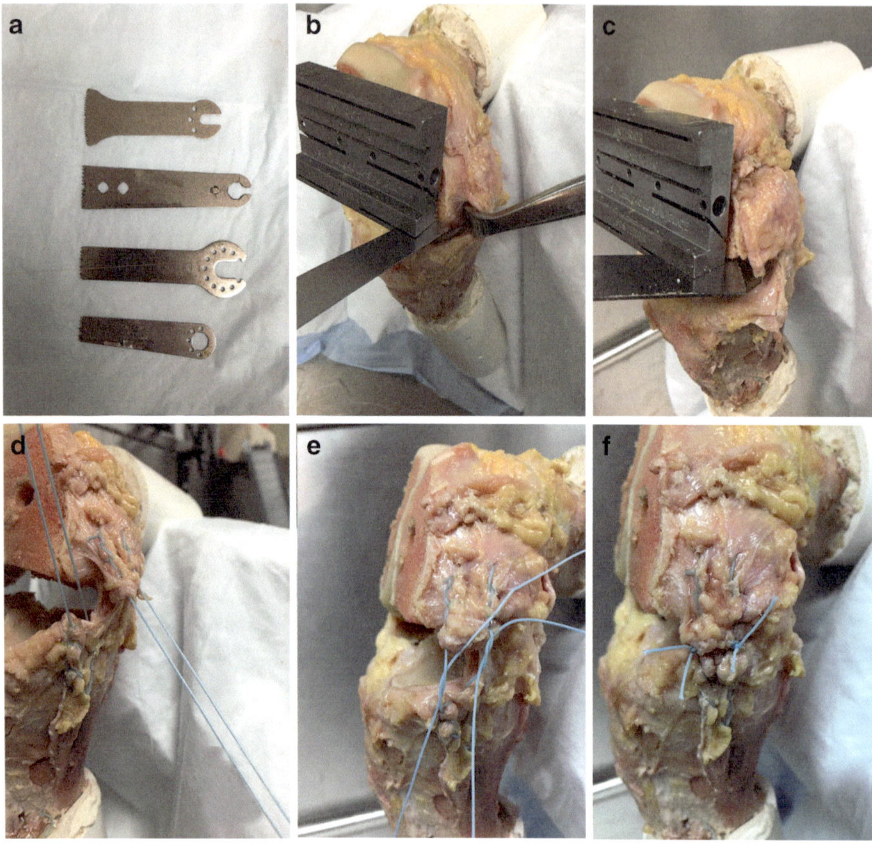

Fig. 19.1 (**a**) Different saw blade sizes. Prefer the ones with less oscillation. (**b**) Adequate saw and proper MCL protection during posterior femoral cut. (**c**) MCL iatrogenic lesion with improper saw blade and protection during posterior femoral cut. (**d–f**) MCL end-to-end repair with 2.0 interrupted nonabsorbable suture using Krackow technique

- The pes anserinus should be preserved.
- Caution with the use of the "Ransall" maneuver (Ranawat + Insall: sublux the tibia forward in flexion and external rotation) on varus knees and avoid this maneuver on valgus knees as the MCL is normally not released and will be at high risk on the way of the tibia subluxation.

Acknowledgments The current chapter was financially supported by FAPESP grant number 2015/10317–7 as the specimens at the figures were primarily used for the grant-related project. Franciozi CES received postdoctoral scholarship from FAPESP supporting his scientific activities at the University of Southern California during 2015–2016. Carvalho RT received financial support while performing his Ph.D. activities at the University of Southern California during 2016.

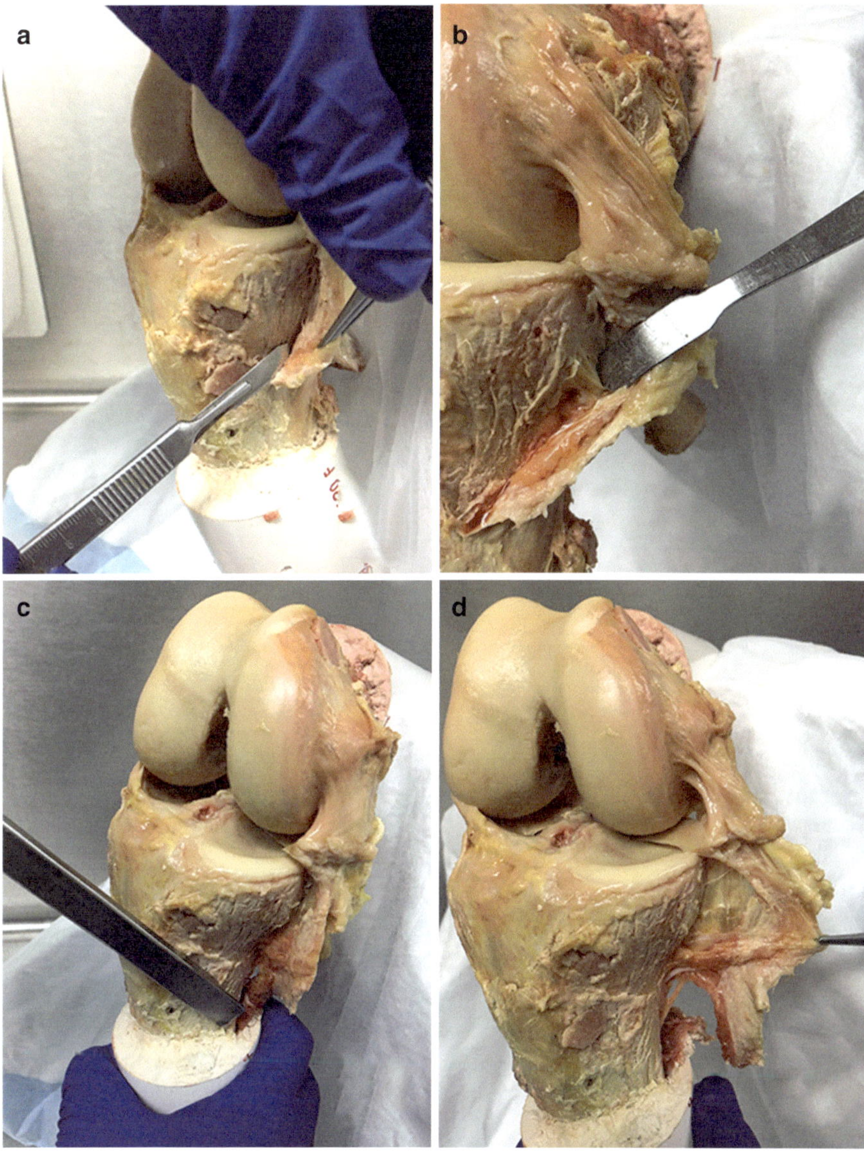

Fig. 19.2 (**a**) MCL distal release with scalpel blade. If not cautious, can cause tibial avulsion. (**b**) MCL distal release maintaining its sufficiency. (**c**) Inadvertent MCL tibial avulsion sample with osteotome. (**d**) Complete MCL tibial avulsion. (**e**) Tibial avulsion anchor reinsertion around 6 cm distal to the joint line. (**f**) Two anchors are inserted at the most distal tibial MCL insertion around 6 cm distal to the joint line adjusted to the remaining tissue as necessary. One anchor is placed more anterior and another one more posterior. (**g**) Suture placement at the remaining tissue. (**h**) Final reinsertion aspect of MCL tibial avulsion

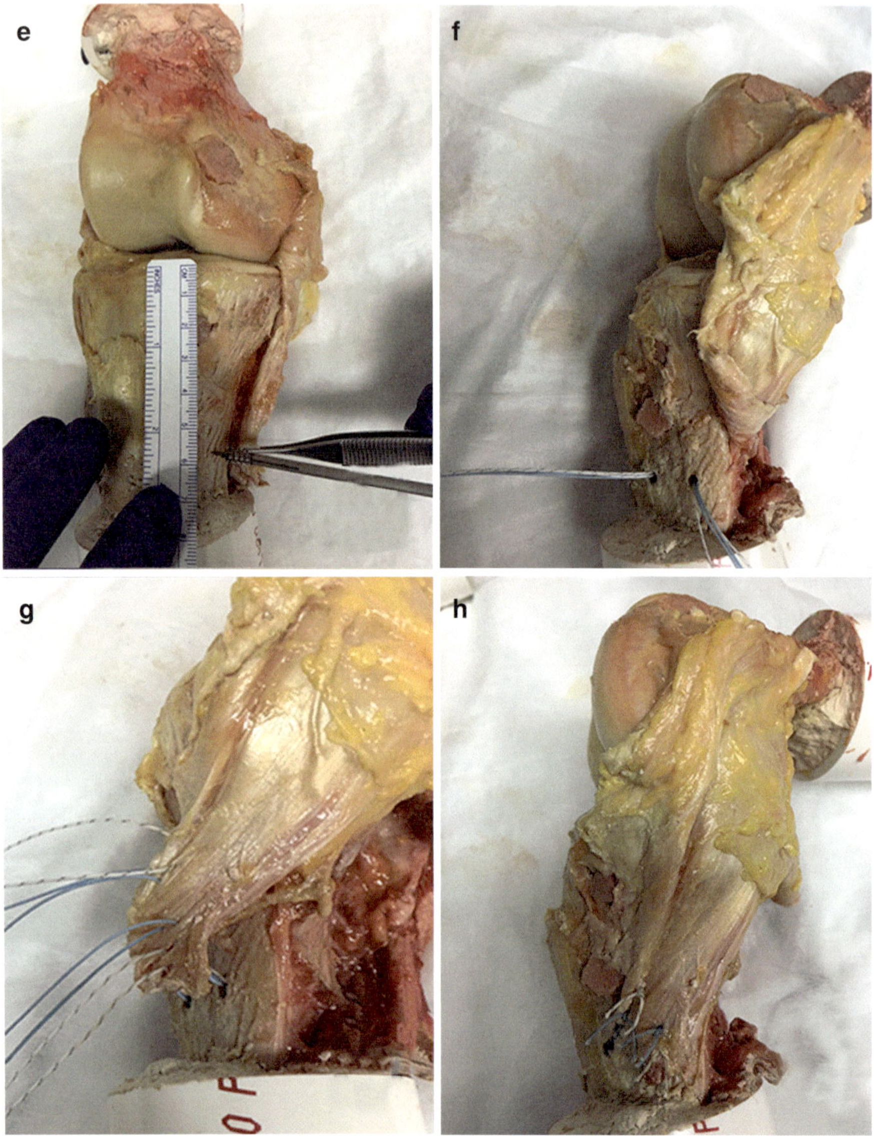

Fig. 19.2 (continued)

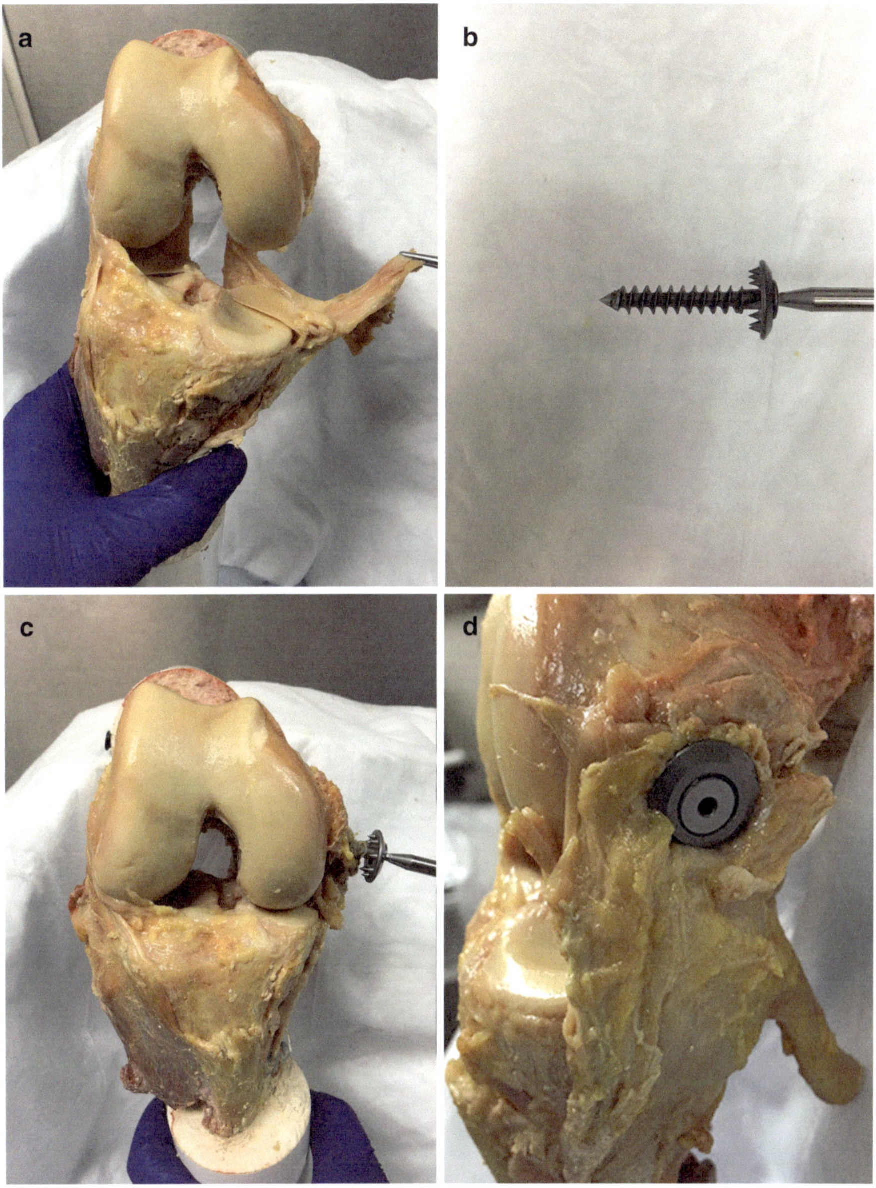

Fig. 19.3 (**a**) Femoral avulsion of the MCL. (**b**) Screw and spiked washer (18 mm). (**c**) Screw and washer insertion. (**d**) Final reinsertion aspect of MCL femoral avulsion

References

1. LaPrade RF, et al. The anatomy of the medial part of the knee. J Bone Joint Surg Am. 2007;89(9):2000–10.
2. Liu F, et al. In vivo length patterns of the medial collateral ligament during the stance phase of gait. Knee Surg Sports Traumatol Arthrosc. 2011;19(5):719–27.
3. Leopold SS, et al. Primary repair of intraoperative disruption of the medical collateral ligament during total knee arthroplasty. J Bone Joint Surg Am. 2001;83-A(1):86–91.
4. Griffith CJ, et al. Medial knee injury: part 1, static function of the individual components of the main medial knee structures. Am J Sports Med. 2009;37(9):1762–70.
5. Winiarsky R, Barth P, Lotke P. Total knee arthroplasty in morbidly obese patients. J Bone Joint Surg Am. 1998;80(12):1770–4.
6. Abdel MP, Haas SB. The unstable knee: wobble and buckle. Bone Joint J. 2014;96-B(11 Supple A):112–4.
7. Adravanti P, et al. Medial collateral ligament reconstruction during TKA: a new approach and surgical technique. Joints. 2015;3(4):215–7.
8. Bohl DD, et al. Repair of intraoperative injury to the medial collateral ligament during primary total knee arthroplasty. J Bone Joint Surg Am. 2016;98(1):35–9.
9. Dragosloveanu S, et al. Outcome of iatrogenic collateral ligaments injuries during total knee arthroplasty. Eur J Orthop Surg Traumatol. 2014;24(8):1499–503.
10. Gardiner JC, Weiss JA, Rosenberg TD. Strain in the human medial collateral ligament during valgus loading of the knee. Clin Orthop Relat Res. 2001;391:266–74.
11. Jung KA, et al. Quadriceps tendon free graft augmentation for a midsubstance tear of the medial collateral ligament during total knee arthroplasty. Knee. 2009;16(6):479–83.
12. Koo MH, Choi CH. Conservative treatment for the intraoperative detachment of medial collateral ligament from the tibial attachment site during primary total knee arthroplasty. J Arthroplasty. 2009;24(8):1249–53.
13. Lee GC, Lotke PA. Management of intraoperative medial collateral ligament injury during TKA. Clin Orthop Relat Res. 2011;469(1):64–8.
14. Petrie JR, Haidukewych GJ. Instability in total knee arthroplasty : assessment and solutions. Bone Joint J. 2016;98-B(1 Suppl A):116–9.
15. Shahi A, et al. Primary repair of iatrogenic medial collateral ligament injury during TKA: a modified technique. J Arthroplasty. 2015;30(5):854–7.
16. Siqueira MB, et al. Outcomes of medial collateral ligament injuries during total knee arthroplasty. J Knee Surg. 2016;29(1):68–73.
17. Song SJ, et al. Causes of instability after total knee arthroplasty. J Arthroplasty. 2014;29(2):360–4.
18. Stephens S, et al. Repair of medial collateral ligament injury during total knee arthroplasty. Orthopedics. 2012;35(2):e154–9.
19. Wierer G, et al. Anatomical MCL reconstruction following TKA. Knee. 2016;23(5):911–4.

Extensor Mechanism Rupture

20

Nicolaas C. Budhiparama, Nadia N. Ifran, Sébastien Lustig, Michel Bonnin, and Sebastien Parratte

Contents

N.C. Budhiparama (✉) • N.N. Ifran
Nicolaas Institute of Constructive Orthopaedic Research & Education Foundation, 12950 Jakarta, Indonesia
e-mail: ncbjr@yahoo.com

S. Lustig
Croix-Rousse Hospital, Albert-Trillat Center, 69004 Lyon, France

M. Bonnin
Centre Orthopedique Santy, 24 avenue Paul-Santy, 69008 Lyon, France

S. Parratte
Institute for Locomotion, Sainte Marguerite Hospital, Aix-Marseille University, Marseille, France

S. Matsuda et al. (eds.), *Soft Tissue Balancing in Total Knee Arthroplasty*,
DOI 10.1007/978-3-662-54082-4_20

20.1 Introduction

Extensor mechanism rupture is one of the most devastating complications after TKA procedures. It occurs in <1% of patients. It more commonly occurs in chronic conditions where the tears are the result of degenerated tissues, major scarring following repetitive operation, or stiffness [1, 2]. Although less frequent, acute injury may occur, usually during exposure in stiff knees. Postoperative injury may occur as a result of falling on a hyperflexed knee, component malalignment, or impingement of the deep structures of the patellar tendon into tibial inserts [3]. Extensor mechanism rupture injury may occur along the extensor mechanism, which include quadriceps tendon, patella bone, patellar tendon, and avulsion of the tibial tubercle. Disruption of the extensor mechanism will compromise knee extension. Conservative treatments are only reserved in patients who are contraindicated to undergo surgery since the outcome may result in impairment and morbidity. Dobbs et al. described partial rupture of quadriceps tendon following total knee arthroplasty (TKA) treated with conservative measures, and result showed satisfactory outcome [4]. Up till today, many techniques have been described; however, the prognosis usually varies and is less than satisfactory. This is due to the nature of the published papers, most of which were case reports or researches with small samples or short follow-up time. With a lack of standardization in methods and adequate follow-up time, it is difficult to determine which technique yields superior outcome.

As surgeons perform arthroplasty either primary or revision, being well prepared to manage the complication intraoperatively and postoperatively is mandatory.

20.2 Brief Anatomy

Extensor mechanism injury consists of quadriceps muscle groups, quadriceps tendon, patella bone, patellar retinaculum, patellar tendon, and tibial tubercle. Through surgical approach and soft tissue dissection, blood supply to extensor mechanism may potentially be damaged and compromised. During medial parapatellar approach, which is the most common surgical approach, all medial vessels may be disrupted, including descending genicular and superior and inferior medial genicular arteries (Fig. 20.1) [5]. Moreover, excision of the lateral meniscus and infrapatellar fat pad may disrupt inferior lateral genicular artery and the recurrent branch of anterior tibial artery. In their study, Pawar et al. [6] did a scintigraphy on 72 knees that had undergone primary knee arthroplasty. Knees which had lateral release showed greater incidence of patellar hypovascularity during early postoperative period.

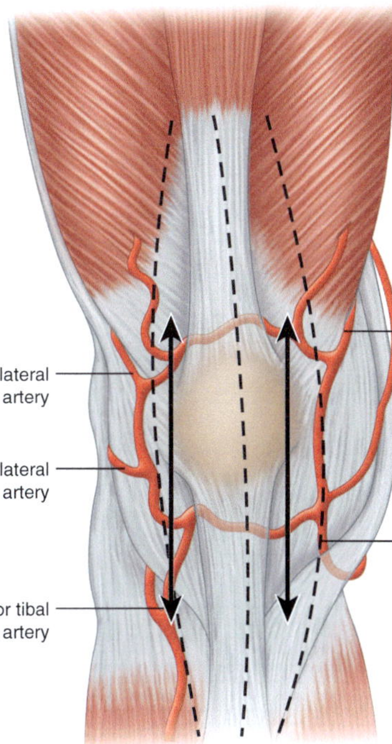

Fig. 20.1 Blood supply to the extensor mechanism (From Pawar et al. [6]. With kind permission from Springer Science and Business Media.) Superior lateral genicular artery, inferior lateral genicular artery, anterior tibial recurrent artery, superior medial genicular artery, and inferior medial genicular artery. Note that whatever the skin incision (*dotted lines*), a medial parapatellar arthrotomy damages medial arteries (superior and inferior medial genicular arteries) and that lateral arthrotomy damages lateral arteries (superior and inferior lateral genicular arteries and anterior tibial recurrent artery)

20.3 Risk Factors

There are many factors contributing to the increased incidence of extensor mechanism injury. Multiple prior operations or revisions resulting in major scarring and stiffness may play a role [7]. Infections are either pre- or post-arthroplasty [8], patella baja [9], and obesity [10]. Rheumatoid arthritis as a cause of arthroplasty may also contribute to extensor mechanism injury, most commonly patella fracture [11]. There are also other systemic pathologies and medications that may predispose patients to extensor mechanism injuries, such as diabetes, hypothyroidism, local corticosteroid injection, and use of floroquinolone [12–14]. These conditions may worsen the soft tissue quality over time, and extensor mechanism injuries may occur long after the arthroplasty. Implant design had also been shown to increase complication rate. As described by Healy et al., metal-backed patellar component has increased risk of complication compared to all polyethylene patellae [15].

20.4 Diagnosis

Diagnosis of compromised extensor mechanism may be easily seen in acute settings such as in trauma or as a result of complication during TKA. Arthrocentesis in acute settings can be done to evacuate hematoma. In a condition where specific incident cannot be identified, high level of suspicion and meticulous examination should be performed. Patients with extensor lag, especially if the lag is more than 20°, inability to lock knee during standing phase in walking, or hyperextended knee to stabilize the knee during walking should raise suspicion. Examination may reveal gap on patellar or quadriceps tendon.

Plain radiograph in anteroposterior (AP) and lateral projections may show patella alta as indirect sign of patella rupture or to rule out other bony abnormalities. An assessment of consecutive lateral x-rays may show progressive patellar migration. If the patellar tendon is distended, then the patellar shows proximal migration and distal migration if quadriceps tendon is distended. Ultrasonography or magnetic resonance imaging (MRI) may help in confirming the diagnosis and the level of injury. Ultrasonography is useful specifically in partial tears when the clinical findings are inconclusive. MRI can be helpful although implant artifacts may hinder readings of the images. In patients with high level of suspicion for muscle weakness, back examination together with the supporting examination should be performed to rule out lower lumbar problems [7, 16].

20.5 Management of Extensor Mechanism Injury

Extensor mechanism injuries may be classified as suprapatellar, patellar, and infrapatellar as described above, but the most challenging to treat is the infrapatellar [17]. Rupture of the distal tendon and avulsion of the tibial tuberosity are also the most common forms of extensor mechanism injury [7, 18].

Management of extensor mechanism injury ranges from conservative management with brace or cast immobilization to repair and/or reconstruction or arthrodesis. Surgery is mainly indicated especially in active person, starting from a simple direct repair up to the incorporation of allograft in a very compromised soft tissue condition. Since high failure rates and poor outcome are often described in direct repair papers [1, 3, 19], soft tissue augmentation of the suture with ipsilateral tendons or synthetic material should be put into consideration. Indications of surgical treatments varied between papers [16]. Rosenberg had described in his paper that extensor lag more than 20° is a cutoff point for surgical management. Successful measures of the intervention also varied among papers, which made it even more difficult to summarize result of papers in this topic. Moreover, the authors of this chapter utilize 20° extensor lag as the cutoff point for surgical indication.

This chapter will point out some of the different techniques that have been described in the literature regarding options of managing extensor mechanism rupture as a complication of TKA procedure, including:

1. Direct repair
2. Soft tissue augmentation
3. Synthetic material augmentation
4. Autograft reconstruction
5. Allograft reconstruction

20.5.1 Direct Repair

Direct repair has a very limited indication. In acute settings, direct repair is still possible; however, in chronic injury where the tendon is retracted or when the soft tissue is not sufficient to perform a good repair, direct repair with augmentation may be a better option [11].

The tendon may be repaired or reattached to the bone with nonabsorbable suture, anchor, or staple. Caution needs to be implemented to position the patella in its normal height. After direct repair, the suture will be protected with cerclage wire that spans from the patella to tibia (transosseous anchor) [11, 20]. Patients' knees are placed in extension with locked brace for 6 weeks postoperative. Afterward, initiate gradual increase in knee flexion while still maintaining mobilization in extension for another 6 weeks.

Studies have shown that direct repair outcomes were less than satisfactory with high failure rate [4, 11]. Therefore, unless the intraoperative result was very convincing, soft tissue augmentation should be considered.

20.5.2 Soft Tissue Augmentation

Surrounding soft tissues that are commonly used to augment the extensor repair are semitendinosus, gracilis and a turned down quadriceps tendon. Several papers have

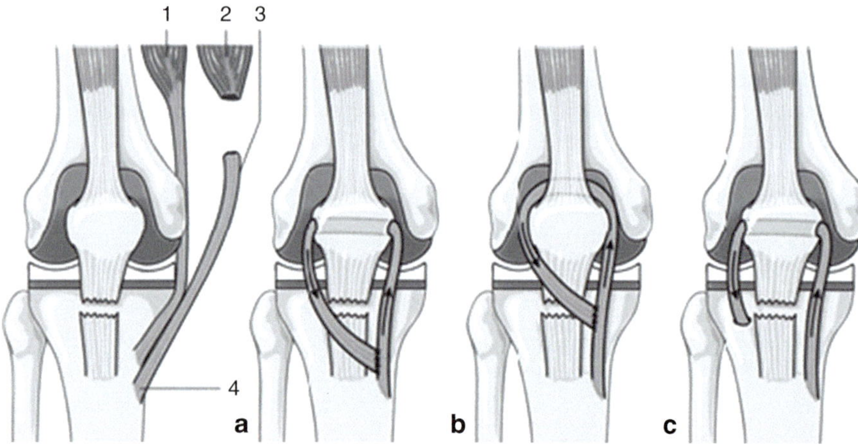

Fig. 20.2 Reconstruction using the semitendinosus tendon (ST) (From Bonnin et al. [41], With kind permission from Springer Science and Business Media.) (**a**) Technique described by Cadambi and Engh [21]. (**b**) Rupture of the patellar tendon, patella too thin to allow creation of a tunnel. (**c**) In the technique described by Jarvela technique [22], the graft is secured distally in a tibial tunnel

described techniques of augmentation in details (Fig. 20.2) [21–23]. Cadambi and Engh [21] harvested the semitendinosus tendon from the ipsilateral leg using tendon stripper and sparing the distal insertion. Then, a 6-mm tunnel was created on the distal third of the patella bone. The semitendinosus tendon was passed from the medial to lateral through the tunnel and sutured to itself. If the patella bone was too thin or too fragile and not possible for creation of a tunnel, then the semitendinosus tendon would be passed through the quadriceps tendon on top of the patella bone. However, quadriceps turndown would be performed to maintain patellar tilt in this technique. In this case, series with follow-up range from 12 to 48 months; all patients had extension lag less than 20°.

Another variation described by Jarvela [22] was to secure the semitendinosus tendon to the tibia on the lateral side. In a short semitendinosus tendon, gracilis or quadriceps tendon might be added to complete the procedure. Utilization of quadriceps tendon was to detach the middle third of the tendon from muscle junction and turn it down to be secured either at the distal end of the patellar tendon or drilled into tibial tuberosity. A case report by Lin et al. described a patient who underwent a quadriceps tendon augmentation showed good result with no extension lag [24].

Another hamstring tendon augmentation used similar technique, except the graft was crossed in the middle to create a figure-of-eight form. Result after average follow-up of 5 years showed no extension lag nor revision [23].

20.5.3 Synthetic Material Augmentation

A biomechanical study [25] showed that augmentation of patellar tendon repair with either cable wire or polydioxanone (PDS™, Ethicon, Somerville, NJ, USA) cord provided higher stability than suture anchor alone. It had higher load to failure and less elongation.

In patients with poor soft tissue conditions, augmentation with synthetic material must be included as one of the treatment options. As in any other ligament/tendon reconstruction, use of synthetic material has the advantages of no donor site morbidity, no additional surgery time for harvesting the donor, free from possible transmitted infection, and no regulatory restriction. However, the disadvantages are the material not being readily available in all countries and prone to infection [26–28].

Leeds-Keio is a scaffold-type artificial ligament. It is expected to work as a ligament until biological tissue is induced around the implant and then subsequently becomes ligamentous tissue and assumes the role of the original artificial ligament [29]. It has been used for different knee ligament reconstructions. Fujikawa and Ohtani, in a retrospective review of Leeds-Keio usage in extensor mechanism injury, found that 19 knees of 18 patients had almost full knee flexion (range of full flexion 140°–160°) with extension lag less than 10° for years after the procedures [30]. No revision was performed.

The procedure was to create a figure-of-eight artificial ligament with distal attachment passing through tibial tunnel posterior to the tibial tuberosity and secured with double staples on the lateral tibial condyle for patellar tendon rupture, or proximal end was sutured to each other and to quadriceps tendon for quadriceps rupture (Fig. 20.3). No drilling was performed on the patella bone, only crossing on top of the patella to prevent fracture of the patella. The artificial graft was passed above (for patellar tendon rupture) or below (for quadriceps tendon rupture) the patella bone [30].

Another synthetic ligament that has been used for extensor mechanism injury is LARS (Ligament Augmentation and Reconstruction System, Orthomedic, Quebec, Canada). This system has been used in other ligament injury, for example, cruciate or collateral ligaments. LARS has advantages as follows: [1] avoidance of donor site morbidity, [2] allowance of early mobilization and quicker rehabilitation due to its mechanical properties, [3] no evidence of tissue intolerance to the artificial material, [4] allowance of fibroblast ingrowth around the artificial ligament bundles, and [5] the possibility of repeating the reconstruction in case of failure [32]. One paper by Naim et al. [33] reported the results of LARS extensor reconstruction in elderly patient, but postoperative range of motion was not stated, and the follow-up time was short (1 year). Another paper by Talia and Tran [34] reported the result of reconstruction on a 26-year-old high-functioning ex-Olympic gymnast who suffered from

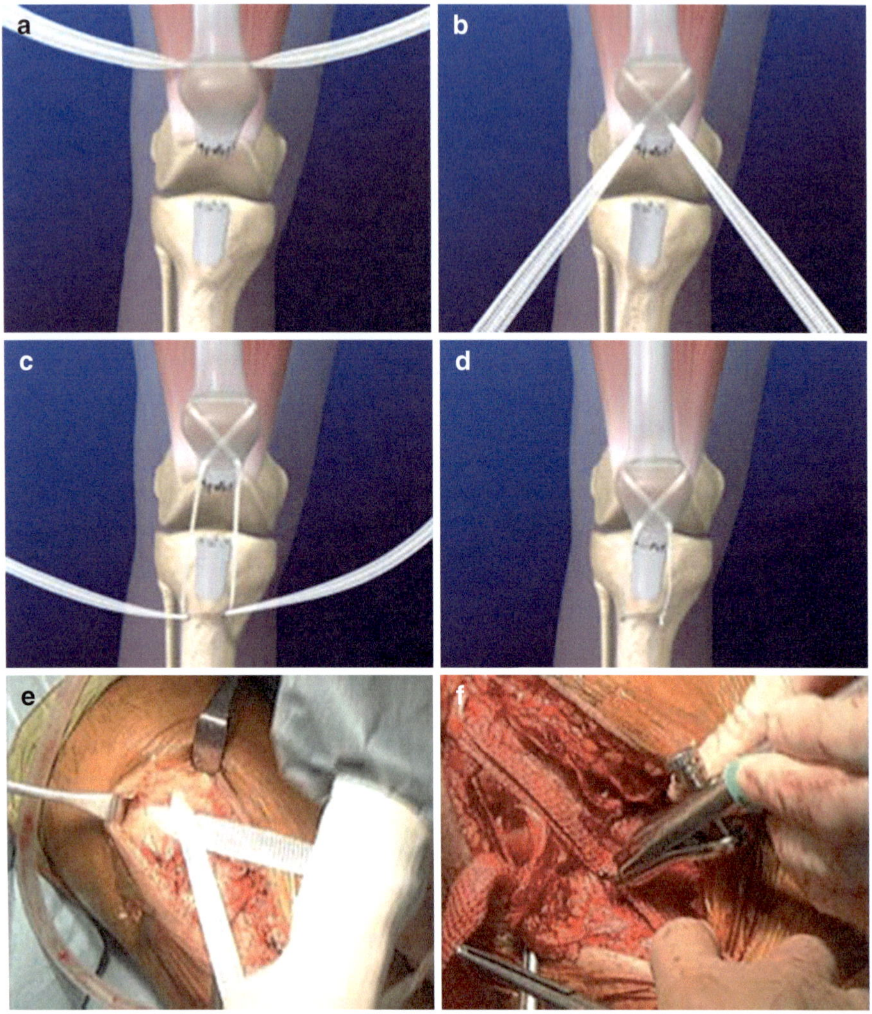

Fig. 20.3 Reconstruction of the patellar tendon rupture with Leeds-Keio artificial ligament. It shows that ligament was passed superior to the patella bone, crossed at the top of the patella, and fixed into tibial tubercle (Courtesy of Hideo Matsumoto)

bilateral patellar tendon rupture and was treated with LARS in figure-of-eight configuration. After 4 years of follow-up, the range of motion was 0–130°, and there was no extension lag. Early rehabilitation started on day 1 for this patient. Although the results were promising, none of these patients were post-arthroplasty patients. Therefore, further studies with large population and longer follow-up are needed.

A technique gaining popularity in the United States and Europe is one standardized by Browne and Hanssen [31] using polypropylene mesh (Marlex mesh, C.R. Bard, Murray Hill, New Jersey) (Fig. 20.4a–c). The mesh is a knitted monofilament polypropylene heavyweight mesh commonly used for hernia and urological procedure. The mesh is folded into several layers measuring 2–2.5 cm wide, and then it is stitched in place with nonabsorbable suture.

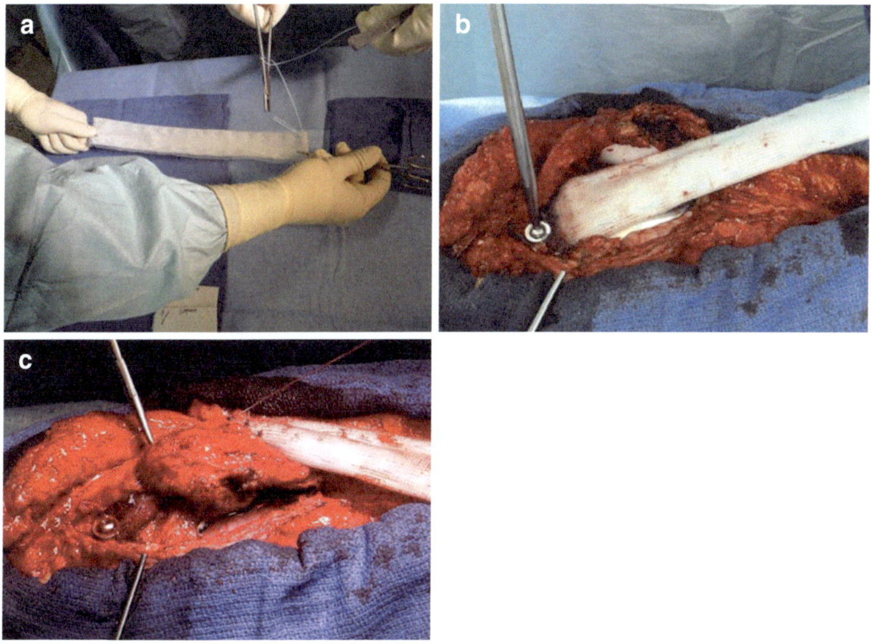

Fig. 20.4 (**a**) The synthetic ribbon is folded into ten layers, which are then stitched together using nonabsorbable suture. (**b**) Fixation to the tibia using cement and a screw. (**c**) The synthetic ligament is passed under the patellar tendon remnant then through a slit in the lateral ligament before being fixed to the patellar and quadricipital tendon

The distal graft is secured into tibial intramedullary slightly medial to the longitudinal axis of the anterior tibial crest. It is incorporated with cement if revision was performed on the tibial stem or fixated with screw and washer. Then, a layer of fibrous tissue is inserted between the graft and the tibial plateau to prevent abrasion of the graft. The graft is passed through the lateral retinaculum and attached to the quadriceps tendon and lateral vastus. Medial vastus is immobilized and positioned on top of the graft. Thus, the graft is located anteriorly from the lateral vastus and posteriorly from medial vastus. The result showed mean postoperative extensor lag of 2.8°, excluding three failure cases [31]. This technique is widely used in the world due to easy access and reasonably priced compared to allograft.

20.5.4 Autograft Reconstruction

Most commonly used autograft for reconstruction is bone-tendon-bone (BTB) patella from contralateral side. The preparation is similar with BTB autograft in anterior cruciate ligament reconstruction. It allows anatomical patellar tendon reconstruction, with its length serving as reference. As described by previous papers [35, 36], quadriceps weakness and anterior knee pain are common complications of this procedure. Another major disadvantage is disruption of normal contralateral knee; however, Shelbourne and Urch [37] showed no impact in its function.

20.5.5 Allograft Reconstruction

Allograft is another one of the options to manage large defect of extensor mechanism. It can be partial (Fig. 20.5) or total (including the whole patella bone with distal insertion and part of quadriceps tendon) (Fig. 20.5b, c). This method may be more suited for patients who have five poor soft tissue or multiple previous operations.

Fresh-frozen Achilles tendon allograft has been utilized in reconstruction of the extensor mechanism. The distal bone was fixed to the tibia with screws in regard to the stem position. The proximal tendon was sutured to the native quadriceps. All cases showed no presence of extension lag [39].

A short follow-up case report described treatment of infected patellar tendon rupture after failed primary repair. In this study, a cadaveric allograft of tendon-patellar tendon-bone graft was used in a sandwich layover type. Result was promising with ROM at the end of the study (9 months) reaching 0–140° [8].

Magnussen et al. [40] performed extensor mechanism allograft in chronic patellar tendon rupture. The graft consisted of tibial bone block, patellar tendon, patella bone, and quadriceps tendon. The patella bone allograft was shaped into an hourglass in coronal plane to be inserted onto the native patella bone (surgical technique initially described by H Dejour and Ph Neyret) (Fig. 20.6). The native patella bone was also prepared for patellar trough, and two coil wires were prepared longitudinally on the patella bone to fix the patella bone allograft in place. After 4 years of follow-up, active knee extensions were noted in all patients. This technique is technically demanding with possibility of patella bone fracture and painful hardware.

20.6 Intraoperative and Postoperative Rehabilitation

Apart from nonuniformity of surgical techniques to repair extensor mechanism problems, follow-up and rehabilitation protocols also have not been standardized.

First, in a chronic condition where obvious marker of previous injury level is difficult to determine, the use of intraoperative imaging to set the level of the patella similar to the contralateral side is needed.

After tensioning the extension mechanism during surgery, Rosenberg [16] opted not to test the range of motion, and his paper stated that the tendon may gradually stretch overtime. However, this practice is not uniformly applied by other surgeons; some may still test the range of motion intraoperatively to see how far the knee may flex. Burnett also discouraged the flexion assessment intraoperatively and performed the tensioning on full extension. This is believed to prevent attenuation of the extensor mechanism and extensor lag [41]. Flexion ability will be aided during rehabilitation process. Bonnin et al. [42] also support that suturing must be performed under tension with the knee in full extension to prevent extension lag postoperatively. They also stated that it is not necessary to test range

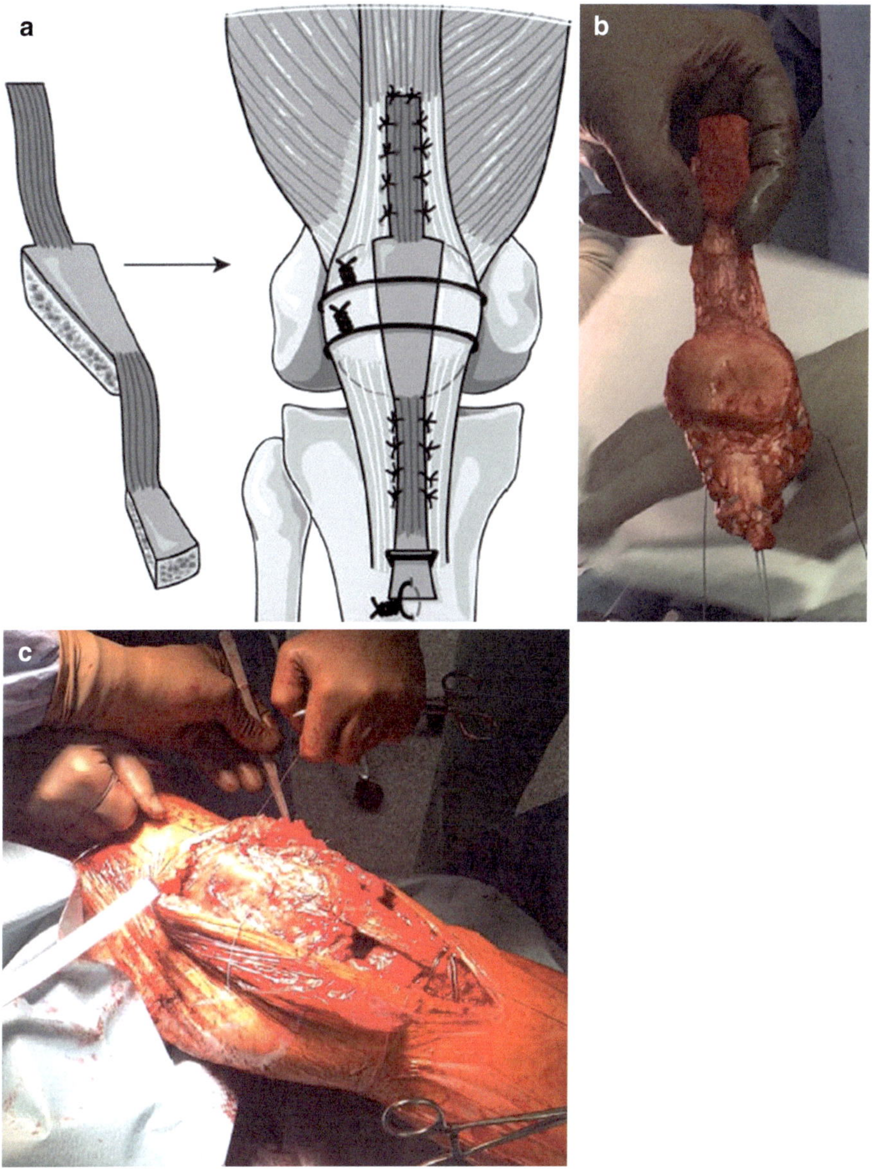

Fig. 20.5 (**a**) Partial extensor mechanism allograft (From Sah [38]. With permission). (**b**) Complete extensor mechanism allograft. (**c**) Complete extensor mechanism allograft in place. The graft is secured distally with two cable wires passed behind the prosthesis stem at the time of the revision. The suture is done proximally with the distal part of the quadriceps with the knee in full extension

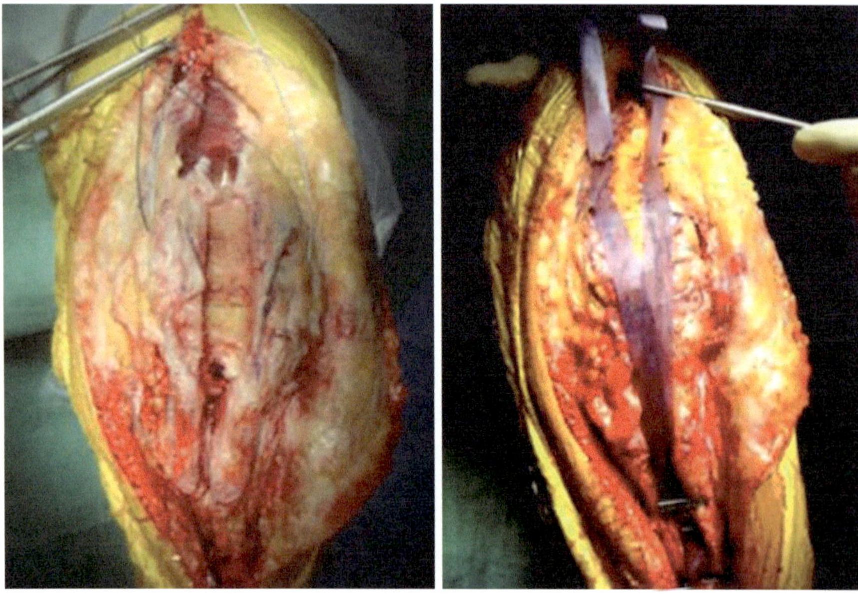

Fig. 20.6 *Left*: 10-mm hourglass-shaped groove in the host patella and 10-mm groove (widening distally) in the host tibia. *Right*: The patellar bony fragment is fixed first, using two or three metal wires. The quadricipital tendon allograft is then sutured to the host quadricipital tendon. A metal wire is passed through the tibial strut then around a screw and washer located more distally. A polydioxanone (PDS™, Ethicon, Somerville, NJ, USA) ribbon is used to augment the graft (Courtesy of Philippe Neyret)

of motion after repair or reconstruction, as the arc of motion will be achieved during postoperative physical therapy. Lastly, it is most importantly to cover the extensor mechanism with adequate soft tissue flaps especially in extensively damaged knee.

After the surgery, patients are put on extension brace for 6–8 weeks, then on the 7th week the brace was set for active flexion up to 30°, and gradually increase each week for 10°. During the 6 weeks of progressive flexion, patients still have to lock the brace on extension during mobilization. Other study applies early passive motion with CPM starting as soon as possible postoperatively. This will depend on what was done during repair or reconstruction. In a stabile and good soft tissue condition or if synthetic graft was used, early range of motion may be initiated, but in a complex revisions cases with poor soft tissue or where allograft was used, complete allograft incorporation is warranted before range of motion can be initiated.

20.7 Repair, Reconstruction, and Rehabilitation Guidelines

Between case reports, prospective and retrospective studies, and review papers, no uniformity was found intraoperatively or postoperatively. No single guidelines has been proven to be the best and most effective. Since the incidence of extensor mechanism is rare, testing guidelines are also troublesome. Below are strategies that may aid in the management of extensor mechanism injury.

20.7.1 Guidelines for Treatment Strategies [42]

- Immobilization usually recommended for partial ruptures of the quadricipital tendon.
- Patients should be aware and be prepared for the high complication risks for any of the treatment options.
- The most complications are infection and skin coverage, so infectious disease specialist and plastic surgeons should be involved.
- For many patients, partial or total knee prosthesis must be changed prior to repair of extensor mechanism which increases the complication risk.
- Suturing carries a high failure rate, so it should always be augmented by either a neighboring tendon or synthetic ligament (higher infection risk).
- Direct repair should be the first option, hence, to be done early prior to retraction of the quadriceps.
- Foreign materials have to be buried as deeply as possible; tendon repair site should be covered by a tension-free skin suture or a muscle flap especially in the area of anterior tibial tuberosity.
- Regardless of the chosen technique, sutures should meet the following criteria:
  - They should be strong – Krakow suture technique preferable.
  - They should perform with maximal tension, while the knee is in full extension and without subsequent knee flexion.
- Immobilization for 6–8 weeks in knee full extension, followed by rehabilitation for gradual increase of flexion. Full weight-bearing is possible early after surgery with the extension brace but should be protected by the use of crutches.
- Scant publication of case series reflects rare cases of knee extensor tendon ruptures. Thus, treatment should be reserved for skilled specialist surgeons who can obtain allografts.
- Knee arthrodesis is the last resort of treatment but should be considered for severe cases. Patello-tibial arthrodesis has been recommended as treatment of exception for patellar tendon rupture.

Conclusion

Difficulties in constructing guidelines for extensor mechanism injury include limitation of good papers especially ones with good research method, large study subjects, standardized study protocols, and long-term follow-up time. From the few papers available, the indications for treatment and objectives of treatment largely varied. A successful treatment in one study might be an unsuccessful result by another study. Thus, this chapter is still unable to conclude that one method of treatment is superior compared to others. Instead, it tried to elaborate on treatments that have been used in different settings and let the readers choose appropriate treatments that are suitable for their cases and technically possible to be performed by the treating surgeons.

References

1. Rand JA, Morrey BF, Bryan RS. Patellar tendon rupture after total knee arthroplasty. Clin Orthop Relat Res. 1989;244:233–8.
2. Cerciello S, Neyret P, Lustig S. Revision total knee arthroplasty: surgical technique in dealing with extensor mechanism failure. In: Rodríguez-Merchán CE, Oussedik S, editors. Total knee arthroplasty: a comprehensive guide. Cham: Springer International Publishing; 2015. p. 267–76.
3. Parker DA, Dunbar MJ, Rorabeck CH. Extensor mechanism failure associated with total knee arthroplasty: prevention and management. J Am Acad Orthop Surg. 2003;11(4):238–47.
4. Dobbs RE, Hanssen AD, Lewallen DG, Pagnano MW. Quadriceps tendon rupture after total knee arthroplasty. Prevalence, complications, and outcomes. J Bone Joint Surg Am. 2005;87(1):37–45.
5. Astur DC, Oliveira SG, Badra R, Arliani GG, Kaleka CC, Jalikjian W, et al. Updating of the anatomy of the extensor mechanism of the knee using a three-dimensional viewing technique. Rev Bras Ortop. 2011;46(5):490–4.
6. Pawar U, Rao KN, Sundaram PS, Thilak J, Varghese J. Scintigraphic assessment of patellar viability in total knee arthroplasty after lateral release. J Arthroplasty. 2009;24(4):636–40.
7. Nam D, Abdel MP, Cross MB, LaMont LE, Reinhardt KR, McArthur BA, et al. The management of extensor mechanism complications in total knee arthroplasty. AAOS exhibit selection. J Bone Joint Surg Am. 2014;96(6):e47.
8. Thakkar SC, Hsu N, Hasenboehler EA. Knee extensor mechanism reconstruction with complete extensor allograft after failure of patellar tendon repair. Am J Orthop (Belle Mead NJ). 2015;44(6):E199–203.
9. Cottino U, Abdel MP, Hanssen AD. Chronic extensor mechanism insufficiency in total knee arthroplasty (TKA). Curr Rev Muscoskelet Med. 2015;8(4):368–72.
10. Goldstein ZH, Yi PH, Haughom BD, Hellman MD, Levine BR. Bilateral extensor mechanism disruption after total knee arthroplasty in two morbidly obese patients. Orthopedics. 2015;38(5):e443–6.
11. Lynch AF, Rorabeck CH, Bourne RB. Extensor mechanism complications following total knee arthroplasty. J Arthroplasty. 1987;2(2):135–40.
12. Emerson Jr RH, Head WC, Malinin TI. Extensor mechanism reconstruction with an allograft after total knee arthroplasty. Clin Orthop Relat Res. 1994;303:79–85.
13. Malhotra R, Garg B, Logani V, Bhan S. Management of extensor mechanism deficit as a consequence of patellar tendon loss in total knee arthroplasty: a new surgical technique. J Arthroplasty. 2008;23(8):1146–51.
14. Stinner DJ, Orr JD, Hsu JR. Fluoroquinolone-associated bilateral patellar tendon rupture: a case report and review of the literature. Mil Med. 2010;175(6):457–9.
15. Healy WL, Wasilewski SA, Takei R, Oberlander M. Patellofemoral complications following total knee arthroplasty. Correlation with implant design and patient risk factors. J Arthroplasty. 1995;10(2):197–201.
16. Rosenberg AG. Management of extensor mechanism rupture after TKA. J Bone Joint Surg Br. 2012;94(11 Suppl A):116–9.
17. Brooks P. Extensor mechanism ruptures. Orthopedics. 2009;32(9) :683–84..
18. Papalia R, Vasta S, D'Adamio S, Albo E, Maffulli N, Denaro V. Complications involving the extensor mechanism after total knee arthroplasty. Knee Surg Sports Traumatol Arthrosc. 2015;23(12):3501–15.
19. Kovacev N, Antic J, Gvozdenovic N, Obradovic M, Vranjes M, Milankov M. Patellar tendon rupture--treatment results. Med Pregl. 2015;68(1–2):22–8.
20. Pagnano MW. Patellar tendon and quadriceps tendon tears after total knee arthroplasty. J Knee Surg. 2003;16(4):242–7.
21. Cadambi A, Engh GA. Use of a semitendinosus tendon autogenous graft for rupture of the patellar ligament after total knee arthroplasty. A report of seven cases. J Bone Joint Surg Am. 1992;74(7):974–9.

22. Jarvela T, Halonen P, Jarvela K, Moilanen T. Reconstruction of ruptured patellar tendon after total knee arthroplasty: a case report and a description of an alternative fixation method. Knee. 2005;12(2):139–43.
23. Maffulli N, Del Buono A, Loppini M, Denaro V. Ipsilateral hamstring tendon graft reconstruction for chronic patellar tendon ruptures: average 5.8-year follow-up. J Bone Joint Surg Am. 2013;95(17):e1231–6.
24. Lin PC, Wang JW. Use of a turndown quadriceps tendon flap for rupture of the patellar tendon after total knee arthroplasty. J Arthroplasty. 2007;22(6):934–8.
25. Schliemann B, Gruneweller N, Yao D, Kosters C, Lenschow S, Rosslenbroich SB, et al. Biomechanical evaluation of different surgical techniques for treating patellar tendon ruptures. Int Orthop. 2016;40(8):1717–23.
26. Burks RT, Crim J, Fink BP, Boylan DN, Greis PE. The effects of semitendinosus and gracilis harvest in anterior cruciate ligament reconstruction. Arthroscopy. 2005;21(10):1177–85.
27. Kustos T, Balint L, Than P, Bardos T. Comparative study of autograft or allograft in primary anterior cruciate ligament reconstruction. Int Orthop. 2004;28(5):290–3.
28. Legnani C, Ventura A, Terzaghi C, Borgo E, Albisetti W. Anterior cruciate ligament reconstruction with synthetic grafts. A review of literature. Int Orthop. 2010;34(4):465–71.
29. Matsumoto H, Fujikawa K. Leeds-Keio artificial ligament: a new concept for the anterior cruciate ligament reconstruction of the knee. Keio J Med. 2001;50(3):161–6.
30. Fujikawa K, Ohtani T, Matsumoto H, Seedhom BB. Reconstruction of the extensor apparatus of the knee with the Leeds-Keio ligament. J Bone Joint Surg Br. 1994;76(2):200–3.
31. Browne JA, Hanssen AD. Reconstruction of patellar tendon disruption after total knee arthroplasty: results of a new technique utilizing synthetic mesh. J Bone Joint Surg Am. 2011;93(12):1137–43.
32. Trieb K, Blahovec H, Brand G, Sabeti M, Dominkus M, Kotz R. In vivo and in vitro cellular ingrowth into a new generation of artificial ligaments. Eur Surg Res. 2004;36(3):148–51.
33. Naim S, Gougoulias N, Griffiths D. Patellar tendon reconstruction using LARS ligament: surgical technique and case report. Strategies Trauma Limb Reconstr. 2011;6(1):39–41.
34. Talia AJ, Tran P. Bilateral patellar tendon reconstruction using LARS ligaments: case report and review of the literature. BMC Musculoskelet Disord. 2016;17(1):302.
35. Dejour H, Denjean S, Neyret P. Treatment of old or recurrent ruptures of the patellar ligament by contralateral autograft. Rev Chir Orthop Reparatrice Appar Mot. 1992;78(1):58–62.
36. Milankov MZ, Miljkovic N, Stankovic M. Reconstruction of chronic patellar tendon rupture with contralateral BTB autograft: a case report. Knee Surg Sports Traumatol Arthrosc. 2007;15(12):1445–8.
37. Shelbourne KD, Urch SE. Primary anterior cruciate ligament reconstruction using the contralateral autogenous patellar tendon. Am J Sports Med. 2000;28(5):651–8.
38. Sah AP. Extensor mechanism allograft: surgical technique. In: Bonin M, et al., editors. The knee joint – surgical techniques and strategies. Springer:Paris; 2012. p. 1049–56.
39. Crossett LS, Sinha RK, Sechriest VF, Rubash HE. Reconstruction of a ruptured patellar tendon with achilles tendon allograft following total knee arthroplasty. J Bone Joint Surg Am. 2002;84-A(8):1354–61.
40. Magnussen RA, Lustig S, Demey G, Masdar H, ElGuindy A, Servien E, et al. Reconstruction of chronic patellar tendon ruptures with extensor mechanism allograft. Tech Knee Surg. 2012;11(1):34–40.
41. Burnett RS, Berger RA, Della Valle CJ, Sporer SM, Jacobs JJ, Paprosky WG, et al. Extensor mechanism allograft reconstruction after total knee arthroplasty. J Bone Joint Surg Am. 2005;87(Suppl 1(Pt 2)):175–94.
42. Bonnin M, Lustig S, Huten D. Extensor tendon ruptures after total knee arthroplasty. Orthop Traumatol Surg Res. 2016;102(1 Suppl):S21–31.

Index

S. Matsuda et al. (eds.), *Soft Tissue Balancing in Total Knee Arthroplasty*,
DOI 10.1007/978-3-662-54082-4

T

V

MIX
Papier aus verantwortungsvollen Quellen
Paper from responsible sources
FSC® C105338

If you have any concerns about our products,
you can contact us on
ProductSafety@springernature.com

In case Publisher is established outside the EU,
the EU authorized representative is:
Springer Nature Customer Service Center GmbH
Europaplatz 3, 69115 Heidelberg, Germany

Printed by Libri Plureos GmbH
in Hamburg, Germany